D1557753

Rheumatology in Practice

José António Pereira da Silva • Anthony D. Woolf

# Rheumatology in Practice

José António Pereira da Silva, MD PhD
Department of Rheumatology
University Hospital
Coimbra
Portugal

Anthony D. Woolf , BSc MBBS FRCP
Duke of Cornwall Department of Rheumatology
Royal Cornwall Hospital
Truro
UK

ISBN 978-1-84882-580-2     e-ISBN 978-1-84882-581-9
DOI 10.1007/978-1-000  [as per e-ISBN]

A catalogue record for this book is available from the British Library

Library of Congress Control Number: 2009938104

© Springer-Verlag London Limited 2010

Previously published in Portuguese by **Diagnósteo** as *Reumatología Prática* by José António Pereira da Silva, 2005.

Printed on acid-free paper

Springer Science+Business Media
springer.com

# PREFACE

This book is intended primarily for medical students, interns, residents in rheumatology, orthopedics and physical medicine (physiatry), and general practitioners interested in improving their ability to deal with rheumatic diseases.

We have essentially chosen to present practical, clinical guidance, departing from the symptoms, signs and clinical patterns, to approach the most appropriate diagnostic strategies and choice of treatment, rather than giving a classical explanation of the different diseases. Our essential goal is to provide our readers with a strategy for clinical investigation and differential diagnosis. The book is therefore based on real clinical experience, and we have attempted to include the methods of clinical reasoning that we consider most helpful.

How well this works will, however, depend on our readers' willingness to collaborate and commit themselves. We suggest that you pay particular attention to the clinical cases and accept the challenge they present. First, read the initial description, think about the questions asked, and then compare your solution with the one that we have adopted. Many of the cases may seem rather exhaustive. We would like to stress, however, that a concise and rigorous presentation of a case represents already the most important task of the physician, which resides in the ability to question, to listen, to observe, to appraise and integrate the information gathered. This is a doctor's most difficult task, and that is why we encourage your active participation as much as possible. This is also why we have avoided the cases that might seem simple and obvious: they are rarely like that in the real world they come from.

Some of the questions we ask about the cases may be too difficult to answer on the first reading, like those concerning treatment, for example. We feel, however, that they will constitute an important contribution to the learning of more experienced physicians, and to training and testing skills during a second reading.

This book is in no way intended to be exhaustive. Fundamental aspects like the pathophysiology of rheumatic diseases, the study of uncommon presentations or complications, or the specialized treatment of each disease are best served by more classical descriptive textbooks. Their inclusion in this book would stand in the way of the pedagogical and practical guidance that we aim to give here. We suggest that any readers who are interested in these aspects should consult some of the wide variety of available books.

In this manual, the different rheumatic diseases have been grouped on the basis of their clinical pattern, and not by the usual classification. The objective is to facilitate recalling of each situation in the appropriate context of differential diagnosis.

The general sequence of the chapters is arranged on a clinical basis. We believe that readers interested in getting a general instruction in rheumatology will reap the greatest benefits if they read the chapters in order. Even if the reader is interested in studying a specific disease, we would advise to start with an integrated approach to the clinical basis of rheumatology, which allows a correct interpretation of signs and symptoms (Chapters 4 and 5), in the context of the classification of common rheumatological syndromes (Chapter 3), and inflammatory arthritidis (Chapter 17).

It is our hope that both you and your patients will take great benefit from this book.

Any criticisms, comments or suggestions on this work are most welcome (jdasilva@ci.uc.pt).

José António Pereira da Silva
Anthony D. Woolf

# TABLE OF CONTENTS

# CONTENTS

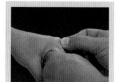

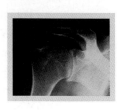

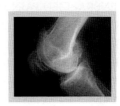

# GUIDE

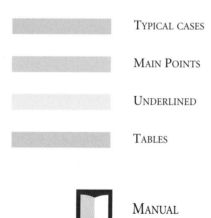

TYPICAL CASES

MAIN POINTS

UNDERLINED

TABLES

MANUAL

# THE IMPORTANCE
# OF RHEUMATIC DISEASES

**1.**

J.A.P. da Silva, A.D. Woolf, *Rheumatology in Practice*, DOI 10.1007/978-1-84882-581-9_1,
© Springer-Verlag London Limited 2010

# 1. THE IMPORTANCE OF RHEUMATIC DISEASES THE SATISFACTION OF CARING FOR THESE PATIENTS

Rheumatology is the branch of medicine that deals with the treatment (preventive, active and rehabilitative) of patients suffering from joint and musculoskeletal diseases, including diffuse diseases of the connective tissue, but excluding trauma.

Rheumatic diseases are the most common chronic sources of pain, suffering and physical disability in humans. They are most common in the elderly, but may affect all age groups.

Independent studies have shown that, at any given time, 30–40% of the population have musculoskeletal signs and symptoms, such as pain, swelling or limited mobility. Most people over the age of 70 have chronic or recurring rheumatic symptoms.

Studies conducted in Portugal and other countries have shown that about 25% of all visits to general practitioners are the result of musculoskeletal complaints, and that about 40% of patients going to see their family doctors have musculoskeletal problems.

They are the main cause of inability to work and early retirement, which emphasizes their enormous social and economic impact.

More than 150 conditions are classified as rheumatic diseases, each with its own pathogenesis, clinical picture, treatment and prognosis. It is essential to identify each condition and its variations if treatment is to be successful.

Currently, we have a wide variety of treatments at our disposal, which, when used carefully, will yield positive results in the vast majority of patients, not only in terms of relieving pain and suffering, but also in preserving long-term articular structure and function. While it is true that rheumatic diseases can rarely be cured completely, there are useful, effective treatments for all of them. Indeed, the inability to "cure" is not specific to rheumatic diseases but is common to almost all areas of medicine. Based on a relatively simple but sound clinical background, a doctor dealing with rheumatic patients can be sure of making an important contribution towards prolonging and improving the quality of the patient's life, which is, of course, the main goal of medical practice. Patients' appreciation of their doctor's intervention is a great source of professional fulfillment experienced by those who devote themselves to this type of pathology.

It is therefore important to eliminate the term "rheumatism" from our medical and everyday vocabulary, not only because it gives an inaccurate, all-encompassing idea of our medical knowledge in this area, but because it is associated with a fatalistic vision of suffering and relentless progression, all of which is far from the truth. We therefore suggest that the different conditions that used to be lumped together under the umbrella term "rheumatism" should be referred to as rheumatic diseases, which helps us to remember that we are talking about a number of different conditions and not just one.

The professional satisfaction of studying and treating rheumatic patients has special dimensions deriving from the very nature of these conditions. The diagnostic approach is essentially clinical. The basis for an accurate diagnosis lies in the doctor's clinical ability, and in the precision and thoroughness he puts into the clinical examination. Here, laboratory tests are merely complementary to our knowledge and skills, giving us full domination of the medical process. Rheumatic diseases are often multi-system, and may involve virtually all the body's organs. Doctors who devote special attention to rheumatic diseases have plenty of opportunity to exercise the holistic and pathophysiological reasoning that constitutes one of the greatest pleasures for those who really love medicine. We cannot, and should not, forget that patients are human beings, and must bear in mind not only their disease, but also its impact on their ability to enjoy life.

Finally, in recent years, rheumatology has achieved extraordinary progress in scientific understanding of rheumatic diseases, with ramifications that involve almost all fields of basic sciences and research, from regulation of the bone and energy metabolism to more advanced immunology and molecular biology. Physicians will find an exceptional opportunity to exercise their scientific curiosity and their taste for technology and advanced research, without losing sight of the actual patient.

# PAIN, DISEASE AND SUFFERING
## AN INTEGRATED PERSPECTIVE

**2.**

J.A.P. da Silva, A.D. Woolf, *Rheumatology in Practice*, DOI 10.1007/978-1-84882-581-9_2,
© Springer-Verlag London Limited 2010

# 2. PAIN, DISEASE AND SUFFERING AN INTEGRATED PERSPECTIVE

Rheumatic diseases are ideal for illustrating the difference between a disease (a confirmed biological or structural anomaly) and the overall impact it has on the patient (illness). At one extreme, let us consider a patient with fibromyalgia who complains of continuous, excruciating, incapacitating pain for which there is no satisfactory anatomical or biological explanation at present, accompanied by anxiety and psychosocial difficulties. At the other extreme, we have a patient with rheumatoid arthritis, involving massive destruction of the joints and marked functional disability who has managed to maintain a good quality of life, because he or she has adapted well to their condition.

The two conditions are completely different. Disease is certainly more severe and obvious in rheumatoid arthritis, but suffering seems much greater in the patient with fibromyalgia. Can a physician separate these two aspects and deal with only one of them?

## UNDERSTANDING PAIN

Pain is the dominant symptom of rheumatic diseases. It is not only the main cause of suffering and therefore the main reason why patients seek medical help, but also the main key to diagnosis. The ability to explore clinically and understand pain is absolutely crucial to diagnosis in rheumatology. Although it seems to be a monotonous symptom that is not worth any thorough investigation, we will see that, when properly analyzed, its minute variations can be extremely useful when making a diagnosis.

Pain is, however, an exclusively subjective manifestation that can only be appreciated in all its dimensions by the person experiencing it, and is not easily verified or quantified. A verbal description of pain, which is naturally essential to the clinical process, depends on a wide variety of factors, including the patient's social background, vocabulary and ease of expression.

For the same person, some pains are easier to describe than others, as we may all have found at one time or another. In addition, due to well-known biological mechanisms, chronic pain that is initially transmitted by site-specific nociceptive pathways tends to become more widespread and diffuse over time. This is due to amplification mechanisms in the spinal cord that eventually cause the areas around the organic lesion to become an additional source of nociceptive stimuli. Afferent signs from these hypersensitized areas will then be perceived as pain at sites where there are no detectable physical anomalies. These processes have been clearly demonstrated in laboratory animals, suggesting that they have nothing to do with the will, personality or emotions of the subject. So when chronic rheumatic patients have trouble pinpointing the exact location of their pain, they are just giving the best possible description of what they actually feel.

Nevertheless, psychological, especially emotional, dimensions play a decisive role in pain perception. Depression increases the perceived intensity of pain and reduces its definition, as pain is inseparable from its emotional implications. In turn, these implications depend not only on the patients' personality but also on their social circumstances (job satisfaction, for example) and on their own interpretation of their pain, i.e. whether they regard it as threatening. It is understandable that a recent-onset back pain will have a completely different significance for someone whose mother always suffered from it without any great functional limitations and for another whose father died from a neoplasm first signaled by back pain caused by metastases.

When we find it difficult to understand the nature and intensity of the pain described by a patient, we must remember that communication is not always straightforward. Patients try to describe a complex, diffuse and often indefinable experience using words they know, influenced by their own culture, emotions and experience of life. As doctors, our job is to decode the message using our own culture and vocabulary while being influenced by our own personality and emotions. It is remarkable that we manage to communicate at all in these circumstances. It is unrealistic to demand total accuracy from patients.

For all these reasons, a clinical understanding of pain requires a safe, accurate methodology, flexibility, patience, time and a capacity for biopsychosocial integration.

## PAIN AS A BIOPSYCHOSOCIAL EXPERIENCE

While focusing on a musculoskeletal diagnosis, doctors have to try to assess the nature and origin of pain as accurately as possible, eliminating any emotional components that color the description. They must also try to understand their patients as a whole and not just their organic disease. Our main goal is to help our patients to get better and improve their quality of life, and to relieve their *suffering* and not only the organic *pain* or the disease causing it. Suffering includes, for example, fear of losing a job, loss of independence, broken dreams or personal plans, sexual difficulties, etc.

It is the *suffering* and not the *disease* that takes the patient to the doctor!

> **Pain should always be regarded as a biopsychosocial experience**
>
> Doctors should consider it as a whole, paying equal attention to all its components. Although we try to consider the organic and psychological components of pain separately, in order to make our diagnosis and treatment more effective, we must also consider them as integral parts of the same process, equally relevant and worthy of attention and care, because they are both causes of the suffering that we want to relieve.

We must resist the temptation to concern ourselves solely with the organic side of pain, as if the emotional aspects were simply voluntary, conscious manipulation on the part of the patient.

Because prevailing medical and general culture can make this concept rather difficult to assimilate, bear in mind that a variety of mechanisms have been scientifically established to explain the intrinsic relationship between these different dimensions of pain. These mechanisms are as biological and "organic" as the metabolism of glucose, relieving the patient of the suspicion that can arise when we separate "physical" from "psychological."

## OBJECTIVES OF DIAGNOSIS AND TREATMENT

The doctor's ultimate goals in relation to a rheumatic patient are:
- a) Relieving pain and suffering
- b) Preserving mobility
- c) Prolonging life

There is nothing to distinguish these objectives from those that we should have in mind in any other area of medicine. The purpose of treatment is length and quality of life and not biological normality at all costs.

We treat high blood pressure not because it is a disease, but because it poses a threat to the patient's length and quality of life. To use all means including corticosteroids to try and bring down a high sedimentation rate with no apparent cause and no suffering would be a crass error. All diagnostic and therapeutic processes, including clinical investigation and additional tests, serve only as essential means to an end. We can't provide effective, safe treatment if we don't know exactly what the problem is. On the other hand, for the patient's sake, we should restrict our investigation to that which is most likely to help achieve these goals.

This may seem to be stating the obvious, but we must always remember it.

## PARTICULARITIES OF CHRONIC DISEASE

Generally speaking, rheumatic diseases are chronic processes often of unknown causes, for which there is no cure. With rare exceptions, patients will have to live with their condition for the rest of their lives. In the absence of appropriate treatment, many of these diseases may result in considerable pain and suffering, progressive deformity, inability to work or earn a living, impaired social relations, dramatic psychological impact, etc.

Even if the disease is diagnosed early, it will have to be considered in all these dimensions in both the short- and the long term. We will try to help our patient as soon as possible, though we must keep in mind the long-term objectives of survival, quality of life and preservation of structure and function for the next 20, 30 or more years.

These factors place great demands on doctors and the doctor-patient relationship. First of all, the dominant symptom, pain, is particularly demanding. If patients do not receive appropriate treatment, they experience pain and suffering and justifiably insist on immediate measures. On the other hand, the preservation of structure and survival often requires prolonged use of medications such as cytotoxic drugs and corticosteroids which, while indispensable, involve risks of serious and potentially fatal toxicity. This aspect means that physicians must be very careful when choosing treatments and try at all times to maintain the difficult balance between efficacy and maximum safety and tolerability. Their scientific knowledge and medical experience will be decisive.

Preserving mobility and relieving suffering (in the broad sense of the word) are the main goals and take precedence over biological normalization or structural preservation, if they are incompatible. It is essential to preserve articular structure, for example, because loss of movement leads to loss of mobility and quality of life. However, there is no point in subjecting patients to the risks of treatment or surgery of uncertain outcome if the function they require from a particular joint in their routine activities is not significantly affected by the disease.

It is very important to be aware of patients' functional ability at any given time and to evaluate the impact that each individual lesion has on that particular patient. A chronic, painless effusion in the knee may not bother an office worker too much but may be a real problem for a model! A little finger may not be too important for a stonemason, but it is essential to a pianist. Subluxation of the interphalangeal joint of the index finger has much more functional impact than ankylosis of the distal interphalangeal joints of the other fingers. A deformed foot does not need surgery if it does not cause pain or prevent the patient from walking.

The social and personal implications of rheumatic diseases and the fact that they are chronic conditions place an immense load and great psychological demands on patients. To understand this better, try imagining your own life differently. Imagine the limited mobility, reduced ability to work, impaired social relations, the fear, if not the reality, of deformity and disability, and the end of personal dreams are an extraordinary source of suffering, in addition to the pain. Patients faced with these prospects, which they will tend to view negatively, even if only from observing patients in more advanced stages of the disease, can do without a pessimistic doctor who doesn't believe in the efficacy of the treatment, who discourages their most enjoyed activities and who envisages them ending up in a wheelchair.

Awareness of these aspects leads to an appreciation of the special care needed in the doctor-patient relationship where rheumatic diseases are concerned. Management plans need to include ways of dealing with moments of discouragement and depression, with the patient's social needs and resources, finding alternative sources of personal satisfaction. In this context, it is essential for doctors to be aware of their patients' psychological state and profile and to involve them actively in their own treatment. It is important to encourage them to commit wholeheartedly to appropriate physical exercise and to enjoying life to the full rather than mourning the loss of abilities. It is vital to make the distinction between *having a disease* and *being a sick person*. We must help patients to focus their attention and energies on the positive results of the treatment, and not on incurable lesions, and to seek the best possible quality of life. It has been shown clearly that patients' psychological attitude and their relationship with their disease and limitations are decisive in the long-term prognosis, not only in terms of mobility and quality of life but also for preserving articular structure.

An attentive doctor must avoid the worst side effect of all: the harm done by words.

# THE STRUCTURE AND FUNCTION OF THE MUSCULOSKELETAL SYSTEM

## SOURCES OF PAIN

3.

J.A.P. da Silva, A.D. Woolf, *Rheumatology in Practice*, DOI 10.1007/978-1-84882-581-9_3,
© Springer-Verlag London Limited 2010

# 3. THE STRUCTURE AND FUNCTION OF THE MUSCULOSKELETAL SYSTEM SOURCES OF PAIN

The musculoskeletal system allows and controls movement. Some parts of the system specialize in providing structure and support: bones, joints, capsules and ligaments. Others are more related to function i.e. movement and its control. This group includes muscles and tendons, which also contribute to stability, and the central and peripheral nervous systems, served by proprioceptors that intervene in the control of the smoothness, fineness, degree and power of movement, and a range of nociceptors whose task is to detect the existence or risk of lesion. Any significant change in any of these components will result not only in pain, which will interfere with the patient's personal and social activities, including work, but also in a loss of quality of life.

The joints are the centre of movement. The joints with the greatest range of movement are synovial joints (diarthroses). Figure 3.1. illustrates their basic structure.

The ends of the bones in these joints are covered with *hyaline cartilage*, whose function is to facilitate gliding and absorb mechanical impact between the bone ends. Hyaline cartilage is composed of collagen fibers and a network of proteoglycans, which are large molecules in the form of a network (Figure 3.2.). The central branch is made up of hyaluronic acid, to which the proteoglycan molecules bind as radiating side branches. This complex structure also binds with water, which enables the cartilage to act as a sponge. Water actually represents 60–80% of the total weight of cartilage. It is the expanding force of the water restrained by the molecular web of proteoglycans and collagen that maintains its form. When the cartilage is subjected to pressure, the water is squeezed out, into the joint space. It is reabsorbed by the cartilage when the pressure is reduced or ceases. This movement of fluids is essential to the nutrition of the cartilage, which contains no blood vessels.

For the most part, collagen fibers are arranged perpendicularly to the surface. In the upper layers of the cartilage, however, they run tangentially to the surface, facilitating gliding and increasing mechanical resistance to friction. The cartilaginous matrix also contains a variety of other molecules with different functions, such as growth factors and the proteolytic enzymes

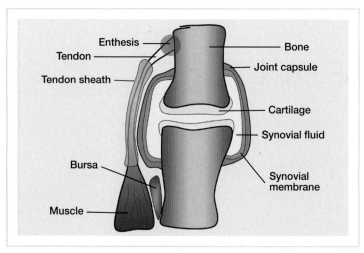

**Figure 3.1.** The synovial joint and periarticular structures.

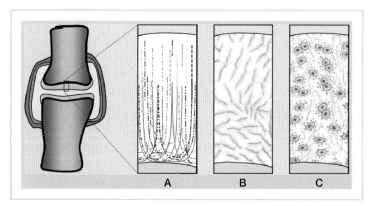

**Figure 3.2.** Articular cartilage: distribution of collagen fibres (**A.**), proteoglycans (**B.**) and chondrocytes (**C.**).

involved in tissue renewal. Dispersed in this matrix are the specialized cells of the cartilage, chondrocytes, which control the formation and degradation of the cartilaginous matrix.

Some joints have additional plates of cartilage that divide the joint space either partially (menisci) or completely (discs).

The *capsule* is a fibrous structure that surrounds the joint, attaching itself to the neighboring bone epiphyses, helping to keep the joint together as a functional unit. Its inner surface is covered by the *synovial membrane (synovium)*, which normally consists of two or three layers of cells with a total thickness of 20–30 μm. This membrane has two basic functions, corresponding to two types of resident cells:

a) Secretion of highly viscous *synovial fluid*, which is fundamental in lubricating and nourishing the cartilage. This function is carried out essentially by type B synoviocytes, derived from fibrocytes. The composition of the synovial fluid also depends on continuous exchanges with the blood and cartilage, and is profoundly altered in the presence of inflammation.

b) Removal of debris and foreign matter. This is done mainly by the type A synoviocytes, which are modified macrophages. Macrophages derive from the circulating monocytes and are largely responsible for the joint's participation in systemic immunological processes, as they act as immunocompetent and antigen-presenting cells. The synovium has a large number of fenestrated capillaries, which facilitates the exchange of cells and molecules between the joint and the blood.

During inflammatory processes, there is a marked synovial proliferation, raising the number of cell layers and the variety of cells present. In some inflammatory diseases, the synovium becomes invasive by forming a destructive tissue, *the pannus*, which causes focal resorption of the adjoining bone, resulting in lesions that are visible in x-rays (erosions). The secretion of synovial fluid increases, resulting in articular effusion, and there is a change in the composition and physical characteristics of the fluid. Inflammatory mediators and proteolytic enzymes in the inflammatory synovial fluid induce cartilage destruction, which shows up in x-rays as loss of joint space. Synovial thickening, local heat and the accumulation of synovial fluid are signs of a clinically detectable inflammatory process.

Articular effusion increases the pressure within the joint. With flexion, the pressure may exceed that of the synovial capillaries, leading to cycles of ischemia and reperfusion. These are ideal conditions for the formation of oxygen free radicals, which exacerbate the inflammatory process and increase its ability to destroy bone and cartilage. An acutely inflamed joint with effusion should therefore be allowed to rest.

*Ligaments* are fibrous bands connecting the ends of the bones, maintaining articular congruence and preventing any excessive movement that might result in dislocation. They may be anatomically independent structures or thicker areas of the capsule. The insertion point of fibrous structures (ligaments, tendons, capsule) in the periosteum and bone is called the *enthesis*. These insertions may be the site of inflammation, enthesitis, which may appear alone or be part of a more generalized disease. The best example of the latter case is seronegative spondyloarthropathy, in which enthesitis is one of the most characteristic manifestations (see Chapter 24).

The **bursae** are liquid-filled sacs that help the periarticular structures to glide smoothly. They are strategically located at friction points between bone and subcutaneous tissue (e.g. the olecranon bursa and prepatellar bursa) or between bones and muscles or tendons (e.g. the subacromial bursa). They are actually located at these sites because the friction causes them to develop. This is why some people have extra bursae, on the first metarso-phalangeal joint, for example.

The bursae are lined with synovium similar to that of the joints, but with no basement membrane. They are often the site of inflammation, which may be local (as a result of repeated trauma, for example) or a local manifestation of a systemic disease.

The **muscles** are inserted at opposite points of the joint and determine its movement. Fine control of movement requires contraction of the agonist muscles and controlled relaxation of the antagonist muscles. The finely coordinated action of these muscles is essential for proper control of the force, degree, smoothness and fineness of the movement. This control requires the intervention of complex proprioceptive mechanisms, which depend on mechanoreceptors in the articular and periarticular structures (Figure 3.3.). Knowing the insertion points of a muscle, allows us to predict in which movements it will act either as an agonist or as an antagonist, plus the range of these movements, thus facilitating the analysis of each clinical case.

The **tendons** anchor the muscle to the bone. Many tendons, particularly those that have a greater range of movement, are surrounded by a fibrous tendon sheath lined by synovium, which enables the tendon to glide smoothly over the adjoining structures. These sheaths are also sites of inflammation (tenosynovitis).

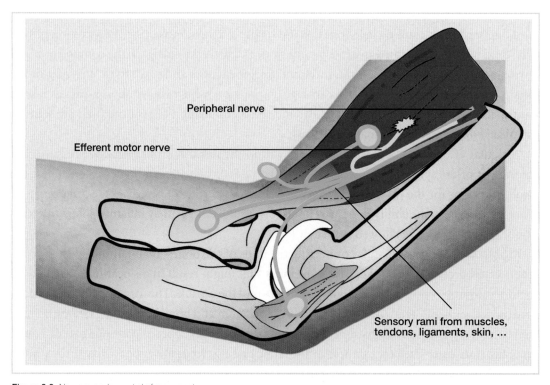

Peripheral nerve

Efferent motor nerve

Sensory rami from muscles, tendons, ligaments, skin, ...

**Figure 3.3.** Neuromuscular control of movement.

The range and type of movement and the stability of each synovial joint vary according to:

- the form of the articular surfaces (a hinge joint, like the humero-ulnar joint for example, only allows flexion/extension, while ball and socket joints, like the scapulo-humeral joints, move in several directions;

- the integrity of the joint's structure (Figure 3.4.);

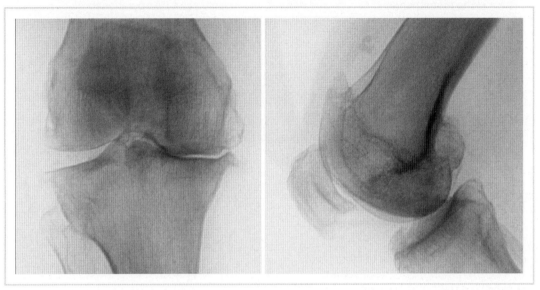

**Figure 3.4.**
Gross changes in the articular structure may result in loss of motion. Radiology of the right knee shows loss of joint space and large osteophytes.

- the strength, but also the distensibility of the capsule (this is why the capsule and its synovium are looser on the extension surfaces of the joints, where they form cul-de-sacs in which surplus synovial fluid will tend to collect)[1];

- the integrity, condition and location of the ligaments (ruptured ligaments result in articular instability, which facilitates the occurrence of dislocation. Patients suffering from hypermobility syndrome have recurring pain related to episodes of subluxation);

- the muscles acting on the joint;

- the presence, malleability and volume of adjoining structures (nearby gouty tophus or accentuated skin sclerosis may limit joint movement);

- age – generally speaking, range of movement decreases progressively with age. This change is not easy to quantify and its evaluation depends on the doctor's experience and a systematic comparison with movement on the opposite side, where applicable.

When addressing the symptoms of each articular structure, we should remember that a complete, smooth movement involves a multiplicity of structures and processes – from the central nervous system to the joint. The movement may be adversely affected by abnormalities in any of the elements involved.

[1] Other joints (than the diarthroses, or synovial joints) have only slight movement. They are called amphiarthroses, of which there are two types: the syndesmoses (e.g. inferior tibio-fibular articulation), and the symphyses (eg. the joints between the vertebral bodies), Others have no movement (the synarthroses).

**Find out for yourself**

Make a list of the conditions needed for a patient to obey an order to bend his right index finger fully.

- He must have no lesions in his central nervous system preventing the generation and transmission of the electric impulse to the peripheral nervous system.
- The motor nerves that carry the order to the muscle must be operational.
- The muscle must be operational.
- The tendons of the flexors and their entheses must be whole (no ruptures, for example).
- The tendons (flexor or extensor) should not have adhered to the neighboring structures (e.g. the tendon sheath).
- The capsule, ligaments and skin must not be stiff.
- The bone ends must not be deformed to the point of blocking the movement.

**And...**

- He must hear the order.
- He must understand it.
- He must be willing to carry it out.

Significant lesions in any of these structures or processes will prevent the patient from carrying out the complete movement. Only a detailed clinical examination will enable us to diagnose the cause and prescribe the most appropriate treatment.

The fineness of the movement also depends on these factors, but it also involves adequate control of the agonist muscles and respective nerve commands and the integrity of the proprioceptive system, which tells the patient the position of the joint, and the resistance and power needed (Figure 3.3.).

And this confirms the old saying that there is nothing in medicine so simple that we can't complicate it! It is obvious, however, that even an inexperienced physician can achieve enough of an understanding of these processes to make a careful or even intuitive clinical evaluation.

## THE PATHOPHYSIOLOGY OF RHEUMATIC PAIN

Pain is caused by the stimulation of so-called nociceptive nerve endings. These endings are dispersed throughout the capsule, ligaments, tendons, bone, periosteum, bursae, adipose tissue and muscles. They do not exist, however, in the synovium or in cartilage. The pain coming from articular pathology is caused by the activation of the nerve endings in the capsule and neighboring structures.

In general terms, we can consider two types of nociceptive receptors: the high-threshold mechanoreceptor, which responds only to strong mechanical stimuli, and the polymodal receptor, with a wide-spectrum response to chemical, thermal and mechanical stimuli.

The nociceptive stimuli generated in the periphery are conducted by afferent fibers that establish synapses in the posterior horn of the spinal cord. There are pathways from there to the thalamus and cortex, where the pain is located and cognitively structured. They also connect to a profusion of short pathways, which link the nerves in adjoining levels of the spinal cord and even with the contralateral posterior horn.

Contrary to what we may think, this is not a mere conduction system like an electrical circuit. Different levels of the system are capable of modulating the response to pain, even before the patient becomes aware of it.

It is especially important to consider some of the pain amplification mechanisms that explain how pain can be so much more severe than would seem biologically plausible.

## Peripheral amplification

Many of the mediators released during inflammatory processes act in the joints as nerve ending sensitizers. In the presence of high concentrations of prostaglandins, cytokines and other inflammatory products, the stimulation threshold of these terminals is reduced considerably (hyperalgesia). Under these circumstances, ordinary, normally proprioceptive stimuli are felt by the patient as nociceptive, i.e. painful stimuli (allodynia). This explains how a small movement or the simple palpation of an inflamed joint will cause pain. In the same way, subclinical inflammatory phenomena may be present in typically mechanical or degenerative conditions, explaining episodes of pain exacerbation that would otherwise be baffling. This is what happens in flare-ups in osteoarthritis or in the inflammation surrounding a compressed nerve root.

These mechanisms partly explain the analgesic efficacy of steroidal and non-steroidal anti-inflammatories.

## Spinal cord amplification

When a particular level of the spinal cord is repeatedly and chronically stimulated by nociceptive impulses, the result is spinal cord hypersensitivity. As a result of this process, the level involved and the adjoining spinal cord levels become hypersensitive and respond with nociceptive (painful) discharges to previously painless stimuli, amplifying further the hyperalgesia produced by the distal nerve terminals. Studies on a single nociceptive fiber in cats have shown that the chronic inflammation of a joint leads to hyperalgesia and allodynia not only of the affected structures but, over time, also of the neighboring structures and even of the contralateral joint! This pain translocation constitutes the second variety of allodynia.

This phenomenon helps us to understand the frequently diffuse, imprecise nature of rheumatic patients' complaints. The above studies have shown that the phenomenon is real and strictly neurophysiological, and does not necessarily involve any of the psychological or social aspects that we are tempted to invoke in clinical practice. Several neuromodulators affect pain, acting on spinal cord excitability, which is increased by prostaglandins and nitric oxide and reduced by opioid agonists and alpha2-adrenergics. The analgesic efficacy of opioids, alpha2-adrenergics and even intrathecal administration of anti-inflammatories shows the importance of these phenomena.

On the other hand, the analgesic efficacy of ordinary physical forms of treatment, such as resting the inflamed joints and the local application of heat or cold can also be related to a reduction in the intensity of the afferent nociceptive stimuli, and therefore of the resulting hypersensitivity.

Nociceptive neurons also establish spinal cord connections with motor neurons in the anterior horn. The aim is to protect the joint, which explains, for example, the rapid reflex action that pulls back a limb when burnt or pricked, or episodes of sudden joint failure in situations of intense pain. In some circumstances, however, a chronic pain stimulus leads to prolonged muscle contractions or even spasms, which, as they are also a source of pain, cause a vicious circle. These mechanisms explain the efficacy of muscle relaxants in treating many cases of musculoskeletal pain and the extensive analgesia achieved with anesthetic infiltration of painful muscle points.

### Central modulation

Another series of neuronal projections descends from the brain to establish a complex network of synaptic connections with the neurons in the spinal cord, especially in the posterior horn. These connections are the basis for the important modulating (excitatory and inhibitive) effects exerted by the central nervous system on the peripheral transmission of pain. They explain the analgesic effects of endogenous opioids (such as endorphins) released at times of stress. This descending modulation system provides the anatomical and neurochemical basis for the influence of psychological factors in the perception of pain. It explains the value of relaxation exercises and other forms of "psychological" therapy in pain control.

The pathophysiology of pain involves more than the system for neuronal transmission and processing of nociceptive stimuli, despite the fact that this alone seems quite complicated! The brain can cause pain in the absence of stimulation from the peripheral nociceptors or the spinal cord. Phantom limb pain and pain in paraplegics are examples of this phenomenon.

It seems, in fact, that the brain has a standardization mechanism or "neuromatrix" capable of superimposing its whole body sensorial knowledge upon the body image while mastering the interaction between them. This new theory, developed by Melzack, holds that a whole body neuronal matrix, which is genetically determined, produces the characteristic patterns of the body's nerve impulses and the multitude of somatosensory "qualities" that we can feel.

A lesion (in the broadest sense) not only produces pain, but also disrupts the brain's homeostatic regulation systems. This results in a stress reaction, which activates complex programs to restore homeostasis. The stress reaction may be activated by a physical, biological or even psychological lesion and involves neuronal, hormonal and behavioral response mechanisms. These programs are selected (from a repertoire that is genetically determined) on the basis of the extent and severity of the lesion. The result is the sequential release of cytokines, adrenaline, cortisol and opioids. This programming is influenced by a wealth of factors such as sexual hormones, emotional state, general health, memory, cultural environment, etc.

The neuromatrix theory takes us from the concept of pain as a sensation produced by a lesion, inflammation or other tissue pathology to a concept of pain as a multidimensional experience resulting from a wide variety of influences.

Neuronal projections connected to the afferent nociceptive system establish a link with sections of the limbic cortex involved in the integration of sensations, cognition, mood, and response selection. The sectioning of these neuronal projections does not eliminate chronic pain but it considerably reduces its most unpleasant side, i.e. suffering.

Recent studies with positron emission tomography and functional MRI have helped us to understand these central mechanisms. These methods have shown that rheumatoid patients undergo a considerable reduction in limbic and frontal lobe response to painful stimuli, suggesting an adaptation of the emotional/cognitive response to chronic pain. Conversely, patients with fibromyalgia show strong activation of the limbic and frontal lobe centers in reaction to pain. The mere expectation and suggestion to which the patient is exposed may change these biological mechanisms. In a recent study of university students, from whom we expected considerable biological objectivity, it was shown that touching the skin with an electrode heated to 10°C caused a CNS response evaluated by positron tomography similar to that of an electrode at 50°, if that was what the subject was told it was.

The physical and psychological aspects are, in fact, inextricably linked.

# DIAGNOSTIC STRATEGY
## THE MAIN SYNDROMES IN RHEUMATOLOGY

4.

J.A.P. da Silva, A.D. Woolf, *Rheumatology in Practice*, DOI 10.1007/978-1-84882-581-9_4,
© Springer-Verlag London Limited 2010

# 4. DIAGNOSTIC STRATEGY THE MAIN SYNDROMES IN RHEUMATOLOGY

## Two-step diagnosis

Differential diagnosis in rheumatology can be compared to a trip to an unfamiliar city that we know is full of interesting places to visit. The aim of our trip is to reach a particular place, i.e. the diagnosis. What we will try to do here is to provide a kind of map that will enable travelers to ask directions, identify the signs leading to their destination, and once they are there, recognize it and distinguish it from other places.

These travelers should first learn how to ask questions and observe their route as they travel along it, so that their search is not random and therefore ineffective. We need to know what we are looking for if we are going to find it!

Our strategy involves two fundamental stages on the route to the diagnosis. We have called this process "two-step diagnosis."

### Step one

Our first goal (or first step) is to define the generic type of pathology in question. We therefore suggest that you consider a set of "main syndromes," i.e. patterns of symptoms.

Our initial interview and observation will be designed to establish the type of problem we are dealing with, i.e. the main syndrome to which the case or complaint belongs. We must try to determine the existence of the typical features of a given syndrome and distinguish it from others. There is not much point in going into details that have no impact on these objectives. On the other hand, it is essential to be as precise as possible in the details that are most decisive in identifying or excluding a particular syndrome.

In rheumatology, these basic sets of symptoms are largely related to the anatomic compartment that is the source of the symptom: articular, periarticular, muscular, systemic, etc.

Going back to the trip analogy, it is as if we know that the city's attractions are in different neighborhoods, like the museum area, the science area, the sports area, etc. Our first goal is to get to the right neighborhood, where we won't be too far from our real destination: a building in that neighborhood, i.e. our final diagnosis.

In order to know what you are looking for in the first step of the differential diagnosis, you must be familiar with the main syndromes (Figure 4.1.).

We need to be especially thorough in the first part of our route. If we get the syndrome (neighborhood) wrong because we have misinterpreted the information or we make assumptions about an uncertain sign, the rest of our search will most certainly be flawed. We can never reach a correct diagnosis of rheumatoid arthritis if we assume that the patient's complaint is muscular in origin. In rheumatology, symptoms and signs are often subjective and imprecise. We tend to assess them more in terms of probability than certainty. To avoid making mistakes, we must always take a critical view of the evidence leading us in one direction or another. For example, edema of the foot with local pain may mean arthritis but it may just be coincidental venous malfunction and some other local pathology. So as we move forward, it must be clear in our minds which signs are absolutely certain and which are still doubtful.

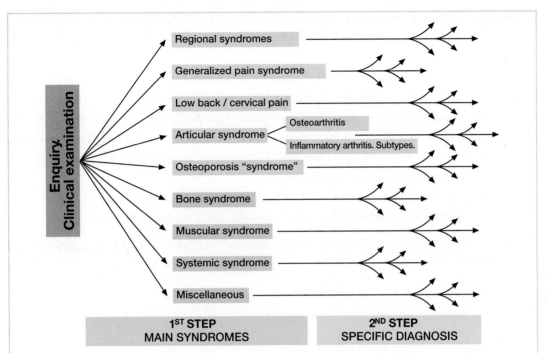

**Figure 4.1.**
Differential diagnosis in rheumatology. First step: main syndromes.

We should remember that a lot of our reasoning is based on key words, as in communication with other people. If we establish at some point that the patient has "arthritis," we must bear in mind the implications of the word. From then on, we will assume that the process is articular and inflammatory. We will no longer consider the possibility of muscle pain or mere arthralgia, which are situations with quite different implications from "arthritis."

At each step of our clinical evaluation, the terms and concepts that we use should be as precise as possible. If we are not yet sure if the pain is due to "*arthritis*," we should base our reasoning on the concept of "*joint pain*," bearing in mind all the conditions that may cause this symptom.

Even when uncertain about the signs, we must still move forward, exploring the road ahead but not forgetting that we may be on the wrong track. If in doubt, we should go back and look into any alternative possibility related to a different interpretation of an ambiguous sign.

Try to get into the habit of doing this exercise Describe your patient with as few, accurate key words as possible. As a rule you will not need more than ten, for example: 1. young man with inflammatory back pain, no systemic signs; 2. Woman with symmetrical, additive, chronic, predominantly peripheral polyarthritis with no axial involvement; 3. Generalized pain with no objective findings.

### Step two

Once we have arrived at a particular set of symptoms ("joint disease," "generalized pain," "bone pain," "back pain," etc.), we then go on to a more detailed investigation to distinguish between conditions that we know can cause these symptoms. Let us call this the second step in differential diagnosis.

Here we will also focus on two aspects. Which features are unique to each condition and which distinguish it from the alternatives? Our exploration of the symptoms should concentrate on these areas. For example, both rheumatoid arthritis and psoriatic arthritis may involve the elbow. Conversely, inflammatory involvement of the lumbar spine or the distal interphalangeal joints is common in psoriatic but not in rheumatoid arthritis. Thus, when we concentrate on the differences between these two conditions, we must be sure whether or not there is spondylitis or involvement of the DIPs, but it does not matter whether the elbow has been affected or not. We will worry about the elbow later, as its involvement may require special therapy, regardless of the underlying diagnosis.

It is in the second step of differential diagnosis that tests play a more important part.

In order to travel the road to differential diagnosis safely, we must (Figure 4.2.):

- Know the characteristics of each main syndrome (see below), so that we know what to look for;

- Know what questions to ask the patient (Chapter 5);

- Know how to conduct a general rheumatologic examination (Chapter 6);

- Know how to conduct a detailed regional examination (Chapters 7–14).

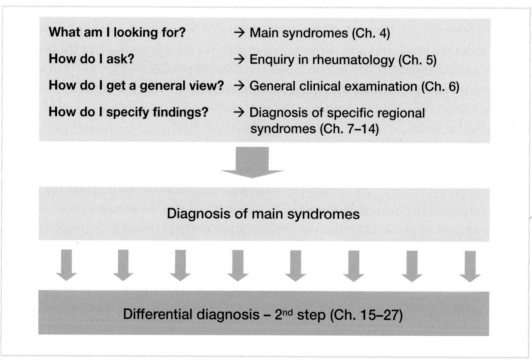

**Figure 4.2.** Differential diagnosis in rheumatology.

A general clinical examination and a complete regional examination of all the affected areas are essential to our final diagnosis. For this reason, we will first discuss the regional syndromes It is the combination of the interview and the findings of the regional examination that will give us the overview we need for a holistic accurate diagnosis.

Once we have completed the interview and the clinical examination, we will have final, specific diagnoses, if the problems are limited to an anatomic area (regional syndromes). The final diagnosis of the pathologies included in the other syndromes involves the second step of differential diagnosis. Each of them has its own strategy, which will be discussed in Chapters 15–27.

Any division and structuring of the clinical reasoning process is necessarily simplistic and therefore open to criticism. We are aware of these limitations. An experienced doctor mixes phases, recognizes patterns and uses shortcuts. This ability is, however, difficult to structure or pass on, and can only be successful and accurate when based on a meticulous model clearly explaining the how and why of our methods. This is the goal with this book and its proposed diagnostic strategy.

You should also remember that rheumatic diseases defy any rigid syndromic classification. Indeed, the presentation of many rheumatic conditions can take many forms and the symptoms may point more strongly to one syndrome or another depending on the patient and the visit. It is important to bear in mind the concept of a *clinical spectrum*, which is well illustrated by systemic lupus erythematosus. The same disease can present with predominantly articular symptoms (as part of the "articular syndrome") or be dominated by a variety of extra-articular symptoms suggesting a "systemic syndrome." A patient with polymyositis will typically suffer from weakness (muscular syndrome), but may present with arthritis (articular syndrome) or photosensitivity (systemic syndrome). The solution is to include these spectra in the map that we are drawing. The map of the arthritis neighborhood should have a sign for lupus, just as the systemic disease neighborhood should have a sign for rheumatoid arthritis, on the border between the two.

Remember that *we all have* a differential diagnosis map in our heads, which is a good thing. If we travel in a strange country without a map, we are bound to get lost. It is very important for us to be aware of the map, and systematically assess its accuracy, and adapt it whenever necessary. The map depends not only on our knowledge but also on the way we structure and store information. If we follow our line of reasoning (i.e. our map) and reach a wrong diagnosis, we have to review our cartography. The same will apply here and there with the strategy that we propose. We urge you to be permanently critical, even of this book!

# The main syndromes in rheumatology

Figure 4.1. shows the main syndromes which constitute the *first step* in differential diagnosis.

The syndromes in blue are by far the most common. They therefore deserve our special care and attention.

The basic characteristics of each syndrome are described below and they should guide our interview and clinical examination.

## REGIONAL SYNDROMES

Regional syndromes are characterized by the patient's complaints being limited to one musculoskeletal area: a joint and its neighboring structures.

The typical patient will deny musculoskeletal symptoms anywhere else. It is not uncommon, however, to find two or more sites affected, which may suggest polyarthropathy. Conversely, patients suffering from polyarticular or even systemic diseases are particularly predisposed to developing regional pathologies, which must be analyzed and treated separately.

As both our history and clinical examination should be complete and systematic, we should have no trouble in identifying the specific aspects of the case in question.

The affected area is, in itself, a clue to the diagnosis, as the relative frequency of articular and periarticular problems varies according to the area in question. In outpatient rheumatology, a pain in the shoulder or elbow almost always corresponds to a periarticular lesion, while in the knee or hip the high prevalence of osteoarthritis makes joint disease more likely.

After our clinical examination, we can divide regional syndromes into four main subtypes:

- periarticular pain;

- neurogenic pain;

- referred pain;

- monoarthropathy.

### *Regional syndromes*
### *Periarticular pain*

For teaching purposes, by "periarticular" or "soft tissue" we mean all structures participating in joint mechanics but located outside the joint capsule: bursae, and tendon sheaths as well as tendons, ligaments, and their insertion points.

These structures are often the site of disease, which is usually inflammatory, as a result of repeated local trauma (e.g. intensive use of the hands or shoulder) or as local manifestations of systemic synovial diseases, like rheumatoid arthritis. Inflammation of the tendon and ligament insertion points may occur in isolation, such as after trauma and occasionally may have no apparent cause. On the other hand, recurrent and multiple tendon insertion inflammation is a typical characteristic of a group of inflammatory joint diseases called *seronegative spondyloarthropathies* (see Chapter 24). Tendons and ligaments may also partially or totally rupture, resulting in pain, loss of active movement or instability of the joint.

This kind of pain is closely related to movements in which the inflamed structure is used or compressed, while other movements of the joint are easy and painless. This aspect, *selectivity of painful movements,* is very useful in distinguishing it from joint diseases in which all movements tend to be painful.

Active movement (i.e. executed by the patient) only causes pain when it requires the use of the affected structure, while other movements are painless. Passive movements (i.e. performed by the examiner on a relaxed patient) have normal amplitude and are usually much less painful than active ones. In the same way, we can trigger pain with resisted movements involving the structure in question. If we ask the patient to carry out a movement that is specific to the affected structure, while we resist that movement, the tendon, bursa or insertion point is put under tension, which causes pain.

There are normally no local signs of inflammation, unless the structure is very superficial, as in olecranon or prepatellar bursitis.

Palpation of the inflamed structure is painful (but not the joint margins, as happens in joint disease).

---

**Note**

These features are easy to predict bearing in mind how joints work. Imagine that you have a synovial inflammation of the shoulder: the inflamed structure is diffusely involved and so it hurts however you move the joint because the inflamed structure is involved in all its movements. The pain is similar whether you carry out the movement (active mobilization) or if someone else does it while you relax (passive mobilization), as the movement of the joint is the same. The joint's mobility may be reduced by the pain or the alteration of its structure, and passive mobilization cannot reduce this limitation.

If, on the other hand, only a tendon is inflamed, for example the supraspinatus tendon, you will only feel pain during abduction, which uses this tendon, but not during flexion of the shoulder, when this tendon is at rest (selectivity of movements). If mobilization is passive and the patient is able to relax, the inflamed tendon remains at rest and the pain is less intense than in the active movement. There is no reason for passive mobilization not to be complete, i.e. with no limitations to its amplitude. In this case, the patient will feel pain if s/he maintains the abduction while resisting the doctor's pressure (resisted mobilization), as the pressure on the tendon increases the pain. There is no reason for this to happen in the former cases, as the joint remains immobile.

Note that in many cases of tenosynovitis, crepitus can be felt over the tendon, which can mislead us into thinking of osteoarthritis, which involves crepitus in the joint.

---

**What suggests periarticular pain?**

Local or regional distribution.

Most frequent sites: shoulder and elbow.

Selectivity of painful movements.

Active mobilization much more painful than passive.

No range limitations in passive mobilization.

Palpation of the structure is painful.

Specific distention or resisted movements painful.

### *Regional syndromes*

### *Neurogenic pain*

Neurogenic pain is caused by the compression or irritation of nerve roots in the spine or entrapment of peripheral nerves. The latter type usually occurs in easily identifiable sites, where the nerves pass through structures that are narrow or subject to repeated compression or friction.

This pain is usually dysesthesic, causing a strange sensation such as tingling, numbness, electric shocks, burnt skin sensation and hyperesthesia (increased local sensitivity).

The distribution of the pain is characteristic and suggestive, coinciding either with a radicular dermatome (radicular compression on the spine) or with an area of sensory innervation of a peripheral nerve.

In radiculopathies, we can expect to find symptoms in the corresponding segment of the spine, and the peripheral pain will usually get worse when this segment moves. For example, in sciatica, the pain affects the lumbar spine, spreads along the L5/S1 dermatome and is worse during flexion of the lumbar spine. Valsava maneuvers, like coughing or sneezing, can exacerbate the pain because they increase the pressure of the cerebrospinal fluid surrounding the nerve roots.

The most common peripheral nerve entrapment is that of the median nerve in the carpal tunnel. The pain or paresthesia affects the palmar aspect of the lateral 3–4 fingers and is worse during the night and early morning. Rheumatologic examination of the painful area is usually normal. Tinel's sign is very useful in peripheral nerve compression – percussion over the compression site causes paresthesia.

A neurological examination appropriate to the affected structure may find impaired sensitivity, strength or myotactic reflexes, but these alterations appear later and should not be considered essential to a diagnosis.

Once again, you do not have to memorize all this, as these characteristics are pathophysiologically intuitive.

---

**What suggests neurogenic pain?**

Distribution in a dermatome or peripheral nerve territory.

Dysesthesic nature of pain.

Most common sites: sciatica, carpal tunnel syndrome, ulnar syndrome.

Normal local osteoarticular examination.

Local alterations in the neurological examination (late onset).

Exacerbation with the Valsava maneuver (in radiculopathies).

Exacerbation with mobilization of the spine (in radiculopathies).

Tinel's sign (in peripheral nerve entrapment).

## *Local and regional syndromes*
### *Referred pain*

Some visceral organ lesions may cause diffuse musculoskeletal pain. Examples include pain in the left shoulder and arm in coronary ischemia, lumbar pain in renal colic, etc.

Degenerative or inflammatory processes affecting a joint may trigger pain that is perceived in a wide area or even in a site far from its anatomical origin. For example, pain or sensitivity to pressure on the knee and thigh muscles may be caused by a lesion of the facet joints of the lumbar spine. Arthritis of the shoulder may cause referred pain on the lateral aspect of the upper arm.

In these situations, our local examination is normal, and there is no apparent local cause for the pain. From this point of view, neurogenic pain is also referred pain.

The pattern of pain referred from another musculoskeletal structure will depend on the use of that structure. For example, a child with Perthes disease (which affects the hip) may complain of knee pain when walking. An examination of the knee will be normal but movement of the hip will cause pain. The periodicity of pain from a visceral origin may be confusing, as it depends on the physiology of the organ in question. A pain in the low back and buttocks that varies with the menstrual cycle may be a sign of an underlying gynecological problem.

So, when musculoskeletal pain is accompanied by a normal local clinical examination, do not forget to investigate the adjacent joints, innervation and organs, whose lesions may cause pain to radiate there.

| **What suggests referred pain?** |
|---|
| Local or regional distribution. |
| Uncharacteristic rhythm. |
| Dysesthesic nature (neurogenic pain). |
| Associated symptoms (neighboring joints, viscera, neurological changes). |
| Normal local examination. |

## *Regional syndromes*
### *Monoarthropathy*

A lesion that affects only one joint, whatever its nature, will cause a regional syndrome.

What distinguishes it from other causes of pain limited to one anatomic area? The pain is usually associated with use of the joint even though the rhythm of the pain may vary depending on whether it is an inflammatory or degenerative process. There is no selectivity of painful movements – any use of the joint tends to cause pain. The local examination confirms that the problem lies in the joint:

- Pain during active mobilization in several directions;

- Painful or mechanical limitation of active and passive movements;

- Crepitus, swelling, effusion or articular heat;

| **What suggests monoarthropathy?** |
|---|
| Local distribution of pain. |
| Typical pattern: inflammatory or mechanical. |
| Pain with all movements of the joint. |
| Crepitus, swelling, effusion or local heat or redness. |
| Pain on palpation along the joint margins. |
| Limited active and passive mobility. |
| Specific maneuvers for periarticular lesions: negative. |

- Pain on palpation along the joint margins;

- Resisted mobilization maneuvers almost or totally pain free.

As we have already mentioned, the coexistence of articular and periarticular lesions is common: a challenge to your diagnostic skills! The use of imaging techniques is often helpful in these cases.

The diagnosis and treatment of the wide variety of causes of regional syndromes are dealt with in the chapters dealing with each anatomic area (Chapters 7–14). Monoarthropathies are also mentioned in the context of arthritis.

## GENERALIZED PAIN SYNDROME

This syndrome is extraordinarily common in clinical practice.

Fibromyalgia is responsible for the vast majority of cases. Its differential diagnosis is dealt with in Chapter 15. It generally affects middle aged and elderly adults, particularly women.

The pain affects different parts of the body diffusely and imprecisely, with little or no focus on the joint. Patients often use or agree with the expression "I hurt all over."

The patient usually describes pain by sliding his or her hand along the limb suggesting that the muscles are also affected. This pain is very often migratory, moving from one place to another in hours or days, without leaving sequelae. In any case, its distribution is "strange" and does not fit with any of the typical patterns of joint disease.

Typically, the pain is exacerbated by exercise, but the patient usually feels worse *after* and not during exercise or work. Coexistent paresthesia is common and is also migratory and transient. The complaints are usually many and varied, and are described dramatically. The patient very often shows signs of marked anxiety, which it is important to consider in this clinical context.

Often the pain occurs mainly at night and in the morning, sometimes with prolonged morning stiffness and a sensation of edema. These aspects may suggest an inflammatory joint disease, which is not confirmed by the clinical examination or lab tests.

Physical, rheumatologic and neurological examinations are normal, except for pain with movement, which is frequently severe. There are no signs of inflammation, deformity or limited mobility. Maneuvers for soft tissue lesions can be misleadingly positive in several locations.

The diagnosis and treatment of generalized pain syndromes are discussed in Chapter 15.

| What suggests generalized pain syndrome? |
| --- |
| Pain "all over". |
| Diffuse distribution with little focus in the joints. |
| Migratory nature. |
| Worse after exercise. |
| Distribution inconsistent with polyarthropathy. |
| Dramatic description. |
| Clinical examination with no objective alterations. |
| Laboratory tests and imaging normal. |

## BACK AND NECK PAIN

If our patient's pain is essentially limited to the lumbar or cervical spine, the situation requires special clinical reasoning and a dedicated diagnostic approach. We should first guarantee that the problem does not originate in other areas, such as the viscera. Once this is certain, go into back or neck pain *mode*, following the strategy described in Chapters 7 and 11, respectively.

## ARTICULAR SYNDROME

Articular syndrome is suggested by the interview and clinical examination, with the possible support of lab tests and imaging.

The clinical elements suggesting joint disease have been described above (monoarthropathy). The presence of these features in different joints will obviously be the basis for talking about oligoarthropathy or polyarthropathy. The distribution of the affected joints is decisive in establishing the differential diagnosis of the specific type of joint disease in question (step two). The number and location of the affected joints is not random; it follows typical patterns.

The signs and symptoms of joint disease are similar in all joints, but we have to adapt our diagnostic technique to each anatomic area. So, when more than one joint is affected, it is only possible to move on to a more accurate diagnosis after examining all the joint areas, using the methodology described in Chapters 7–14.

Joint disease can be classified into two main types:

- *Inflammatory joint disease* (arthritis).
  In these situations, the synovial membrane is the site of an inflammatory process with suggestive signs and symptoms, leading to the progressive destruction of the cartilage and subchondral bone. Examples include rheumatoid arthritis, gout, septic arthritis, etc.

- *Degenerative joint disease* (osteoarthritis and associated conditions).
  This is characterized by focal loss of cartilage with a reaction of the subchondral bone. Occasionally, mild inflammation of the synovial membrane may also occur.

- *Clinical assessment gives us the elements we need to distinguish between the two types.*
  We start with the diagnosis of joint disease, based on the indicators presented for monoarthropathy. We now have to consider two other elements: 1. timing of the pain and stiffness, and 2. the clinical examination of the joints.

### The timing of the pain and stiffness

In degenerative joint disease, the pain tends to have a so-called "mechanical pattern." It worsens with the continuous use of the joint. The patient feels worse at the end of the day or after a few hours of walking or work. Rest brings considerable relief and there is rarely any pain during the night. Remember that we also move around in bed, so if the patient mentions nocturnal pain we have to find out whether the pain occurs only when the patient moves or also when s/he is immobile, and whether it is possible to find a pain-free position (typical of mechanical pain).

Conversely, in inflammatory joint disease, the pain tends to have an "inflammatory pattern." The patient feels worse in the morning and the pain is relieved by continued use of the joint. Nocturnal pain is common and does not depend on movement, and so there are no pain-free positions.

All joint diseases may be accompanied by stiffness after long periods of immobility of the joint. This stiffness eases with repeated use of the joint. What distinguishes mechanical from inflammatory disease is the *duration of stiffness*. Usually, in untreated inflammatory joint disease, morning stiffness lasts for more than 30 minutes, while in degenerative joint disease it ceases after 5–10 minutes. Post-rest stiffness (e.g. after meals) may last more than 5 minutes in inflammatory joint disease, while it lasts only a few seconds in osteoarthritis (Table 4.1.).

| Inflammatory pattern | Mechanical pattern |
|---|---|
| Worse in the morning | Worse in the evening |
| Improves with movement | Worsens with movement |
| Pain at rest, no pain free position | Eases at rest, pain free positions |
| Prolonged morning stiffness (> 30 minutes) | Short morning stiffness (< 10 minutes) |
| Stiffness after rest > 5 minutes | Stiffness after rest < 2–3 minutes |

Table 4.1.
Mechanical and
inflammatory
rhythms of pain.

After we have confirmed these aspects with patience, care and repeated questioning, we can say whether we are dealing with *inflammatory joint pain* or *mechanical joint pain*, but we still cannot say whether it is arthritis or osteoarthritis. This diagnosis requires us to look for signs of joint inflammation in our clinical examination.

### Clinical examination of the joints

In clinical examination, arthritis is characterized by articular swelling of a *firm rubbery consistency*, which is a sign of an inflamed, engorged synovium. As the synovium is limited by the capsule, this swelling is uniform, and is spindle shaped and globular in superficial joints. On the other hand, the swelling in osteoarthritis is localized, and of a *bony consistency*, as it reflects the presence of osteophytes, which are bony excrescences at the edge of the joint. Palpation of the articular margins during movement may detect signs of friction, called crepitus, which are typical of osteoarthritis.

Both forms may be accompanied by clinically perceptible articular effusion. Palpation of the joint margins may be painful: diffusely in the case of inflammatory arthritides, and more irregularly in osteoarthritis. Acute arthritis is accompanied by local increases in temperature by comparison with the contralateral joint or adjoining areas. Rubor is rare. Note that osteoarthritis may have short inflammatory flare-ups in which it may acquire some of the characteristics of arthritis.

In more advanced stages or during acute inflammation, there may be painful restriction of active and passive movements. If there are no lesions of the soft tissue, the limitation is the same in both types of movement (Table 4.2.). Tests, especially acute phase reactant proteins and x-rays, will help confirm our diagnosis and clear up any doubts.

| Arthritis | Osteoarthritis |
|---|---|
| Firm, rubbery swelling | Stony swelling |
| Spindle shaped swelling | Irregular, nodular swelling |
| Pain along the joint margins | Focal pain along the joint margin |
| No crepitus (or fine crepitus) | Rough crepitus |
| Signs of inflammation | No signs of inflammation* |
| Extra-articular signs are common | No related systemic signs |
| Any joint | Predominantly in weight-bearing joints and hands |

**Table 4.2.** Main features of inflammatory arthritis and osteoarthritis, on clinical examination.
*Osteoarthritis may be associated with inflammatory signs during acute flares. Longstanding inflammatory arthritis may result in secondary osteoarthritis: thus features from both conditions may coexist.

If the pain has an *inflammatory pattern* and we detect signs of articular inflammation, we know we are dealing with "arthritis" and can limit our differential diagnosis to this type of disease. Until we have demonstrated articular inflammation, we should talk only of "inflammatory joint pain," and remain open to the possibility of this type of pain being caused by something other than arthritis.

The second step in the differential diagnosis between the different types of osteoarthritis and inflammatory arthritis is dealt with in Chapters 16 and 17.

## THE OSTEOPOROSIS "SYNDROME"

The osteoporosis syndrome is worth our attention.[1] Although it is a bone disease, we do not include it in the bone syndrome for two reasons:

1. Osteoporosis is an extraordinarily common disease;

2. The ideal time for intervention is before any symptoms occur, at a time when we can only identify the disease by assessing its risk factors.

---

[1]As you will see, the use of the word "syndrome" here is rather inappropriate as there are usually no symptoms. However, we use it for the sake of clarity.

Ideally, we should think of the disease before it manifests itself. This means considering the risk factors and taking proactive measures. The manifestations of osteoporosis are bone fractures sustained after low impact trauma. They indicate that we have missed the optimum opportunity to take preventive action.

Table 4.3. shows the main risk factors for osteoporosis and the manifestations that should lead us to consider the disease.

| Risk factors | Manifestations |
|---|---|
| Post-menopausal women | • Whenever a patient of any age presents a history of low-impact fractures i.e. fractures caused by falls of less than his/her own height, whether it manifests itself clinically or radiologically, in a spinal x-ray for example |
| Early menopause | |
| Late menarche | |
| Low weight and height | |
| Family history of osteoporosis | |
| Prolonged corticosteroid therapy | |
| Sedentary lifestyle | |
| Insufficient intake of dairy products | • Whenever an x-ray suggests low bone mass (radiological osteopenia) |
| Diseases causing osteoporosis: malabsorption, hyperthyroidism, hyperparathyroidism, chronic alcoholism, liver disease ... | |

**Table 4.3.** When should we think of osteoporosis?

The appropriate approach to the problem is discussed in Chapter 26.

## BONE SYNDROME

Pain originating exclusively in bone is rare in clinical practice. It may appear in association with bone tumors (primary or metastatic), metabolic diseases (e.g. Paget's bone disease) or inflammation of the periosteum. It is usually described as deep, unlocalized, continuous pain, occurring night and day, and unrelated to movement. It is most common in the spine, pelvis and the proximal segments of the limbs. A local examination is usually normal. If there is no suggestion of referred pain, we should request appropriate tests for this type of disease (see Chapter 27).

## MUSCULAR SYNDROME

The pathological involvement (inflammatory or metabolic) of muscles is most commonly reflected by *predominantly proximal weakness and muscular atrophy*. Proximal predominance helps to distinguish it from weakness caused by neuropathy, which is chiefly distal. Myopathic patients may have difficulty going up and down stairs, getting up from a low chair or combing their hair but their handshake is firm and they can walk on tiptoe. The opposite is the case in patients with polyneuropathy. In some myopathies, weakness only occurs after repeated movements, though it is normal initially. Muscular atrophy also varies depending on the type of muscle disease.

It is not uncommon for a rheumatic patient to complain of "weakness." This symptom also often accompanies depression. Localized weakness (e.g. foot drop) is more likely to be significant than generalized weakness. In either case, however, the "weakness" requires a neurological examination to assess its significance.

Muscle pain, whether it is spontaneous or triggered by palpation, often accompanies general inflammatory conditions like flu, but it may also be due to muscular inflammation (myositis) as part of a systemic rheumatic condition (Chapter 25). However, systemic rheumatic diseases are quite rare in unspecialized clinical practice.

Of course, we must remember that muscles may be altered as a result of nerve or articular processes causing disuse atrophy. Pain originating in joints is often diffuse and involves the neighboring muscles. Referred pain is often felt in muscles. Patients with fibromyalgia (see Chapter 15) describe muscular weakness and generalized pain that may involve the muscles, without any physical changes.

## SYSTEMIC SYNDROME

All inflammatory rheumatic diseases may be accompanied by extra-articular manifestations, involving other organs and systems. The best example is systemic lupus erythematosus, which can affect practically all the body's structures and functions. Looking into these extra-articular clinical manifestations is therefore a compulsory part of our investigation of a rheumatic patient's symptoms, especially if the preliminary interview suggests inflammatory polyarthropathy. If we fail to do this, we run the risk of missing essential diagnostic clues or of leaving potentially fatal conditions untreated.

Table 4.4. shows the extra-articular manifestations most commonly associated with rheumatic diseases.

In many cases, these manifestations occur together with polyarthritis, which may constitute the basis for our subsequent differential diagnosis. In others, extra-articular manifestations predominate, sometimes discreet but often multiple, and they are important to consider, particularly in young patients. It is essential to recognize their possible association with a connec-

| | Associated diseases (in descending order of frequency) |
|---|---|
| • **Constitutional manifestations** <br> Fever <br> Weight loss <br> Severe fatigue | Systemic lupus erythematosus <br> Systemic sclerosis <br> Rheumatoid arthritis <br> Mixed connective tissue disease <br> Vasculitis… |
| • **Skin and mucosal manifestations** <br> Photosensitivity <br> Skin rash <br> Purpura, ulcers <br> Hair loss <br> Oral and genital aphthae <br> Dry eyes and mouth <br> Red eye <br> Balanitis … | Systemic lupus erythematosus <br> Rheumatoid arthritis <br> Psoriatic arthritis (psoriasis) <br> Sjögren's syndrome <br> Systemic sclerosis <br> Reactive arthritis <br> Behçet's disease and other vasculites… |
| • **Serositis** <br> Pleurisy/pleural effusion <br> Pericarditis | Connective tissue diseases |
| Raynaud's phenomenon | Idiopathic Raynaud's phenomenon <br> Systemic sclerosis <br> Systemic lupus erythematosus… |
| Dysphagia | Systemic sclerosis |
| Dyspnea | Connective tissue diseases |
| Lower limb edema, hypertension | Connective tissue diseases |
| Lymphadenopathy | Connective tissue diseases |
| Muscular weakness | Myositis, overlap syndromes |

**Table 4.4.**
Main systemic
manifestations of
rheumatic diseases.

tive tissue disease and begin a differential diagnostic process based on the concept of a systemic syndrome (Chapter 25).

Identifying these syndromes is the first step towards a final differential diagnosis. Going back to our travel analogy, we could say that, having identified the syndrome, we know which neighborhood we are in and that we are not far from our final destination, an exact diagnosis, a building in the neighborhood. Just as all roads lead to Rome, we can follow many roads to reach our exact diagnosis, depending on the predominant manifestations in a systemic disease.

Note, however, that we cannot skip any of the stages without running the risk of making a mistake. Diagnosis of the syndrome or the disease itself always requires a thorough, well planned interview, and may not be possible without a careful general and regional examination of all the areas presenting symptoms. Do not forget to examine also those areas whose affection could be important for your diagnosis, even if assymptomatic. This methodology is described in the next 3 chapters.

# THE STANDARD ENQUIRY IN RHEUMATOLOGY

5.

J.A.P. da Silva, A.D. Woolf, *Rheumatology in Practice*, DOI 10.1007/978-1-84882-581-9_5,
© Springer-Verlag London Limited 2010

# 5. THE STANDARD ENQUIRY IN RHEUMATOLOGY

*TYPICAL CASES*
**5.A. RHEUMATIC FEVER (I)**

Maria Helena, an 18 year-old student, came to the surgery with her mother. She said that she was being treated for rheumatic fever with monthly injections of penicillin, but had shown no improvement. She described three episodes of joint pain, the first of which had affected her right ankle some years previously. The other two episodes involved her knees. According to the patient, there had been joint swelling, and the skin over the affected joint was hot, red and itchy. On each occasion, the symptoms had lasted one to two weeks then disappeared without a trace. She had had repeated measurements of anti-streptolysin antibodies, which were always high. Her clinical examination on that day was completely normal.

The case continues at the end of this chapter.

*TYPICAL CASES*
**5.B. "RHEUMATOID ARTHRITIS" (I)**

Joaquim Fernandes was sent to us by his family doctor with a diagnosis of rheumatoid arthritis.

According to the letter of referral, he suffered from continuous pain, which persisted at night and was not relieved by non-steroidal anti-inflammatories. His serology was strongly positive for rheumatoid factor.

The case continues at the end of this chapter.

## The doctor's attitude: controlling and focusing the enquiry

Together, the patient's history and the clinical examination are the essential pillar of diagnosis in rheumatology, and in many cases additional investigations are not required.

Whether we are aware of it or not, we begin our differential diagnosis with our first question and then test out, reinforce or eliminate hypotheses as the enquiry goes on. To make the enquiry work, therefore, we must be aware of the value and degree of certainty of each answer, question each partial conclusion and be aware of its impact on our reasoning.

When interviewing a patient, we must divide ourselves in half. One part of us is focused on the interaction with the patient, maintaining and reinforcing empathy, while the other part is constantly questioning the validity and accuracy of the answers, the certainty of our interpretation and the influence these conclusions will have on our differential diagnosis. Going back to the trip analogy – one part of us asks for directions in the street, while the other looks at the map and finds the most probable route, on the basis of the information we are given.

If our enquiry is to be productive, we must make constant use of our knowledge of possible pathologies. We should try to identify a pattern of symptoms (a syndrome) that fits with the patient's complaints, paying equal attention to the characteristics that are typical of the syndrome and to those that distinguish it from others.

The enquiry must therefore be as thorough, oriented and consistent as possible, to make it more productive and economical. Politely respecting the patient's answers, we should clearly and surely take charge of the enquiry, focusing it on the aspects that make a difference to our reasoning.

While adapting to individual circumstances, our enquiry should try to answer some essential questions:

- *What is the affected structure or origin of the pain?*
- *Soft tissue (tendons, ligaments, muscles, nerves …)*
- *Joints*
- *Viscera*

**Within the articular lesions:**
- *What is the probable nature of the condition: inflammatory, degenerative, post-traumatic, etc?*
- *Which joints are affected?*
- *What is the pattern of onset and progression?*

**Symptoms suggesting multi-system development.**

**What medication has been given and with what results?**

**What is the functional and psychological impact of the disease?**

**What are the patient's beliefs, expectations and fears related to the disease?**

Pain is the predominant symptom of rheumatic diseases. It is a subjective experience and the communication difficulties inherent in the nature of the symptom require persistence, patience and insight. It is often necessary to ask the patient about the same feature in several different ways, until we are certain how to interpret the symptom.

### *Location of the pain*

The mere fact that the pain is limited to the cervical or lumbar region identifies a syndrome that will lead us to a particular diagnostic strategy.

When pain is limited to a single area, the probability of soft tissue lesions increases, as joint disease often affects more than one joint. The relative probability of periarticular (as opposed to articular) lesions varies according to the area in question. Regional shoulder pain should be considered periarticular in origin until proven otherwise because it is extremely common, while isolated disease of the shoulder joint is quite rare. Conversely, pain affecting only the knee usually derives from a joint lesion, as the prevalence of knee osteoarthritis is high, as is mechanical disruption of this joint.

Carpal tunnel syndrome is also very common in clinical practice and should always be considered whenever the patient mentions symptoms localized to the hand, particularly if it is unilateral.

Keep in mind that visceral pain can radiate to the musculoskeletal system and mimic rheumatic disease.

Table 5.1. shows the most common situations of referred pain of visceral origin. This possibility should be considered whenever pain affects the indicated areas, especially if the local clinical examination is normal.

Our suspicions, systemic enquiry and clinical examination may be decisive.

| Visceral origin | Location of referred pain |
|---|---|
| Retroperitoneum | Upper lumbar region |
| Biliary tree | Right shoulder |
| Heart | Left shoulder and arm |
| Urinary tract | Lumbar and inguinal regions |
| Genital organs | Sacral region |
| Pleura | Thoracic wall |
| Esophagus | Dorsal region and sternum |

Table 5.1.
Most common causes of musculo-skeletal pain referred from visceral origin.

- *How many joints have been affected?*
  We use the terms **mono**arthropathy when only one joint is involved, **oligo**arthropathy for two to four joints and **poly**arthropathy when five or more joints are involved.

- *Is the involvement predominantly **proximal** (shoulders, elbows, hips and knees) or **distal** (hands and feet)?*

- *Is the cervical and/or lumbosacral spine involved?*

- *Is the distribution of the affected joints **symmetrical** or **asymmetrical**?*

As we will see, these elements are essential to differential diagnosis between different arthropathies.

For example, rheumatoid arthritis is normally peripheral and symmetrical, while psoriatic arthritis is often asymmetrical and may affect the lumbosacral spine. The former spares the distal interphalangeal joints, but they may be affected by the latter. Symptoms localized to the upper and lower limb girdles are highly suggestive of polymyalgia rheumatica.

The pattern of affection of the small joints in the hands is particularly important. The patient often tells us quite simply that "all" the joints of the hand hurt. Given that different joint diseases tend to affect different joints in the hands, we should try to be specific, asking the patient to point out exactly which joints are painful or swollen (rarely "all" of them!).

Keep in mind that the patient may present an association of a number of soft tissue lesions in different places, with a distribution that may suggest a more generalized process suggesting joint disease. Careful clinical examination will be the key to the diagnosis in such a case.

## Radiation of the pain

Patients with articular or periarticular lesions can usually localize the pain quite accurately, pointing to the most affected area. Patients with joint pain usually indicate the affected joint precisely. Often, in inflammatory conditions, the pain is demonstrated around the whole circumference of the joint. When pain is located at a specific point on a joint, the possibility of a localized periarticular lesion such as tendonitis or bursitis, should be considered.

We should bear in mind that pain originating in deep joints may be felt some way away from the joint. Shoulder pain is sometimes referred to the lateral aspect of the upper arm, for example. Hip pain is generally localised to the groin but may be felt deep in the buttock too. Pain in the sacroiliac joint is normally located in the lumbosacral region with radiation to the buttocks. In children hip disease may present as knee pain.

Conversely in generalized pain syndromes, which are very common in clinical practice, the patient describes diffuse pain in many different areas, often varying over time and not clearly localised to the joints. The distribution of pain does not follow any particular pattern. It is interesting to note that, as a rule, patients with joint disease point to the painful area by running their hands around the joint, while sufferers from generalized pain run their hand along the limb, suggesting muscular pain.

Pain radiating along the territory of a nerve root or peripheral nerve naturally suggests neurogenic pain. In these cases, it is often dysesthetic and described as burning, tingling, numbness, etc. Radicular pain is typically affected by movements of the corresponding spine segment, which is also usually painful.

Pain originating in bone is deep and ill-defined and usually presents in the axial skeleton and the proximal parts of the limbs.

## The rhythm of pain

We distinguished above (Chapter 4) between inflammatory and mechanical pain. This is an essential aspect that ought to be thoroughly and accurately assessed with every patient. Our aim is not only a differential diagnosis, but also an assessment of the degree of activity of the inflammatory joint disease.

These characteristics need to be defined more accurately, in order to avoid errors of interpretation.

If we take rheumatoid arthritis as a characteristic example of an inflammatory joint disease, a typical untreated patient, if asked the right questions, may say that the pain is worst first thing in the morning and improves afterwards as the joints are used. Morning pain is accompanied by stiffness which also decreases with continued use of the joints. If untreated, this stiffness lasts for more than 30 minutes and often for several hours, from when the patient gets up until he feels "his best."

The duration of morning stiffness is an important factor, not only for differential diagnosis, but also for assessing the degree of inflammatory activity of the disease and its response to treatment. We should therefore be as precise as possible when evaluating it, trying to ensure that the patient understands exactly what we need to know. Patients should be told at their first visit to assess this parameter regularly to help evaluate the progression of their disease and the response to therapy.

When the disease is active, a patient with inflammatory arthritis will describe pain even when at rest and during the night. It is usually a duller, less defined pain, sometimes taking the form of discomfort or feeling unwell. Pain when at rest is a sign of intense inflammatory activity and is among the first to disappear with appropriate medication. The presence of nocturnal pain is an indication that the inflammatory process is not being controlled properly. The same applies to the duration of morning stiffness.

Usually, in active inflammatory joint disease, the patient also has joint stiffness after periods of rest, for example while eating or waiting to see the doctor. This stiffness lasts long enough to be noticeable when the patient enters the doctor's room.

On the other hand, a typical osteoarthritis patient describes pain with movement that gets worse with continued, repeated use. These patients feel worse at the end of the day and improve when they rest the joint and at weekends. Even here, our questions and interpretation of the answers must be careful. When asked if they feel better with rest, osteoarthritis patients often say, "Certainly not; I feel worse" meaning that they become stiff and find it difficult to move again after resting ("gelling"). which is often quite marked. This post-rest stiffness in osteoarthritis is usually of short duration, lasting no more than five minutes. These patients may also experience morning stiffness, but it does not usually last more than half an hour.

Questions about night pain can also cause misunderstandings. When asking patients about night pain, we think about pain at rest but we must remember that people still move in bed. So, when patients with osteoarthritis describe nocturnal pain, we have to find out whether it hurts when they are lying still or when they move in bed. And when they move can they find a pain-free position? The answer will usually be "no" to the first question and "yes" to the second, unlike patients with inflammatory arthritis.

We have been talking about typical patients. In practice, clinical descriptions are often less precise, associating characteristics of both types. This is what we call mixed rhythm. Whether we consider the condition to be more inflammatory or mechanical will depend on the relative weight that we lend to the arguments in favor of one of the interpretations.

This superimposition may be the result of the patients' difficulty in expressing themselves, but some rheumatic conditions may be associated with mechanical and inflammatory processes whose predominance may vary over time.

In osteoarthritis there may occasionally be flare-ups associated with synovitis. In these phases, the patient may mention nocturnal pain or longer morning stiffness, possibly accompanied by increased swelling. In the same way, in rheumatoid arthritis, the intensity of the inflammatory symptoms indicates the degree of inflammatory activity. In controlled phases, the inflammatory symptoms may disappear altogether though mechanical symptoms corresponding to the structural sequelae in the meantime may persist. The evaluation of the more or less "inflammatory" nature of the patient's complaints not only helps our differential diagnosis, but also our assessment of the degree of inflammatory activity at any given moment, i.e. the efficacy of the treatment in inflammatory joint disease...

### *Rhythm of back pain*

If the patient complains of pain affecting a number of joints, whose onset and progression suggest the same disease, we do not need to ascertain whether it is inflammatory or mechanical in each separate joint. We can assume that it is part of the same process. There is one exception, however.

Inflammatory back pain is a "red flag" that we must not ignore for several reasons. Firstly, it points strongly to a large arthritis group, the seronegative spondyloarthropathies: secondly, it may indicate more sinister pathologies such as infections or neoplasms. Back pain is so common, however, that we will find patients with peripheral arthritis also have back pain, by chance alone.

> **Note**
>
> The distinction between inflammatory and mechanical pain is particularly important when dealing with joint disease or back pain (inflammatory back pain always needs attention!). In other conditions, it may even be misleading if we are not careful. Although tendonitis is inflammatory, it may cause pain only with movement and not be accompanied by morning stiffness. In generalized pain syndromes, patients often say that they feel worse during the night and morning and may describe prolonged morning stiffness. A careful physical examination will exclude joint inflammation, however. In carpal tunnel syndrome the pain is usually worse at night and in the morning even when there is no inflammation. Bone pain has little or no relationship with movement or rest and tends to be continuous day and night. Systematic questioning is once again of vital importance.
>
> Be alert. Inflammatory pain does not necessarily mean an inflammatory process.

When dealing with peripheral arthritis, we should always ask about back pain and, if the patient suffers from it, characterize its rhythm separately from the other joints. In most cases, we will find mechanical pain which means peripheral arthritis coinciding with common low back pain. If the back pain is also inflammatory, we must consider seronegative spondyloarthropathy or other pathologies.

### *Inflammatory signs*

Signs of inflammation described by the patient are an indication of an inflammatory lesion, but should be assessed carefully. It is important to note that redness of the skin overlying the joint rarely occurs in rheumatic diseases. It is usual-

> **Note**
>
> In cases of oligoarthritis or polyarthritis we must ask the patient about the coexistence of back pain, and characterize its rhythm separately.

ly found in microcrystal joint diseases such as gout, and in septic arthritis. It was often seen in cases of rheumatic fever, which is now very rare in the developed world. Note, however, that redness is rare in rheumatoid arthritis, for example, even in the presence of highly active synovitis. Active-phase psoriatic arthritis is often accompanied by a mauve color over the joints.

A feeling of heat over inflamed joints is much more common, but its significance is doubtful if not accompanied by other manifestations, though anxious patients often mention it.

Complaints of joint swelling suggest effusion or synovitis. They can, however, be misleading, as the presence of swelling of the feet, for example, may indicate heart or venous impairment more often than arthritis. Swelling of the hands may suggest arthritis, but it is also common in healthy women, frequently associated with water retention as part of the premenstrual syndrome. Patients with carpal tunnel syndrome often describe swelling of the hands, especially in the morning. In some cases, the swelling is only perceived and is not visible to the external observer, but some patients describe difficulty in removing rings. In many other cases, no cause can be found. The swelling is usually diffuse without the typical spindle-shaped deformation of the fingers, seen in the presence of synovitis (in these conditions, the inflammatory process is contained by the joint capsule).

Swelling described as located in major joints like the elbow or the knee is much more reliable as an indication of a local inflammatory process. Note, however, that joint effusion with swelling is not synonymous with arthritis, as it may arise in, for example, bursae as well as advanced osteoarthritis of the knee and lesions of the meniscus, for example. Progressive bone deformity, typical of osteoarthritis, is more persistent than effusion, and can be better assessed by clinical examination.

### *Aggravating and mitigating factors*

As expected, almost all pain of musculoskeletal origin is exacerbated by the use of the affected structures, i.e. by movement. There are, however, details of these aspects that are worth a closer look.

As we have seen, when a joint is affected, all its movements tend to be painful. When a specific movement is particularly painful (selectivity of movements), we should consider the possibility of periarticular lesions (tendons, bursae, ligaments). The selectivity of painful movements should be especially investigated when the patient's complaints are limited to one articular area, such as the shoulder. In either case, the pain worsens when the joint is used. This does not preclude the fact that pain arising from inflammatory joint disease tends to ameliorate with continued movement.

Patients with generalized pain will usually say that the pain is worse with exercise, but, typically, it is particularly bad after they stop (that night or the next day). Cold and stress also exacerbate pain in fibromyalgia.

If back pain worsens with Valsava's maneuvers (like coughing or defecating), this strongly suggests nerve root irritation.

Occasionally the pain may have a strange rhythm that is unrelated to the use of the painful structure. In this case, think of bone pain or referred pain! Is it related to respiratory movements (pleurisy, pericarditis)? Is it influenced by meals, as in biliary or peptic lesions? With menstruation? With urination? Pain in fibromyalgia may also not be exacerbated by use of the affected area.

## Form of onset and progression

The onset of some rheumatic diseases is acute, reaching its active phase in hours or days. This is the case with post-traumatic lesions, gout and other microcrystalline joint diseases, septic arthritis and reactive arthritis.

Others are more insidious in their onset, manifesting themselves over weeks, as is the case with most periarticular lesions, rheumatoid arthritis, psoriatic arthritis and other seronegative spondyloarthropathies, connective tissue diseases, etc.

In other cases, the process develops insidiously over months or years before the patient seeks medical attention. This is typical of osteoarthritis, ankylosing spondylitis, fibromyalgia, and many cases of chronic back pain.

To put it simply, we can classify pain on the basis of its onset into **acute, subacute and insidious** (which is preferable to "chronic," as this is also related to the duration of the condition).

Where progression over time is concerned, the pattern is often atypical at the beginning, and it is sometimes necessary to wait a few weeks or months for the disease to assume a clearer, definitive profile.

Here, we can consider several patterns that are particularly useful in classifying joint disease.

## Additive versus migratory

In many joint diseases, new joints are successively added to the originally affected site. In others, one of the patient's joints is involved, then it improves before another is affected. The pain and inflammation move from one joint to another. We call the former "additive," and the latter "migratory." The first pattern is characteristic of rheumatoid arthritis, psoriatic arthritis, lupus, etc. The second strongly suggests rheumatic fever or other forms of reactive arthritis. It is also the typical pattern in gout and other types of microcrystal arthritis, but, in these cases, there are usually symptom-free periods between episodes.

## Recurring versus persistent

In rheumatoid and psoriatic arthritis, lupus and other inflammatory joint diseases, once the process has started, its development is usually persistent. The patient may undergo periods of relapse and remission while never being completely asymptomatic. In other cases, the patient mentions episodes of arthritis ("crises") separated by disease-free intervals. This pattern is highly suggestive of microcrystalline joint diseases or reactive arthritis. In these situations, the intervals tend to get shorter over time until the disease becomes continuous, though there is always a typical recurrent pattern at the beginning.

## Treatments and their results

The patient's response to non-steroidal anti-inflammatory drugs, corticosteroids or even simple analgesics is of very little use in differential diagnosis, given the non-specific nature of these medications. The response to other treatments may, however, be helpful.

A rapid, clear response to colchicine during an articular crisis, will lend support to a diagnosis of microcrystalline arthritis, because, as a rule, other inflammatory joint diseases do not respond to this therapy. A marked improvement after an extra-articular injection will reinforce the possibility of a periarticular lesion. An improvement in generalized pain with hot baths is very common and suggestive of fibromyalgia.

On the other hand, if an apparently suitable medication has failed in the past, we should reconsider the dose, regimen and duration of the treatment.

Of equal importance is the patient's tolerance of the medications used: a history of peptic ulcers, gastrointestinal hemorrhage, hypertension or asthma after taking non-steroidal anti-inflammatories requires great care with any subsequent use. A history of intolerance to other anti-rheumatic drugs must also be taken into consideration.

It is important to know about any concomitant medication, not only because it gives us a clue as to associated diseases, but also because we have to consider the possibility of drug interactions. In addition, many medications can have musculoskeletal side effects. For example, fluoroquinolones have been associated with tendonitis; colchicine, statins and zidovudine, among others, can cause myositis; antidepressants may simulate Sjögren's syndrome; and there are several medications that can cause conditions similar to systemic lupus erythematosus (e.g. isoniazid, hydralazine, diphenylhidantoin, carbamazepine, sulfasalazine, ...), etc.

A long history of the use of psychotropic drugs is indicative of an important psychosomatic component, and is common among fibromyalgic patients.

### Functional and psychological status

Maintaining functional capacity is one of the basic goals of treatment in rheumatic diseases, as it is essential to the patients' quality of life.

For this reason, our enquiries should consider their functional capacity at each visit and attempt to identify any limitations requiring attention. Patients' mobility can be assessed in an accurate and reproducible way by means of validated instruments designed to quantify the difficulty they experience when carrying out different tasks. Some of these instruments are disease-specific, i.e. they have been designed for the particular features of a certain condition. Examples of these are the Arthritis Impact Measurement Scale (AIMS) and the Health Assessment Questionnaire (HAQ) for rheumatic diseases. Others are generic, i.e. they can be used for a variety of conditions, such as the Sickness Impact Profile (SIP) and the Index of Well Being (IWB).

Although these tools are extremely useful in scientific research and are even applied routinely at certain rheumatology units, their use in clinical practice is time consuming and requires experience.

At ordinary visits we should still ask patients about any difficulty they may have in everyday activities, such as getting dressed, washing, combing their hair, eating, walking, doing housework, carrying things, etc. What other activities do they have trouble with? When there are limitations, it is important to find out whether the patient can get help from other people in doing essential tasks.

Our clinical study and choice of treatment should be governed by the most significant limitations *for the individual patient,* i.e. those that represent a significant conflict between what they want to do and what they are actually capable of doing. The same limitations can have very different impacts on quality of life, depending on the patient's occupation or leisure activities.

It is very important to make a direct or indirect assessment of the psychological impact of the disease on patients and to assess their attitude to the pain, limitations and demands of their condition. It is easy to understand that a patient may feel depressed, discouraged or bitter, when faced with a diagnosis of a serious, chronic and potentially incapacitating disease. If these reactions are not kept under control, they will affect his or her quality of life much more than necessary and may in themselves become more serious than the rheumatic condition itself. Overcome by these feelings, the patient will find it difficult to comply with the treatment or cooperate with the doctor. The patients' interpretation of their symptoms and their expectations from the treatment also affect their attitude.

As a result, we must consider these aspects and regard controlling them as one of the main aims of treatment. The attitude of family and friends to patients, their limitations and their needs may also require the doctor's attention.

## SYSTEMATIC ENQUIRY

After asking patients about the musculoskeletal complaints that brought them to the doctor in the first place, we must then question them about each system in order to identify any relevant extra-skeletal manifestations.

For a number of reasons:

- Many rheumatic conditions, especially connective tissue diseases, are perfect examples of multi-systemic diseases, which can involve almost all the organs and systems in the body. In these conditions, the identification of extra-skeletal manifestations is important not only for the diagnosis but also for selecting the most appropriate treatment.

If, in the case of a patient with symmetrical, additive polyarthritis, we do not ask about the existence of photosensitivity, mouth ulcers or hypertension, we run the risk of mistaking a case of lupus for rheumatoid arthritis, giving free rein to the renal involvement that will determine the prognosis. If we do not identify and pay attention to alterations in bowel habit accompanying arthritis, we may miss a diagnosis of inflammatory bowel disease, the treatment of which may ameliorate both symptoms. Note that the patient may not describe these systemic manifestations spontaneously as s/he does not associate them with joint pain.

- There may be musculoskeletal involvement in many primarily extra-articular conditions, such as metabolic diseases, and these manifestations may be the primary expression and even the key to the diagnosis. In addition, the treatment of the rheumatic manifestations must involve the underlying systemic condition.

For example, joint disease is one of the first and most common manifestations of hemochromatosis and an early diagnosis will enable us to begin treatment to prevent liver cirrhosis and heart failure. Patients with gouty arthritis often have renal lithiasis or hyperlipidemia. One may treat the gout whilst ignoring the renal and cardiovascular risk but we would not be providing good medical care. Diabetic patients are particularly prone to periarticular lesions and carpal tunnel syndrome. Hypothyroidism can cause myopathy, diffuse pain and compression of the median nerve…

- In the case of referred pain of visceral origin, our systematic enquiry can be crucial to our pinpointing the organ in question.

- Treatment of rheumatic diseases often has to be adapted to concomitant pathologies and therapy. There are many examples of this. In patients with a history of peptic ulcers, anti-inflammatory treatment may be contraindicated. This kind of treatment must be carefully monitored in cases of hypertension, kidney failure and asthma. Diabetes requires special care when using corticosteroids.

- Our approach to patients should always be global and holistic, and this involves the interpretation, diagnosis and treatment of each of their health problems, considering their relative importance to the quality and duration of life. Patients have the right to expect this from their doctor.

Our systematic enquiry should be structured and address all the systems, in sequence. Our questions should be open-ended and chosen to detect the most common diseases. If we find anomalies, we will go on to more specific questions to identify the nature and importance of the problem. Our questions should be adapted on the basis of the patient's previous history. As the systematic enquiry progresses, we should make a mental review of any manifestations in that area that may be related to the clinical condition in question and include them in our questions. Important possibilities that have not been considered in the musculoskeletal enquiry will often arise here.

You can use a method that consists of imagining a horizontal plane running downwards over the patient and asking the questions inherent in the system that the plane touches (Table 5.2.).

As you can see, almost all the questions that would be asked in a systematic enquiry in internal medicine can be significant in the context of rheumatic diseases. We have to follow the thorough, consistent methodology that is compulsory in any branch of medicine.

### Past medical history

Questioning patients about their past medical history is obviously an integral part of the clinical assessment. Depending on the context suggested by the previous enquiry, however, some aspects are particularly important in rheumatology. Here, we will only present a few examples.

The possibility of osteoporosis should be considered before any fractures occur, i.e. by taking into account appreciable risk factors in the patient's past and present clinical history. Osteoporosis is more common in post-menopausal women of low weight who smoke and have

| General | Known associated diseases |
| | Fever? |
| | Recent weight loss? |
| Skin | Skin problems? |
| | Rash? Psoriasis? |
| | Nodules? |
| | Skin sensitivity to light? |
| | Hair loss? |
| Eyes and mucous membranes | Aphthae or mouth ulcers? |
| | Genital ulcers? |
| | Gritty eyes (as if they had sand in them?) |
| | Painful red eyes? |
| | Dry mouth? |
| | Loss of vision? |
| Respiratory tract and circulatory system | Shortness of breath? |
| | Cough? |
| | Chest pain? |
| | Lower-limb edema? |
| | Raynaud's phenomenon? |
| Digestive tract | Dysphagia? |
| | Dyspepsia? |
| | History of gastric ulcers? |
| | Diarrhoea? |
| Urinary tract | Change in urine color? |
| | Kidney stones? |
| Genitalia | Discharge? |
| | Dyspareunia? |
| Nervous system (peripheral and central) | Dysesthesia? |
| | Weakness? |
| | Convulsions? |
| | Alterations in behavior? |
| Global | Any other concerns that we have not talked about? |

Table 5.2. Some relevant questions in the systematic enquiry in rheumatology.

a positive family history. Insufficient intake of dairy products and lack of physical exercise, especially in adolescence, increase this risk. Prolonged treatment with corticosteroids or anticonvulsants, late menarche or early menopause, liver disease or malabsorption (for any reason), and signs of hypogonadism, among others, are indicators of a risk of osteoporosis that should lead to further investigation.

Previous articular trauma or joint infection may explain osteoarthritis in an atypical location, for example.

A history of pleuritic pain, possibly caused by non-specific pleurisy, mouth ulcers or recurring skin eruptions may suggest a connective tissue disease underlying the polyarthritis or polyarthralgia that have prompted the patient's visit to the doctor.

A history of repeated miscarriages, venous or arterial thromboses may suggest the possibility of antiphospholipid syndrome.

A history of recurring monoarthritis may point to gout as the cause of acute polyarthritis, though this diagnosis is not apparent at the start. The same may occur with a long history of kidney stones.

A history of significant peptic disease requires special care in the use of corticosteroids or non-steroidal anti-inflammatory drugs.

A history of anterior or posterior uveitis may indicate seronegative spondyloarthropathy, sarcoidosis or Behcet's disease. Alterations in bowel movements may be a sign of inflammatory intestinal disease, malabsorption or Whipple's disease.

In a case of acute-onset arthritis, it is particularly important to ask about the patient's recent history, which may point to an infection. Arthritis of this kind, especially in young people, may raise the possibility of reactive arthritis due to an infection in the preceding two or three weeks. Infections most often related to this type of pathology are gastrointestinal (diarrhea, dysentery), oropharyngeal (tonsillitis, odynophagia, rhinorrhea) and genitourinary (urethritis, vaginal discharge, dyspareunia). These types of arthritis are sometimes associated with fever, conjunctivitis, urethritis, skin eruptions, mucosal ulcers or lymphadenopathy that the patient may not mention spontaneously.

### *Family history*

There are very few rheumatic diseases that can be considered to have simple Mendelian genetic transmission. In most cases, there is polygenic inheritance meaning that the family history increases the risk of having the same disease without determining it from a Mendelian point of view. Family history is therefore important but usually has no definitive impact on diagnosis and should be considered merely as a pointer.

Common rheumatic conditions within a family include seronegative spondyloarthropathy (linked to HLA-B27), rheumatoid arthritis, systemic lupus erythematosus, nodal osteoarthritis, osteoporosis and gout. In the presence of arthritis with a pattern suggesting psoriatic arthritis but without skin lesions, a family history of psoriasis makes it much more likely.

Some aspects of the patient's family history may be relevant as they affect the treatment or monitoring of rheumatic diseases. A history of breast cancer before the age of 50 in a patient's mother or sister indicates a higher risk of this disease in the patient herself and is a relative contra-indication to hormone replacement therapy. A substantial family history of lymphoid neoplasm requires special monitoring for lymphoproliferative disease in patients with Sjögren's syndrome, and in patients being treated with immunosuppressants. A family history of glaucoma or diabetes requires closer monitoring of the side effects of corticosteroids.

### Age and gender

This general information may have a substantial influence on the probability of different diagnoses.

Table 5.3. shows the most common rheumatologic diagnoses per age group and gender. We must remember, however, that none of these distinctions are clear cut. We may find osteoarthritis in a young adult, though it is rare, or the onset of lupus at the age of 70 or over.

| | Women | Men |
|---|---|---|
| Children 0–16 | Trauma<br>Post-viral arthritis<br>Hip lesions<br>Scoliosis<br>Juvenile idiopathic arthritisl | |
| Young adults 17–35 | Fibromyalgia<br>Rheumatoid arthritis<br>Systemic lupus erythematosus | Soft tissue lesions<br>Reactive arthritis<br>Ankylosing spondylitis<br>Rheumatoid arthritis |
| Middle-aged 36–65 | Fibromyalgia<br>Soft tissue lesions<br>Osteoarthritis<br>Rheumatoid arthritis<br>Systemic lupus erythematosu | Soft tissue lesions<br>Gout<br>Osteoarthritis<br>Rheumatoid arthritis |
| Elderly >65 | Osteoarthritis<br>Osteoporosis<br>Rheumatoid arthritis<br>Polimyalgia rheumatica<br>Gout and pseudogout | |

Table 5.3.
The most common diagnoses per age group and gender.

*TYPICAL CASES*
### 5.A. "RHEUMATIC FEVER" (Epilog from page 5.2)

We were not convinced by the diagnosis of rheumatic fever. The pain was certainly articular and its migratory nature was suggestive. These aspects only enable us to identify "migratory joint pain," while rheumatic fever requires the presence of arthritis! The patient certainly described swelling and redness over the painful joints, but pruritus was not to be expected in arthritis! The episodes of arthritis were not preceded by oropharyngeal infections as would be expected in rheumatic fever and our systematic enquiry did not come up with any associated manifestations suggesting carditis, erythema marginatum, etc.

So we asked more questions and found out that Maria Helena had an atopic history, with asthma and itchy, transient skin lesions. Could it be urticaria?

On the other hand, rheumatic fever is exceptional these days and requires prolonged treatment. It was essential to be sure about the diagnosis.

We asked the patient to stop all medications and to come back as soon as she had a "crisis." Two months later she had a painful knee. The skin was very red and infiltrated but only over the medial aspect of the knee. There was no synovitis. So she did not have either arthritis or rheumatic fever. She was suffering from chronic urticaria with a predilection for periarticular areas!

We treated her with anti-histamines.

This case is an example of the error of taking uncertain information as definite without considering the implications that this will have on the diagnosis, treatment and the patient's life. It is also an example of the need for systematic questioning and patience. It stresses the importance of a proper clinical examination at the time the lesions are present.

*TYPICAL CASES*
### 5.B. "RHEUMATOID ARTHRITIS" (Epilog from page 5.2)

When we asked Joaquim about his rheumatic complaints he only mentioned continuous pain in the lumbar region, which kept him awake and was not related to effort. He had never had any other joint complaints. This goes completely against a diagnosis of rheumatoid arthritis.

Our systematic enquiry revealed marked weight loss (about 12 kg in 6 months). He complained of dyspepsia and a bad cough, which he attributed to the fact that he was a heavy smoker.

A clinical examination excluded any inflammation of the small joints. His lumbar spine was painful on palpation over L3.

We hospitalized the patient. Unfortunately the diagnostic tests showed two neoplasms: one pulmonary and the other gastric. The former had spread with a metastasis in L3.

This case shows how our questions need to be guided by a minimum knowledge of the possible pathologies. The condition had nothing to do with rheumatoid arthritis. It did not justify a test for rheumatoid factor and even if this is positive, a diagnosis of rheumatoid arthritis is not possible if, at the very least, there is no arthritis. The rhythm of the lumbar pain suggested that it originated in bone. The weight loss forced us to take a completely different view!

Once again, this shows the decisive importance of carefully directed, critical questioning and the constant need for a systematic enquiry and integrated/holistic approach to every patient.

# THE GENERAL CLINICAL EXAMINATION

6.

J.A.P. da Silva, A.D. Woolf, *Rheumatology in Practice*, DOI 10.1007/978-1-84882-581-9_6,
© Springer-Verlag London Limited 2010

# 6. THE GENERAL CLINICAL EXAMINATION

The prevalence of rheumatic diseases in the general population justifies including a rheumatologic screening examination in the routine clinical examination of every patient. In this chapter, we will suggest a methodology for general clinical examination that includes all the organs and systems, with a generic assessment of the musculoskeletal system. The idea of the proposed sequence is to combine economy of time and effort with the greatest possible sensitivity. In rheumatology, this global examination serves as a screening method and is aimed at detecting any significant anomalies. We suggest using it systematically on all patients, regardless of the reason for their visit.

This general screening is followed by a detailed examination of each area (regional examination) in which the patient has mentioned symptoms or in which we have detected abnormalities. The regional examinations are described in the following chapters, together with the pathologies located there.

We feel that it is essential to use a thorough, standardized method for every patient, without exception. A complete examination of all patients, regardless of their complaints or our suspected diagnosis, will often turn up unexpected clues, correct mistaken interpretations that may have arisen during the enquiry and give us an overall view of the patient, which is essential for an accurate diagnosis and subsequent choice of treatment.

This method naturally means that, most of the time, the examination will be perfectly normal. We believe that this is one of the most valuable features of the method. It is only by knowing exactly what is normal that we can detect even small degrees of abnormality! If we just assume that something not mentioned during the enquiry is normal, we are liable to make mistakes.

Please be critical of this methodology, adapting it to your own needs and clinical leanings and even creating your own method. The important thing is to have a good systematic method!

Before examining any patient, it may be useful to write the following headings in your clinical notes.

| | |
|---|---|
| • Skin | • Mucosae |
| • Lymphadenopathy | • Thyroid |
| • Auscultation of heart | • Auscultation of lungs |
| • Abdomen | • Lower limbs |
| • Blood pressure | • Musculoskeletal |

If the enquiry suggests any other potentially relevant aspects, write them in as well. For example: neurological examination, retinal examination, lumbar auscultation, rectal examination, shoulder examination, Tinel's sign, fibromyalgia points, etc.

By doing this, you avoid leaving out something important. After observing the patient, write in the answer to each question and add any other relevant findings.

The examination of the patient should be organized and oriented in the same way whenever possible, so that actions become automatic.

The methodology and sequence proposed for the general clinical examination are described below.

**The patient should be asked to undress down to underwear.**

## PART I

Ask the patient to take a few steps in a straight line away from you and come back. Observe the ease, symmetry and coordination of his movements. If the patient's gait is antalgic, ask him to pinpoint the pain – it may give clues for the examination.

If the enquiry suggests the possibility of neurological lesion of the lower limbs or the involvement of the lumbar spine, ask the patient to walk first on heels and then on toes. This enables the assessment of the integrity of L5 and S1 roots. You can also ask the patient to crouch down and stand up without using hands, which will help to evaluate proximal lower limb muscle strength, together with the mobility of the hips and knees

The examination continues with the patient standing with his/her back to us, with feet in line with the shoulders. ***Before going any further, ask the patient to describe any pain or difficulty during any particular movement.***

In this position, you can examine:

- ***Spinal alignment*** – abnormalities in the physiological curvatures in the frontal or sagittal (anteroposterior) planes.

- ***Balance of the shoulders and the pelvis*** – It helps to put your index fingers on the patient's shoulders and then on the iliac crests (Figure 6.1.). An unbalanced pelvis suggests asymmetry of the lower limbs, which is commonly associated with scoliosis and back pain;

- ***Position of the hips and knees*** – Complete extension? Fixed flexion deformity? Hyperextension of the knees? Deviation outwards (varus) or inwards (valgus)?

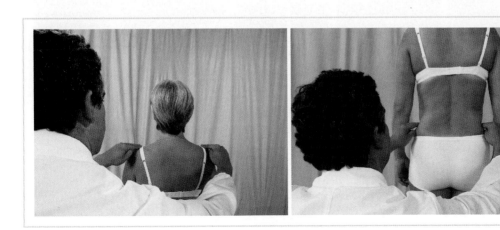

**Figure 6.1.**
Alignment of shoulders and iliac crest. It is useful to confirm alignment by placing fingertips on shoulders and iliac crests.

- *Inspection of the visible skin*, including the scalp;

- *Palpation of the thyroid gland*;

- *Palpation of the* submandibular, submental, anterior and posterior cervical, and supra-clavicular *ganglia*;

- *Mobility of the cervical spine* – Ask the patient to touch his right shoulder with his right ear and his left shoulder with his left ear. Then ask him to rotate his chin as far as he can to one side and the other. Now, standing beside the patient, ask him to touch his chest with his chin, which tests the flexion of the spine, and then ask him to look up at the ceiling (Figure 6.2.);

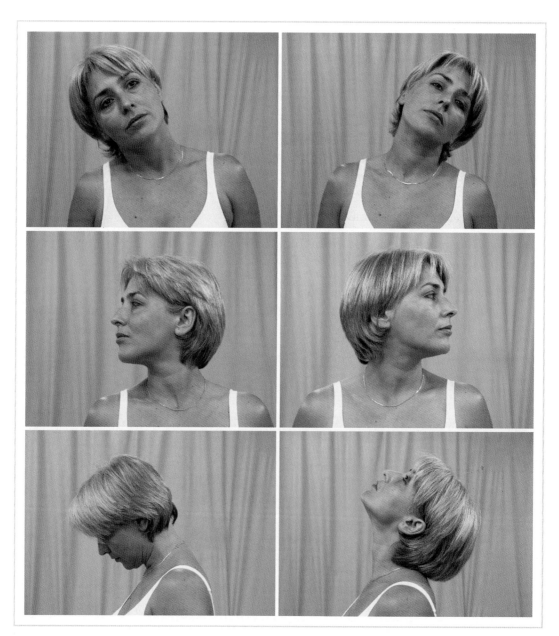

**Figure 6.2.**
Assessing cervical
spine mobility.

- ***Mobility of the lumbar spine*** – Put two fingers on the spinal processes of L4 (immediately above the line joining the iliac crests) and L2 and ask the patient to bend forward and try to touch the floor with his fingers, keeping legs straight (Figure 6.3.). The distance between your fingers indicates the degree of flexion of the lumbar spine.[1]

  The patient then bends backwards as far as possible, and then flexes laterally, to each side. Do not let the patient bend his knees during these maneuvers, so as not to confuse the site of the movement.

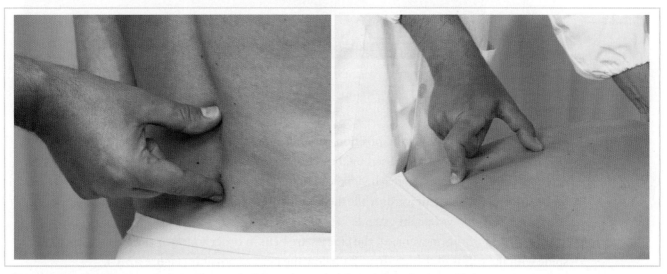

**Figure 6.3.** Assessment of lumbar spine flexion. The separation between the examiner's fingers indicates the degree of flexion.

## PART II

In this part, the patient stands at ease and we observe the following aspects from the front.

- ***Skin***, with special attention to the areas usually exposed to sunlight;

- ***Colour and hydration of the conjunctiva***;

- ***Oral mucosa and teeth*** – a suspicion of connective tissue diseases or Behçet's disease justifies closer inspection;

- ***Mobility of the shoulders and elbows***.

We suggest that you make the following movements, asking the patient to repeat them and tell you if there is any pain or difficulty.

---

[1]Bending forwards requires flexion not only of the lumbar spine but also limited flexion of the thoracic spine and particularly of the hips. Limited movement of the lumbar spine can be masked by good flexibility in the hips. By placing our fingers on the lumbar spine, we can assess the spine separately.

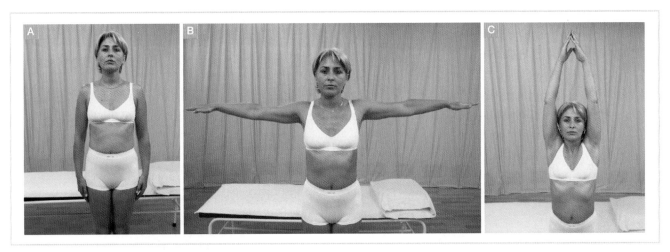

**Figure 6.4.** Appreciation of shoulder abduction and elbow extension.

The arms start from a relaxed position hanging at the sides with the palms facing the thighs (Figure 6.4A.). The arms are raised in abduction, at the side of the body, keeping the elbows extended, until the shoulders reach 90° abduction (Figure 6.4B.).

Now turn your palms upwards while the shoulder movement continues up to 180°, i.e. above your head. The elbows remain extended (Figure 6.4C.).

At the limit of this movement, the elbows are bent in order to touch the thoraco-cervical spine with the palms of the hands, as far below the neck as possible (Figure 6.5A.).

The arms are then lowered to touch the thoraco-lumbar region as high up as possible with the backs of the hands (Figure 6.5B.).

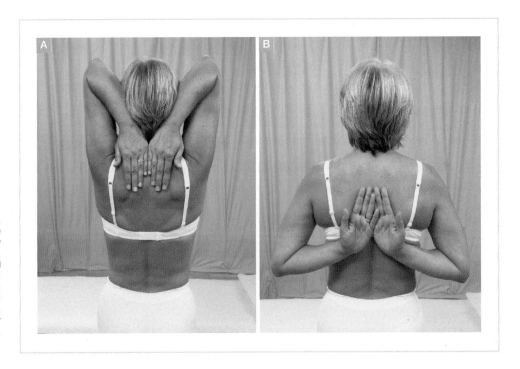

**Figure 6.5.**
General evaluation of the mobility of the shoulder, elbow and radio-ulnar joints. **A.** Shoulder: abduction and external rotation. Elbow: flexion. Radio-ulnar joints: supination. **B.** Shoulder: adduction and internal rotation. Elbow: Flexion. Radio-ulnar joints: pronation.

## HOW DO WE INTERPRET THESE MOVEMENTS?

These maneuvers assess the amplitude of movement of the shoulders, elbows and upper and lower radioulnar joints. Try them yourself!

When the palms touch the back, the shoulder is in complete abduction and total external rotation. The elbow is in complete flexion and the hands in supination (a movement that depends on the radioulnar joints).

To touch the lumbar region with the backs of the hands, the shoulders are in complete adduction and internal rotation, the elbows are in flexion and the hands in total pronation. The complete extension of the elbows is observed in the intermediate movements.

All that is left is the flexion (anterior elevation) of the shoulder, but this is rarely affected if the other movements are free. If the patient complains of pain in his shoulder, it is essential to conduct a more detailed examination of this region, even if the clinical examination was normal.

This examination also has the advantage of observing movements of great functional relevance; we need them for washing, for example.

Why do we ask patients to repeat our movements rather moving them passively? Periarticular diseases are much more common than articular diseases in the shoulder and elbow. One of the characteristics of this type of pathology is that passive movements are much less painful than active movements. When completely relaxed, a patient with subacromial bursitis, for example, may not feel pain in passive abduction of the shoulder but the active movement is hardly ever pain-free because it places the structure under tension. Active movements of the upper limbs are therefore much more likely to be sensitive in detecting disease than passive mobilization.

## PART III

The patient is now asked to sit down facing the examiner.

**Examining the wrists and hands:**

- *Inspection* – looking for deformities and deviations, changes in the color and integrity of the skin and nails, muscular atrophy;

- *Passive mobilization* – passively move the patient's wrists into full flexion and extension (Figure 6.6A. and B.)

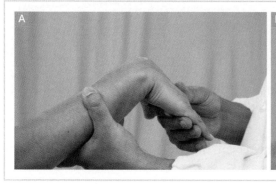 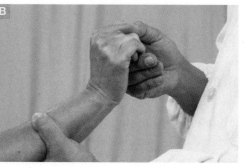

**Figure 6.6.**
General evaluation of the mobility of the wrist. **A.** Flexion. **B.** Extension.

• *General palpation of the joints* – The metacarpo-phalangeal, proximal and distal inter-phalangeal joints are palpated transversally to see if this causes any pain (Figure 6.7.)

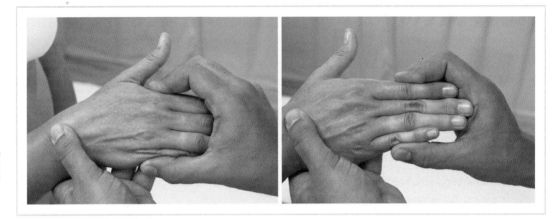

**Figure 6.7.**
Squeezing of metacarpo-phalangeal and proximal interphalangeal joints. General examination.

• *Active mobilization* – Finally, ask the patient to bend and extend his fingers and watch for any limitation in mobility or triggering.

If anomalies are detected, we will have to examine the wrists and hands more closely, as described in Chapter 10. The same will be the case if the patient has complained of anything in this area during the enquiry, even if the screening is normal. The hands can give us an extra-ordinary amount of information in a variety of rheumatic diseases.

### Mobility of the thoracic spine

Ask the patient to fold arms across his/her chest and, keeping the pelvis still, rotate the shoulders round to one side and then the other. This movement depends on the rotation of the thoracic spine, and allows detection of any pain or range limitations.

### Auscultation of the heart and lungs

We then auscultate the heart and lungs according to normal procedures. Our cardiorespiratory examination will naturally also include palpation, percussion, etc. if the auscultation or enquiry suggests any anomalies.

## PART IV

In this phase, we examine the abdomen and lower limbs with the patient lying on their back.

### Abdominal examination

Relaxed, lying on his back with hips and knees bent, the patient is in the ideal position for a standard examination of the abdomen.

### Examination of the lower limbs

We now ask the patient to extend his lower limbs and relax them. All the following movements will be passive and the patient should remain relaxed and tell us of any pain or difficulty.

- **General inspection** – We first assess the alignment of the thighs and lower legs, checking for muscle wasting, articular deformity or changes in the skin or nails. When at rest, the posterior aspect of the knee should touch the examining table. If it does not, we should explore a possible limitation to extension of the knee.

- **Stretching of the sciatic nerve** – If our enquiry suggests the possibility of compression of the lumbar roots we can take the opportunity to stretch the sciatic nerve (roots L5 and S1) by passive elevation of the lower limb while keeping the knee extended (Figure 6.8.). A positive test results in pain radiating from the lumbar region down the posterior face of the thigh and leg and requires a more detailed neurological examination.

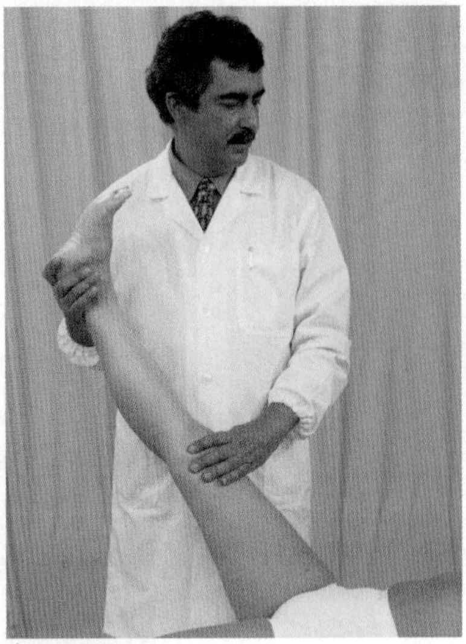

- **Mobilization of the hip joint** – Place one hand on the patient's knee while the other holds the lower third of the leg. All movements are carried out on both sides. It is always important to assess symmetry.

  - *Flexion and extension*
    With the patient relaxed, induce complete flexion of the hip joint and the knee, followed by extension. Repeat these movements (Figure 6.9.).
    The hip should flex to about 120° over the pelvis. During this movement, observe the contralateral thigh. The patient should keep the other knee in contact with the table, by extending the contralateral hip joint. If the left knee rises when we induce complete flexion of the right thigh, this suggests limited extension of the left hip joint (Thomas's test) (Figure 6.10.).

**Figure 6.8.** Sciatic nerve test: passive elevation of the lower limb keeping the knee extended.

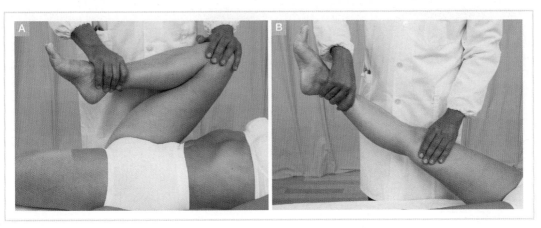

**Figure 6.9. A.** Hip and knee flexion. **B.** Knee extension.

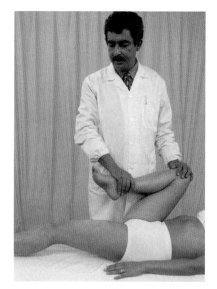

**Figure 6.10.** Thomas' test – simple evaluation of the extension of the contralateral hip.

The maximum degree of extension is not assessed in this test, but this shows sufficient mobility for the patient to walk without difficulty.

• *Internal and external rotation*

Now flex the hip joint to 90°, while also maintaining the knee flexed to 90° then induce internal rotation (the foot rotates outwards, normal about 30° – Figure 6.11A.) and external rotation of the hip joint, (the foot rotates inwards, normal about 60° – Figure 6.11B.). These movements are limited very early in osteoarthritis of the hip, sometimes before the appearance of spontaneous pain.

• *Adduction and abduction*

Now hold the leg by its lower third in a neutral position with the knee extended. Place the other hand on the iliac crest on the opposite side so that you can detect any movement of the pelvis.[2]

The leg is then passively moved into total abduction of the hip joint (outward deviation, normal: about 45° – Figure 6.12A.) and total adduction, passing over the other limb (Normal: about 30° – Figure 6.12B.).

**Figure 6.11.**
Assessment of hip mobility.
**A.** Internal rotation.
**B.** External rotation.

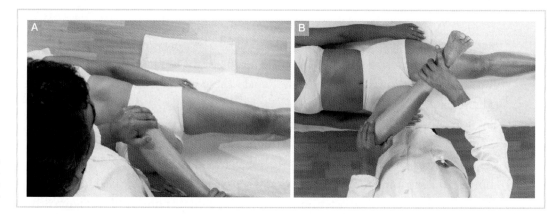

**Figure 6.12.**
Assessment of hip mobility.
**A.** Abduction. **B.** Adduction.
The hand placed on the opposite iliac crest controls for movement of the pelvis.

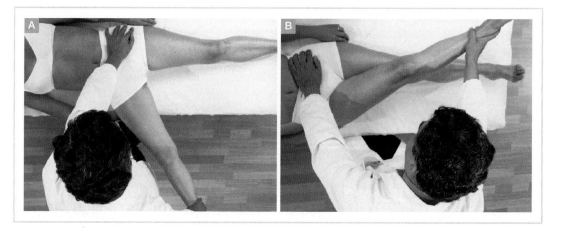

[2]When we force adduction or abduction, the pelvis swings to the same side. This movement apparently increases the lower limb's amplitude of movement, but should not be attributed to the hip!

- *Mobilization of the knee* – At the same time the hip is flexed and extended, the knee is placed in total flexion (normally about 130°) and then total extension (normally 0 to −10° – Figure 6.9.). By doing this, we check amplitude of movement and pain. The hand on the knee checks for crepitus (a sensation of coarse friction) and snapping of the joint. It is useful to repeat the flexion and extension of the knee several times.
These movements are then repeated with the opposite limb.

- *Mobilization of the ankles and feet* – With the patient in the same position, ask them to flex and extend ankles and feet as far as possible (Figure 6.13A. and B.). This allows a general assessment of the movement of the tibiotalar and tarsal joints as well as the small toe joints.
Then ask him to rotate his feet inwards (inversion) and outwards (eversion) (Figure 6.13C. and D.). These movements depend on the subtalar, midtarsal and tarsometatarsal joints, which are common sites of osteoarthritis and inflammatory joint disease.

If there are limitations or pain in any of these movements, we must study the affected area in more detail.

If indicated, we can test for the *godet* sign to check for edema of the lower limbs.

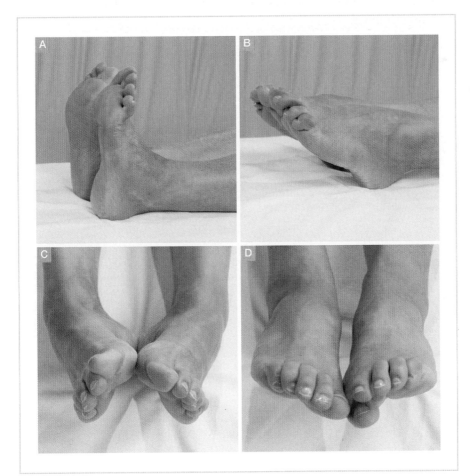

**Figure 6.13.**
Summary evaluation of ankle and foot mobility. **A.** Flexion. **B.** Extension. **C.** Inversion. **D.** Eversion.

Finally, while the patient is lying on his back, you can take the opportunity to examine the sacroiliac joints and perform a neurological examination, if the clinical context so warrants. In our experience, it is not necessary or productive to do this with all patients.

If the lumbar or thoracic spine requires further attention, we will ask the patient to lie face down for a thorough local examination.

## PART V

If the enquiry suggests a generalized pain syndrome, now is the ideal time to check the typical tender points of fibromyalgia, with the patient standing with his back to us (see Chapter 15). We do not do this at the beginning, because the diagnosis of fibromyalgia is one of exclusion, which we should only consider if the general musculoskeletal examination has failed to demonstrate any objective changes capable of explaining the symptoms.

We should also take this opportunity to weigh our patient and measure his height.

The local and regional examinations that prove necessary after the enquiry or clinical examination can easily be included in this sequence, as we will see.

After going through these steps, we can ask the patient to get dressed while we write up and think about our notes.

# REGIONAL SYNDROMES
## NECK PAIN

7.

J.A.P. da Silva, A.D. Woolf, *Rheumatology in Practice*, DOI 10.1007/978-1-84882-581-9_7,
© Springer-Verlag London Limited 2010

# 7. REGIONAL SYNDROMES NECK PAIN

Pain in the cervical region (neck pain) is very common in clinical practice. Young people are often affected by episodes of acute neck pain, which are usually transient, but the most common condition is chronic pain with acute, recurring episodes in adults and the elderly. Although this is rarely the case, neck pain may be of sinister origin, which it is important to exclude.

## FUNCTIONAL ANATOMY

The cervical region is the most mobile part of the spine. It is a complex structure and its mobility and congruence are maintained by a multiplicity of structures, all of which can cause pain. It consists of seven vertebrae joined by intervertebral disks and by the joints between the articular processes of adjacent vertebrae – facet joints (Figure 7.1.).

The disks consist of a fibrous peripheral ring and a gelatinous central core, which makes them flexible and compressible. The fibrous ring adheres to the upper and lower surfaces of the adjacent vertebral bodies, forming a synchondrosis (a joint without a synovium and with interposed cartilage). The disk does not take up the whole platform of the vertebral body, leaving a space on each side for a small synovial joint.

Facet joints are diarthroses, which have synovium and are therefore prone to involvement in systemic inflammatory processes. They are often the site of osteoarthritis with the formation of osteophytes.

The atlanto-axial joint, C1–C2, is very special. The vertebral body in the atlas (C1) is replaced by a bony arch, whose posterior face articulates with the odontoid process of the axis, which projects upward from the body of this bone (C2) (Figure 7.2.). A fibrous band, the transverse ligament of the atlas, keeps the odontoid process of the axis congruent with the ring of the atlas

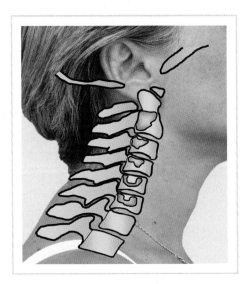

**Figure 7.1.** Cervical spine.

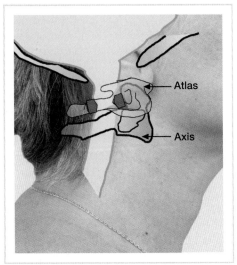

**Figure 7.2.** Atlanto-axial joint and its relation to the spinal cord.

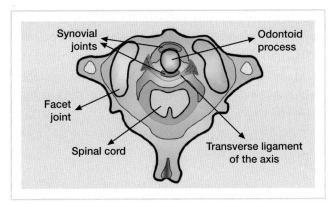

**Figure 7.3.** Atlas, odontoid process of the axis and spinal cord.

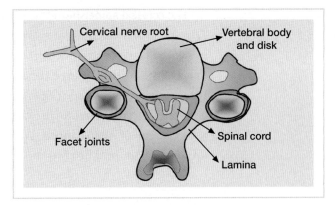

**Figure 7.4.** Origin and anatomical relations of nerve roots.

(Figure 7.3.). This forms a synovial joint. The spinal cord is immediately behind this joint and can therefore be readily affected by local instability (Figure 7.2.).

The atlanto-occipital and atlanto-axial components are responsible for an important part of the flexion, rotation and lateral inclination of the cervical spine.

The cervical roots emerge from the spine through the intervertebral foramina, which are delimited anteriorly and internally by the intervertebral disk and posteriorly and externally by the facet joints (Figure 7.4.). Changes in the form or stability of these structures can cause irritation and compression of the nerve routes, resulting in neurogenic pain. When a disk herniation occurs, the gelatinous core usually protrudes in a posterior, external location, i.e. directly in contact with the root.

The cervical nerve roots are responsible for the innervation of the scalp overlying the posterior aspect of the head and the whole surface of the shoulder and upper limb (Figure 7.5.). The root of C1 emerges above the first cervical vertebra, hence the presence of eight (and not seven) cervical roots, with C8 emerging below C7 (Figure 7.6.). The root called T1 (of the first thoracic nerve) emerges below the T1 vertebral body. The C6 root is therefore in the vicinity of disk C5/C6.

The stability of this column is maintained by the intervertebral synchondroses and the facet joints, and also by a multiplicity of paravertebral muscles and ligaments, which are commonly a source of pain. Trauma or inflammation affecting nerve or muscle bundles may cause reflex muscle contraction that exacerbates and extends the pain, further limiting mobility.

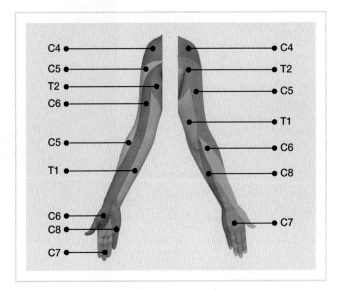

**Figure 7.5.** Sensory territory of nerve roots – dermatomes.

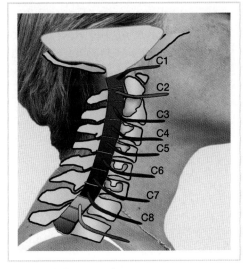

**Figure 7.6.** Nerve root exits.

The cervical spine should be studied using anteroposterior and lateral radiographs (Figure 7.7.). When viewing the anteroposterior film, note the alignment of the vertebrae and possible presence of lytic or sclerotic bony lesions. Sclerotic changes in the facet joints are sometimes visible. On the lateral film, vertebral alignment in the AP plane is observed and the intervertebral spaces may be examined. The disk height should be the same from C1 to C7 and the vertebral endplates should be uniform, with no sclerosis. The joints between the articular processes, a common site of osteoarthritis, are clearly visible. The density of the vertebral bodies should be uniform and appear brighter at the edge, by the cortical bone.

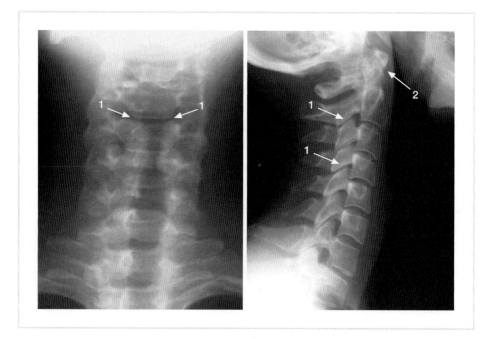

**Figure 7.7.** Normal radiology of the cervical spine. **1.** Facet joints. **2.** Atlanto-axial joint.

Oblique views (Figure 7.8.) give a better impression of the intervertebral foramina. Osteophytes located here can cause root compression but this must be confirmed by compatible clinical manifestations.

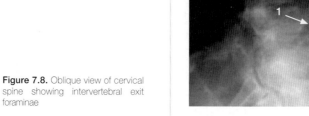

**Figure 7.8.** Oblique view of cervical spine showing intervertebral exit foraminae

## COMMON CAUSES OF NECK PAIN

In most cases the pain has a mechanical rhythm. It is triggered by movement and relieved by rest. In adults, most of these conditions are caused by spondyloarthrosis. In many other cases, particularly in young people, there is no apparent cause for the pain, and it is thought to be the result of mild articular instability and irritation of the nerves and muscle bundles leading to painful reflex muscle contractions. Both situations should be treated conservatively, aiming to relieve the pain and restore function, without any specific etiological intervention.

In a few cases, the pain may be neurogenic, inflammatory, neoplastic or psychogenic in origin. These cases require a specific cause-oriented diagnostic and therapeutic approach.

The main aim of our primary diagnostic approach is to distinguish the few potentially serious causes of neck pain, which require specific treatment, from the many sources of non-specific mechanical pain.

Table 7.1. shows the general clinical aspects of the most common causes of neck pain.

| Etiology | Clinical clues |
|---|---|
| Trauma | History of trauma |
| | Occupational factors |
| | Bad posture |
| | – Often causes acute attacks in young people |
| | – Diagnostic tests usually normal |
| Spondyloarthrosis | Pain usually mechanical |
| | Chronic or recurring pain |
| | Can be associated with neurogenic manifestations, arising from the nerve roots or spinal cord |
| | – The most common cause of neck pain in adults and the elderly |
| | – Suggestive x-ray features |
| Inflammatory joint disease | Pain tends to be inflammatory |
| | Usual association of manifestations of arthritis in other locations |
| | – Rheumatoid arthritis, seronegative spondyloarthropathies and juvenile idiopathic arthritis often affect the cervical spine |
| Infection | Acute or chronic infections of the vertebral bones or disks, like tuberculosis or brucellosis, may, on rare occasions, affect the neck |
| Metastases | Tumors in the thyroid, lung, breast, kidney and prostate may metastasize to the cervical spine |
| | Multiple myeloma can affect this region |
| | Primary bone tumors are rare |
| Referred pain | Special attention to the shoulder, pulmonary vertex and heart |
| Non-musculoskeletal pain | Lymphadenopathy caused by oropharyngeal infections |
| | Thyroiditis |
| | Meningitis and meningism |

**Table 7.1.**
Common causes of neck pain and associated clinical clues.

## THE ENQUIRY

The enquiry should try to identify the type of pain and find clues to its most likely cause. Age is an important factor. A history of recent trauma or the appearance of pain as a result of a prolonged, forced position indicates this etiology.

In cases of pain that develops more slowly, the rhythm is an important clue. An inflammatory rhythm suggests infection, inflammation or neoplasm. In this case, the onset of pain is usually insidious and progressive. The pain is often continuous, not relieved by rest, and may be accompanied by morning stiffness. It is important to look for symptoms and signs of arthritis in other locations. The systematic enquiry will try to identify signs of systemic disease (such as fever, weight loss, cough, or hematuria) or an oropharyngeal infection.

Pain due to spondyloarthrosis is normally triggered by movement and relieved by rest. It often radiates to the shoulder or upper arm, even in the absence of any demonstrable neurological compromise. The location of the pain gives an indication of its most likely point of origin (Figure 7.9.).

Real neurogenic pain indicating root compression is intense, dysesthesic ("electric shock" or "pins and needles") and follows a dermatome distribution (Figure 7.5.).

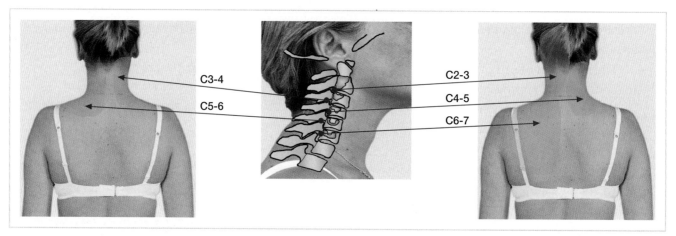

**Figure 7.9.** Radiation of pain originating at different levels of the cervical spine.

## REGIONAL CLINICAL EXAMINATION

### Observation

An inspection of the cervical region and surrounding areas may show clear deformity, such as accentuation or attenuation of physiological lordosis, localized angular kyphosis, interscapular fat pad caused by corticoids, scoliosis and lateral deviation, atrophy of the shoulder muscles, localized swelling, etc.

## Palpation

Palpation can detect extra-skeletal anomalies such as lymphadenopathy or goitre, which may indicate the origin of the pain. Where musculoskeletal pain is concerned, palpation is not very informative, as the structures are deep set. It is common to find pain on palpation of many muscular points, even without any apparent local lesion. The muscle spasm associated with a stiff neck is sometimes easily perceptible. Pain that is clearly located over one or two spinous processes may suggest infection or neoplasm. Apart from these particular circumstances, cervical palpation is non-specific and should be interpreted with caution.

## Mobilization

Amplitude and freedom of movement of the cervical spine are assessed with the maneuvers shown in Figure 7.10.

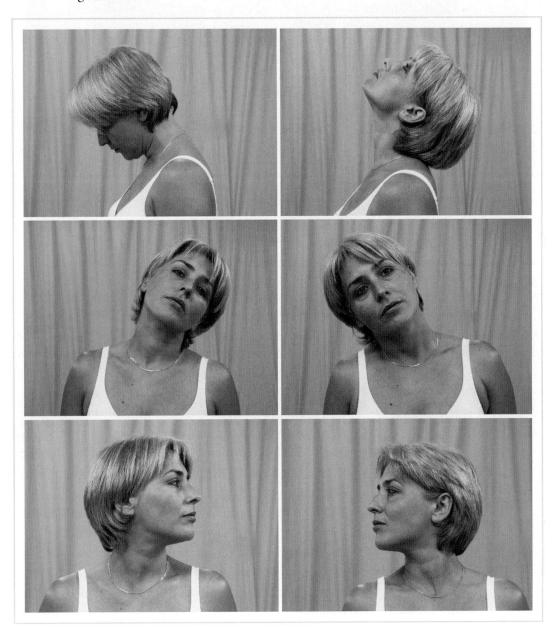

**Figure 7.10.**
Clinical evaluation of cervical spine movements.

If we wish to be more precise, we can ask the patient to hold a pencil between his teeth to make it easier to quantify the angles of movement (Figure 7.11.) or measure distances, such as that between the chin and the sternal notch during flexion and extension.

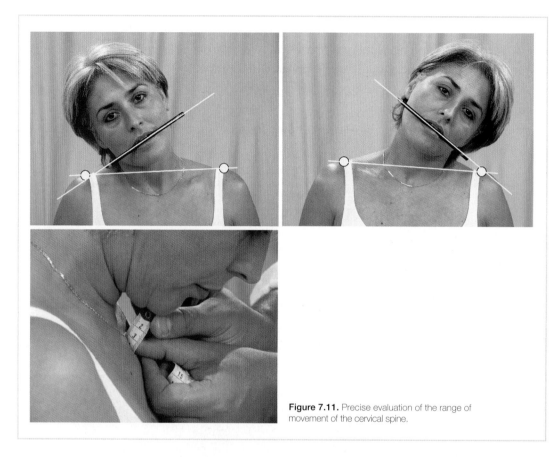

**Figure 7.11.** Precise evaluation of the range of movement of the cervical spine.

When compared to previous assessments in the same patient, these measurements can be useful for detailed evaluation of treatment. They are not, however, essential in routine clinical practice. Amplitude of movement varies considerably from one person to another. It can be affected by physical training, and decreases significantly with age in normal people. In clinical practice, measurements of the range of movement tend to be qualitative, looking for a significant reduction in mobility associated with functional impact and local pain, or for pain radiating with movement. Experience acquired during repeated examinations is our best guide.

When there is root irritation, forced inclination of the neck to the opposite side can trigger symptoms similar to the spontaneous ones, as it distends the roots ("cervical Lasègue" – Figure 7.12.). These symptoms will be more important if they are dysesthesic and show typical root distribution.

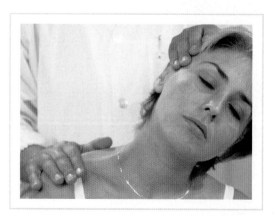

**Figure 7.12.** Cervical Lasègue test: forced inclination of the neck to one side. The test is considered positive if neurogenic pain is felt on the contralateral side.

### Neurological examination

If we suspect root or spinal cord compression, a detailed neurological examination of the upper limbs is called for. Evaluation of touch and pin-prick sensation will follow the dermatomes described in Figure 7.5. Muscle strength and reflexes can be assessed as shown in Table 7.2. The lower limbs and sphincters should also be assessed.

|  | Muscle strength | Myotactic reflexes |
|---|---|---|
| **Shoulder** | C5 (abduction) | |
| **Elbow** | C5 (flexion) C7 (extension) | C5 (biceps reflex) |
|  |  | C7 (triceps reflex) |
| **Wrist** | C6 e C8 (extension) | C6 (supinator reflex) |
| **Fingers** | C7 e C8 (extension) | C8 (finger jerk) |
|  | T1 (spreading fingers; opposition of thumb) | |

**Table 7.2.** Nerve root origin of muscle strength and tendon reflexes in the upper limbs.

---

## *TYPICAL CASES*
## 7.A. CHRONIC NECK PAIN (I)

Maria de Jesus was 68 years old. She was a housewife and farm worker. She went to the doctor because of pain affecting the cervical and upper thoracic region. The pain had begun insidiously when she was about 40 and had been getting progressively worse. In the first years of the disease, the pain appeared occasionally at times of strenuous physical work. As the years went by, it became more frequent and appeared with less and less effort until it was almost constant, with flares. During such exacerbations, which lasted up to a week, the pain extended to the whole cervical area, and also involved the shoulders. The pain was worse with exercise (such as carrying heavy items in her arms) and was relieved by rest. She had no pain at night except when she moved in bed. When asked, she described occasional pain and tiredness in her arms but denied any paresthesia or weakness. The pain was not exacerbated by Valsava's maneuver. Maria de Jesus also had similar pain in the lumbar region and in her knees. She denied any relevant systemic manifestations. She had a history of peptic ulcer, which was attributed to anti-inflammatories taken for the neck pain.

Our clinical examination showed reduced lateral inclination and rotation of the neck, with pain at the extremes of movement. There was pain on palpation of different muscular points on the posterior and lateral aspects of the neck. A screening neurological examination of the upper limbs showed normal power, reflexes and pain sensation. There was no muscle atrophy. Cervical Lasègue to the right revealed pain on the left side of the neck extending to the shoulder. Her weight was 76 kg, and her height was 156 cm.

*Think about this case:*

*What are the probable diagnoses and why?*

*What diagnostic tests would you request?*

We requested lateral x-ray of the cervical spine. It showed a reduction in the intervertebral space from C2 to C7, with osteophytes and sclerosis of the vertebral endplates (Figure 7.13.). There were no significant changes in the bone structure or vertebral alignment.

*Reconsider your diagnosis.*

*What treatment would you recommend?*

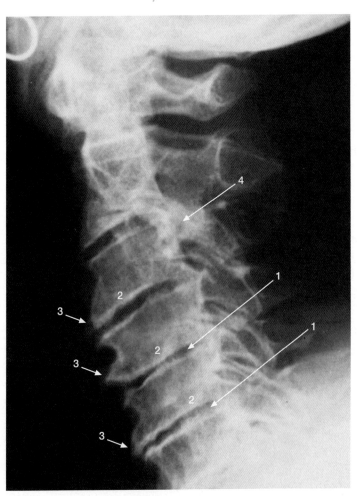

**Figure 7.13.** Osteoarthritis of the cervical spine. Note intervertebral joint space loss (**1**), sclerosis of the vertebral endplates (**2**) and anterior osteophytes (**3**) from C2 to C7. Facet joint osteoarthritis is also visible (**4**).

In view of these findings, we reassured the patient as to the cause of her pain, explaining that it was not likely to get much worse. We encouraged her to stay active in spite of the pain and suggested that she did regular relaxation exercises, mobilizing and stretching the muscles. We advised her to avoid strenuous activities that put a strain on her neck, such as carrying heavy loads and effort in forced positions. A trolley for shopping might help relieve the pressure on her spine. We also suggested that progressive loss of weight might help the pain considerably, as would a low, well-adjusted pillow.

We prescribed a selective COX-2 inhibitor to take as necessary for the pain, a firm cervical collar for her to wear during painful exacerbations, and intermittent active mobilization exercises. During these flares she might find that the local application of heat (a hot shower or hot, damp towels, for example) relieved the pain and relaxed the muscles. In the future, if an acute, incapacitating crisis persisted for some time, we could resort to physiotherapy.

## CHRONIC NON-SPECIFIC NECK PAIN
### *MAIN POINTS*

This is a very common condition in the elderly.

The pain is usually insidious and chronic, with exacerbations. It may also involve the scapular region though it has no neurogenic characteristics. Manifestations or signs suggesting actual neurological involvement require a more detailed study.

As a rule, neck movements are limited (especially rotation and lateral inclination). Pain on flexion or extension and limitation of these movements suggest neurological involvement. There may be pain on palpation at different paravertebral points.

Spondyloarthrosis is the most common underlying cause, but the correlation between x-ray, clinical examination and response to treatment is very unreliable. X-rays are often unnecessary and there is no need to repeat them often.

Even in an apparently typical situation, it is important to rule out any neurological signs, relevant systemic manifestations and inflammatory pain.

Investigation should be limited to the essential.

Treatment is conservative.

Avoidance of excessive effort should be combined with a program of regular mobilization and relaxation exercises. Analgesics, mild anti-inflammatories and muscle relaxants may be necessary during flare-ups, when a properly adjusted cervical collar may aid recovery.

It is essential to reassure patients and encourage them to keep active in spite of the pain. Dramatic, pessimistic interpretations should be avoided at all costs.

Prognosis varies but the pain tends to be persistent, with significant improvement in response to the right measures.

### *TYPICAL CASES*
### 7.B. NECK PAIN with radiation

During 2 years of follow-up, Maria de Jesus, our previous patient, was very pleased with her response to treatment. Although she still had some pain, it was more tolerable. Exacerbations were now rare and related to effort.

This time, she came back to us because of exacerbation of the pain, which was no longer responding to the usual measures. The pain was particularly intense and involved the left arm and forearm as far as the thumb. She described this radiated pain as "an electric shock" and had noticed that it appeared especially when she turned her neck to the right. A slight cough that she had had for a few days made the pain unbearable, as it increased the radiated pain, causing the pins and needles to last longer.

*What could be happening?*

*What aspects of the clinical examination need further attention?*

Our local examination found that the pain worsened during active and passive mobilization of the neck, which was more limited, with associated muscle spasm. Forced lateral flexion of the neck to the right (cervical Lasègue – Figure 7.12.) caused the pain to radiate to the lateral aspect the left forearm. Vertical compression of the head towards the neck (Spurling's maneuver) caused local pain without radiation. A neurological examination showed reduced pin-prick sensation over the thumb and radial side of the left forearm. There were no apparent changes in muscle strength. Tinel's and Phalen's signs for carpal tunnel syndrome were negative (see Chapter 10).

*What treatment would you suggest for this patient?*

She had already been wearing a cervical collar for about 2 weeks, associated with an anti-inflammatory and the application of local heat, but to no avail.

We advised her to keep wearing the cervical collar, and added a muscle relaxant. We asked for a new profile lateral x-ray of the cervical spine, which excluded the existence of cervical dislocation or any other alterations in the bone, besides the signs of spondyloarthrosis of which we were already aware.

The patient was sent to physical therapy for muscle relaxation treatment and careful traction of the cervical spine, which resulted in a considerable improvement, thus avoiding surgery, which was an option in view of the severity of the symptoms.

## CERVICAL NERVE ROOT COMPRESSION
### MAIN POINTS

Cervical nerve root compression should be suspected whenever there is dysesthesic pain in the territory of a root and exacerbated by cervical movements. Sensory or motor deficiencies may ensue.

The roots C5–C7 are most often affected.

Root compression may accompany the onset of cervical pain, especially in young people, suggesting a disk lesion, or develop insidiously in the presence of a chronic degenerative condition such as spondyloarthropathy.

Lasègue's cervical maneuver, Spurling's maneuver and a neurological examination of the upper limbs are the key to the diagnosis.

Treatment should be conservative, using analgesics, anti-inflammatories, muscle relaxants and a cervical collar. Physical therapy by experienced professionals may be useful.

The persistence of incapacitating symptoms or progressive neurological alterations over a few months in spite of appropriate conservative treatment may justify assessment by an experienced surgeon.

Electromyography and MRI (Magnetic Resonance Imaging) may be indicated when the persistence or severity of the situation may warrant surgery.

*TYPICAL CASES*
## 7.C. ACUTE NECK PAIN

João Manuel was a 19-year old university student. He came to us because of intense cervical pain, mainly on the right side of his neck, which had begun without apparent cause on the morning of the day before. The pain worsened considerably with any attempt to rotate or laterally flex his neck, especially to the right. He denied any recent trauma and had noticed no changes in his health. He did mention having felt some discomfort in his neck in the last few weeks after studying for a few hours, though it went away after a hot bath.

On direct enquiry, he said that he had been sleeping poorly in recent weeks not only because he was anxious about his exams but also because he had been sleeping in an unfamiliar bed.

He described similar episodes at the same time in previous years, but never as intense as this. He led a sedentary life and did not take regular exercise of any sort.

When we examined the patient, his neck was stiff and strongly inclined to the right, with painful blocking of practically all movements. Palpation of the neck showed muscle spasm of the muscles on the right side, which were firm and painful. Active mobilization of the upper limbs triggered cervical pain but there was no apparent loss of sensation and the reflexes were normal.

*Think of the most probable causes of this situation.*

*What treatment would you suggest?*

We recommended bed rest for 24–36 hours with locally applied heat. We reassured the patient as to the benign, transient nature of the problem, relating it to stress, lack of sleep and a possible unsuitable position during the night. We prescribed analgesics and muscle relaxants, while drawing his attention to the impairment in concentration these drugs may cause. We suggested gentle, regular, gradually intensified exercise, especially after the application of local heat.

We saw João again a week later. He had no pain and his cervical movements were also free and painless. We discussed the cause of the symptoms with him, emphasizing the relevance of stress and the advantages of regular physical exercise and posture.

## NON-SPECIFIC ACUTE NECK PAIN
### MAIN POINTS

Most episodes of acute neck pain are likely to resolve spontaneously in days or weeks, but they tend to recur.

They appear more often in young people, without any previous pathology.

They may sometimes be part of fibromyalgia.

The pain is usually unilateral, but may be bilateral and involve the scapular regions.

Its origin is unclear, but muscle spasm seems to play an important role.

Muscle spasm is often obvious on examination, and tender points can be found on palpation. In some cases, there are trigger points which, when pressed, cause distant pain or pain radiating to the whole spontaneously painful area.

Bad posture, emotional stress and unusual exercise favor these episodes.

In the absence of other symptoms or signs, no further investigation is justified.

Treatment is conservative and based on analgesics, muscle relaxants and gentle mobilization and relaxation exercises, facilitated by local heat. Physiotherapy may be necessary and is especially effective if applied early.

*TYPICAL CASES*
### 7.D. CHRONIC NECK PAIN (II)

Natércia, aged 48, was being followed up at our clinic for rheumatoid arthritis that had begun 3 years before. She was being treated with anti-inflammatories and methotrexate with highly satisfactory results on her peripheral arthritis.

At a follow-up appointment with her family doctor nothing seemed to have changed, with the exception of the patient's complaint of neck pain for the first time. She put it down to working long hours at the computer and some stress. A more detailed enquiry revealed that the pain was in the upper cervical area and sometimes involved the occipital region. It was worse at the end of the working day, but improved very little with rest. The pain was there when she woke up, and she experienced moderate morning stiffness of the neck lasting for about 2 hours. She denied any neurogenic manifestations in the upper limbs or her body.

Her sedimentation rate was somewhat higher than in previous months.

Her family doctor sent the patient to our clinic for an urgent appointment.

*Give a brief summary of this condition*[1]

*Could this situation be related to her rheumatoid arthritis? How?*

*How would you confirm your suspicions?*

Our examination revealed painful restriction of neck movements, but neurological examination was normal. We requested an x-ray of the cervical spine, asking for a lateral view focusing on C1 and C2, in flexion and extension. We also asked for a transoral x-ray of the odontoid process.

These x-rays showed that the distance between the posterior edge of the arch of the atlas and the anterior edge of the odontoid process during flexion was enlarged to 7 mm (Figure 7.14.). There was no ascending migration of the dens. The transoral x-ray showed an erosion of the axial dens, which was well centered between the masses of the atlas.

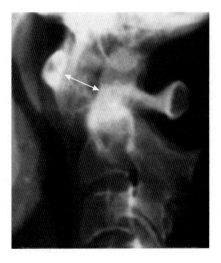

**Figure 7.14.**
Atlanto-axial subluxation. The distance between the anterior aspect of the odontoid process and the posterior aspect of the arch of the atlas is more than 5 mm.

*Does this confirm your suspicions?*

*What is this complication called?*

*What would you do?*

In view of these findings, which show cervical inflammation and atlantoaxial subluxation, we decided to reinforce immunosuppressive therapy and advised the patient to wear a cervical collar when there was risk of trauma, such as when travelling by car. We regularly monitored this situation clinically and radiologically, as any aggravation of the dislocation or of

[1]Neck pain with a mixed rhythm and no neurological manifestations in a patient with rheumatoid arthritis.

the symptoms might expose the patient to the risk of spinal cord lesion and require stabilizing surgery.

---

**INFLAMMATORY NECK PAIN**
*MAIN POINTS*

Inflammatory cervical pain should always be considered an alarm signal justifying careful clinical investigation and diagnostic tests.

Pain of metastatic origin may have an inflammatory rhythm, although it tends to be more constant and unrelated to movement or rest.

The possibility of cervical involvement should always be borne in mind and actively investigated in patients with rheumatoid arthritis, juvenile idiopathic arthritis and seronegative spondylarthropathy. On rare occasions, cervical involvement may be the first manifestation of these diseases.

Infections of the cervical vertebrae and disks (spondylodiscitis) are relatively rare but should always be considered, especially in a clinical context suggesting tuberculosis or brucellosis.

The systematic enquiry makes an essential contribution to this diagnosis.

Clinical examination may be non-contributory in the initial phases.

X-rays should be performed and acute-phase reactants measured together with tests specific to the clinically suspected causes.

Cervical infection or metastasis requires urgent referral to a specialized centre.

---

## DIAGNOSTIC TESTS

Only rarely are diagnostic tests necessary to investigate neck pain.

### Imaging

Given the poor correlation between radiology, the clinical examination and response to treatment, plain radiographs have little to offer in most cases of simple, acute or chronic mechanical pain. They may be justified when more serious non-degenerative lesions are suspected.

In standard x-rays, the lateral view is most informative. It enables us to see the platforms of the vertebral bodies and the height of the disk spaces. A reduction in these spaces, associated with subchondral sclerosis and osteophytes, suggests spondyloarthrosis.

In the lateral view, we can also assess the alignment of the vertebral bodies, identifying the presence of dislocations (listheses – dislocation of a vertebral body over another) (Figure 7.15.).

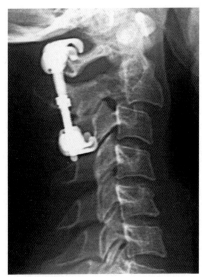

**Figure 7.15.** Cervical lysthesis (after surgery). Note the anterior dislocation of C2 over C3.

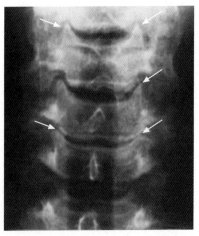

**Figure 7.16.** Osteoarthritis. Note the joint space loss and subchondral sclerosis (*arrows*).

Metastases take the form of lytic or sclerotic lesions in the vertebral bodies. Disk and bone infections result in the suggestive images discussed in Chapter 11.

Arthritic involvement of the cervical spine can produce complex images, which will be addressed in the appropriate chapters.

A frontal view x-ray is very difficult to interpret, because of the superimposition of images. Radiologists often describe the presence of facet joint degenerative change (Figure 7.16). Its relationship with symptoms can vary considerably and should only be interpreted as an indicator of local degenerative changes. Their relevance can only be assessed by clinical examination. Provided that they are properly executed, oblique views can give a good image of the intervertebral foramina, but can never take the place of a careful neurological examination.

Investigation of atlantoaxial subluxation, which is especially important in the context of rheumatoid arthritis, requires the special views indicated in the clinical case and should ideally be interpreted by a doctor with experience of this pathology.

MRI and CT scans have very specific indications related essentially to neurological signs. It might be argued that scans are indicated only if surgery is contemplated.

### Other investigations

An electromyogram of the upper limbs can be decisive in the case of inconclusive abnormalities in the neurological examination as it clarifies the existence of and aids in the location of lesions.

Other tests may be indicated if the clinical examination suggests the possibility of an infectious, inflammatory or neoplastic lesion.

## TREATMENT

Only a very small percentage of patients with neck pain present lesions that require specific treatment. A general practitioner's first concern should be identifying these cases and referring them to a specialist.

In most cases, the pain will be due to a degenerative or merely functional condition (with no identifiable underlying pathology). In these circumstances, the aim of treatment is to reduce the pain and discomfort, restore function, avoid exacerbations and, above all, prevent progression to chronicity. We should bear in mind that psychological factors related to personality, anxiety, or work-related and other problems, may play a decisive role in resolution or progression to chronicity.

Treatment is essentially conservative.

**Educating the patient** – Patients should be reassured as to the significance of their pain and its prognosis. We should make sure that our assessment and explanation of the problem focus on function and not the pain, and even less on the underlying structural lesion. We should educate patients about potentially harmful postures and activities. Any possible relationship between pain and stress should be addressed and dealt with. Patients should be encouraged to remain as active as possible.

It is essential for patients to follow a program of regular, gentle exercise suited to their condition. Leaflets are extremely useful here. Teaching patients exercises to do at home should be considered an integral part of any physiotherapy program. Local heat applied at home is also very effective.

**The cervical collar** – This can be very useful in exacerbations of chronic neck pain. Patients should be taught how to put it on so that it is comfortable but effective (Figure 7.17.).

**Medication** – Analgesics are very important in relieving pain and, in doing this, interrupting the vicious circle of pain and reflexive spasm. Anti-inflammatory drugs should be reserved for cases that do not respond adequately to analgesics. Muscle relaxants can be important adjuvant therapy when muscle spasm seems to play a significant role in maintaining the symptoms. Antidepressants can be useful in modulating chronic pain. Local friction with anti-inflammatory gel or cream can help to relieve the symptoms.

Where secondary care is concerned, local injection of an anesthetic and/or corticosteroid aimed at painful points or particular anatomical structures may be useful in relieving the symptoms and identifying their origin.

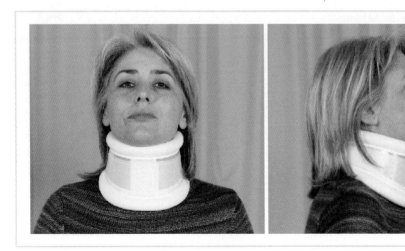

**Figure 7.17.**
Hard neck collar. Adequate height and positioning of the collar are very important for treatment success.

**Physiotherapy** – This is a valuable resource in cases in which the symptoms are still incapacitating in spite of other measures. In cases of acute, intense symptoms, early physiotherapy or manipulation can be highly worthwhile.

**Surgery** – The need for surgery is exceptional, and limited to situations with incapacitating symptoms and significant neurological signs, in spite of appropriate conservative treatment.

---

### WHEN SHOULD THE PATIENT BE REFERRED TO A SPECIALIST?

Almost all cases of neck pain should be managed by general practitioners. Some situations justify sending patients to a specialist (rheumatologist, orthopedic surgeon, neurosurgeon, physiatrist or even a specialist in internal medicine, as the case may be):

• Reason to suspect an infectious or neoplastic lesion

• Neck pain as part of polyarthritis

• Manifest cervical instability or deviation

• Neurological signs in the nerve roots or spinal cord

• Intense symptoms that are resistant to conservative treatment

---

## ADDITIONAL PRACTICE
### REGIONAL SYNDROMES. NECK PAIN

10.A. PAIN IN THE HANDS (I)                                          PAGE 10.22

# REGIONAL SYNDROMES
## THE PAINFUL SHOULDER

**8.**

J.A.P. da Silva, A.D. Woolf, *Rheumatology in Practice*, DOI 10.1007/978-1-84882-581-9_8,
© Springer-Verlag London Limited 2010

# 8. REGIONAL SYNDROMES THE PAINFUL SHOULDER

Pain in the shoulder region is a common reason for seeking medical attention. When shoulder pain presents as an isolated problem, the cause is usually periarticular disease that can be diagnosed accurately by clinical examination. It is not uncommon for shoulder pain to be referred from adjacent areas or internal organs. While isolated affection of the glenohumeral joint is rare, this joint is often involved in a variety of polyarthropathies.

Shoulder pain is often extremely incapacitating. Conservative treatment is usually highly satisfactory.

## FUNCTIONAL ANATOMY

The shoulder is an extremely complex structure.

Take a moment to imagine a mechanical structure capable of carrying out all the shoulder's movements: adduction, abduction, flexion (anterior elevation) and extension in an arc greater than 180°. The hand can reach any point within more than half a circle with a radius similar to the length of the upper limb! In addition, this mechanical structure should be able to rotate round its own axis – internal and external rotation – and to provide considerable force. This mobility requires considerable strength from the soft supporting structures, which results in considerable risk of instability. If we add all this to the need for a control system capable of conducting all these movements smoothly and accurately, we are looking at an amazing structure! There is no way it could be simple.

The shoulder consists of three bones and three joints. The proximal end of the humerus, the scapula and the lateral end of the clavicle come together here (Figure 8.1.).

The humerus articulates with the glenoid surface of the scapula, amplified by a cartilaginous ring (the glenoid labrum), making the glenohumeral joint, which has a synovial lining and is strengthened by a fibrous capsule and ligaments. It is the most mobile joint in the whole body and is involved in rotation, flexion, extension, and a substantial amount of adduction and abduction (between 0 and 120°).

Above the glenohumeral joint is the acromioclavicular joint, which joins the lateral end of the clavicle to the internal edge of the acromion. Anteriorly, the coracoacromial ligament continues coverage of the head of the humerus and adjacent structures.

The scapula glides over the subscapularis muscle and the muscles of the posterior thoracic wall, suspended by muscles

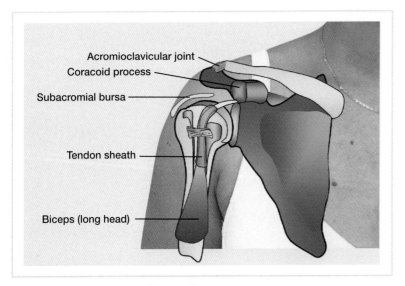

Acromioclavicular joint
Coracoid process
Subacromial bursa
Tendon sheath
Biceps (long head)

**Figure 8.1.** Functional anatomy of the shoulder.

responsible for elevation and internal and external rotation: the elevator muscle of the scapula, serratus anterior, trapezium and rhomboids, among others. It thus constitutes what we call the scapulothoracic joint, which plays an important part in all the movements of the shoulder: abduction between 120 and 180°, and part of extension, and internal and external rotation.

The shoulder is served by a complex set of muscles. Externally, the deltoid arises from the lateral third of the clavicle, the border of the acromion and along the spine of the scapula. Below,

it inserts into the lateral aspect of the humerus. It is divided into three parts: anterior, external and posterior, which induce flexion, abduction and extension, respectively. It is responsible for abduction of the arm between 30 and 90°. Over 90°, abduction is the result of the contraction of trapezius, which elevates the scapula and clavicle.

The first 30° of abduction depend on the contraction of the supraspinatus. This muscle is part of the so-called rotator cuff of the shoulder. This is the name given to the musculotendinous structure that results from the junction of the tendons of four muscles joining the scapula to the humerus: the supraspinatus, infraspinatus, subscapularis and teres minor. The tendons of the muscles in the rotator cuff are inserted externally along the anatomical neck of the humerus (Figures 8.2. and 8.3.). The supraspinatus tendon inserts in the greater tuberosity of the humerus, a bony prominence lateral to the head of the humerus. The infraspinatus inserts posteriorly and induces external rotation with the support of the teres minor, with slightly more distal insertion in the posterior aspect. The subscapularis inserts in the lesser tuberosity of the humerus along the internal border of the bicipital groove of the humerus. Its contraction induces internal rotation of the shoulder.

Anteriorly, the predominant muscle is biceps brachialis. It inserts inferiorly via a common tendon in the radial tuberosity. The upper part of the biceps is divided in

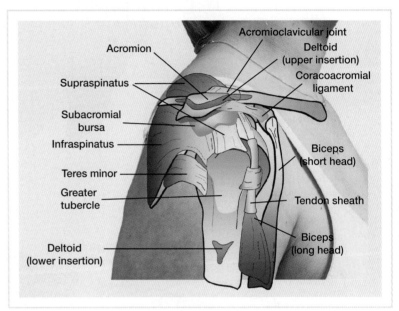

**Figure 8.2.** The rotator cuff of the shoulder and its anatomical relations.

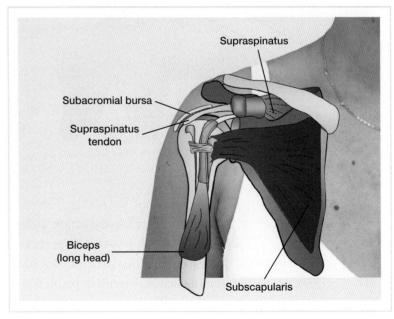

**Figure 8.3.** Functional anatomy of the shoulder. Internal rotation.

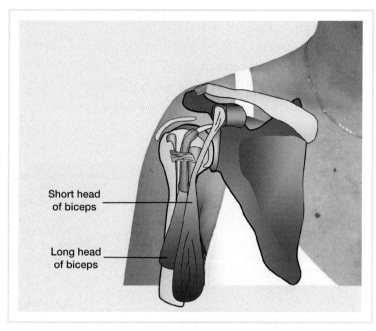

**Figure 8.4.** Functional anatomy of the shoulder. Short and long head of biceps.

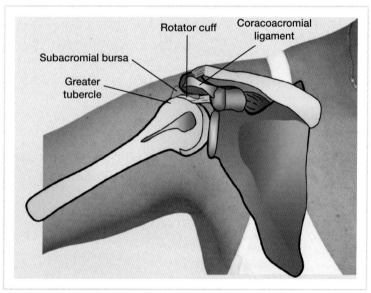

**Figure 8.5.** Subacromial impingement.

two. The inner part, the short head of the biceps, inserts in the coracoid process of the scapula. The long head of biceps becomes a long tendon that runs on the anterior aspect of the humerus (the intertubercular sulcus or bicipital groove) and through the glenohumeral joint to insert in the upper aspect of the glenoid cavity of the scapula. This tendon is coated with a long synovial sheath along the upper third of the humerus, which is a common site of inflammation (Figure 8.4.).

Contraction of the biceps naturally induces flexion of the humerus at the shoulder and flexion of the forearm on the upper arm. Given that the radial tuberosity is located in the medial aspect the radius, the biceps promotes the supination of the hand and forearm.

Other muscles are involved in the movements of the shoulder: the pectoralis major and latissimus dorsi, which are responsible for adduction, and the teres major. The triceps and rhomboid support the swinging movements of the scapula.

The upper outer quadrant of the shoulder is a problem area, with frequent conflicts of space. Above, the acromion forms a rigid, unyielding ceiling. Below, is the supraspinatus tendon, which pulls the head of the humerus upwards every time it contracts, reducing an already limited space. In addition, complete abduction means that the greater tuberosity enters the space.[1]

There is a synovial bursa that helps these structures to glide more easily: the subacromial bursa. Understandably, this structure, together with the rotator cuff, is exposed to the repeated friction trauma that may result in painful, incapacitating local inflammation (Figure 8.5.).

[1]Try elevating your arms in abduction up to 180°, keeping the palms of your hands facing down. Did you manage? Congratulations! Many people cannot do it without rotating their palms upwards when they reach about 90° abduction because there is not enough subacromial space to accommodate the greater tuberosity. They are therefore forced to induce external rotation of the humerus, moving the greater tuberosity behind the acromion.

### *Radiological anatomy*

An anteroposterior x-ray of the shoulder in a neutral position (Figure 8.6.) enables us to assess the regularity of the glenoid cavity of the scapula, the head of the humerus and the greater tuberosity and any calcification of the rotator cuff or subacromial bursa. Acromioclavicular osteoarthritis may require a special view. The distance between the lowest point of the acromioclavicular joint and the highest point of the head of the humerus should be at least 5 mm. Any less suggests a rupture of the supraspinatus tendon. The view in internal rotation (Figure 8.7.) makes it possible to assess the rest of the head of the humerus: sphericity, regularity, and the subchondral bone. In both views, look for possible lytic or sclerotic lesions.

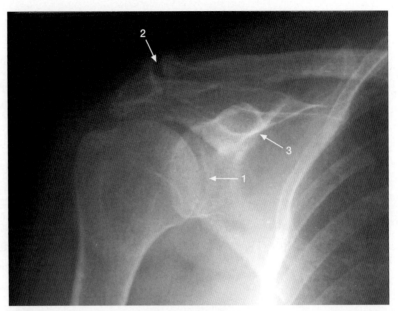

**Figure 8.6.** Normal radiology of the shoulder (right shoulder in neutral position). **1.** Gleno-humeral joint. **2.** Acromio-clavicular joint. **3.** Coracoid process of the scapula.

## COMMON CAUSES OF SHOULDER PAIN

Until proven otherwise, isolated pain in the shoulder is likely to be of periarticular origin. Periarticular lesions of the shoulder are extremely common, while isolated disease of the glenohumeral joint is rare

Disease of the shoulder is most common in people whose occupation or leisure activities involve repeated movements with the arms raised: cleaners, teachers, agricultural workers, factory workers, professional swimmers etc.

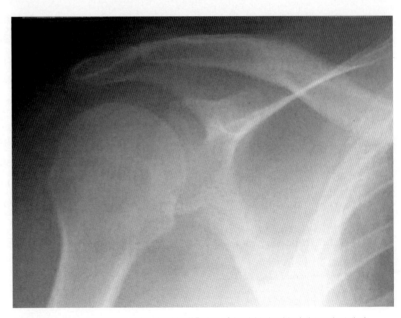

**Figure 8.7.** Normal radiology of the shoulder (AP view of the right shoulder in internal rotation).

Provided that they are thorough, the enquiry and clinical examination are extremely rewarding, as, in most cases, they allow an accurate diagnosis without the need for diagnostic tests. On the other hand, most of these lesions, which are highly incapacitating, can be treated effectively with simple techniques, which is very rewarding both for the patient and the doctor.

Table 8.1. shows the most common causes of shoulder pain.

| Etiology | Clinical clues |
|---|---|
| Tendonitis of the supraspinatus or infraspinatus and subacromial bursitis. | Localized pain in the shoulder or upper arm.<br>Worse during abduction<br>Nocturnal pain common – unable to sleep on same side<br>Specific maneuvers in the clinical examination |
| Tendonitis of the long head of the biceps. | Pain mainly in the anterior aspect of the shoulder<br>Worse during flexion<br>Specific maneuvers in the clinical examination |
| Adhesive capsulitis ("Frozen shoulder"). | Diffuse shoulder pain<br>Limitation of all movements during active and passive mobilization* |
| Complete tear (rupture) of the supraspinatus. | Pain similar to tendonitis of the supraspinatus<br>Complete active abduction impossible |
| Referred pain. | Diffuse<br>Unrelated to movements of the shoulder<br>Normal local and regional clinical examination |
| Glenohumeral arthritis. | Inflammatory pain<br>Pain on active and passive mobilization<br>Limited active and passive mobility<br>More joints usually involved |
| Acromioclavicular disease and instability. | Pain in the upper aspect of the shoulder<br>Mechanical pain<br>Worse during extreme abduction |
| Glenohumeral instability | Most common in young people<br>Recurring |

**Table 8.1.** Common causes of shoulder pain
*NB: capsulitis has clinical characteristics suggesting joint disease.

## THE ENQUIRY

The first aim of the enquiry is to find out whether the problem is limited to the shoulder or is part of a more widespread disease. Knowing the patient's occupational and leisure activities and assessing any chronic concomitant diseases such as diabetes mellitus, sequelae of a cerebrovascular accident, previous heart surgery or myocardial infarction, etc. can give us important clues. A history of trauma or a fall is particularly relevant.

The onset of periarticular lesions tends to be sudden or subacute, quite often related to a precise moment or gesture. Rupture of the supraspinatus is usually preceded by prolonged suffering with repeated episodes of pain.

Selectivity of painful movements is highly suggestive of a periarticular lesion and even of its type. Is the pain worse with movement? Is there a particularly painful movement? Abduction? Flexion? Patients with a periarticular lesion often say that the pain is worse at night, especially when lying on the same side. This is common to arthritis however and is not much use to differential diagnosis.

If the pain does not get worse during movement of the shoulder, we should look for causes of referred pain. Neurogenic radiated pain (of cervical origin) is suggested by dysesthesia and concomitant neck pain radiating to the shoulder and/or upper limb. As a rule, in these cases, movement of the neck exacerbates the pain in the shoulder. Questions about coronary, respiratory and biliary problems are mandatory.

If the pain also affects other articular areas, we must ascertain their nature, exploring the possibility polyarthropathy with shoulder involvement. We should not, however, ignore the fact that the association of periarticular lesions, of the shoulder and hand, for example, is quite common and can be misleading. Shoulder pain is also common in patients with fibromyalgia, but there is usually generalized pain, which is suggestive of this diagnosis.

## REGIONAL EXAMINATION

### Observation

Surface observation of the shoulder is relatively unproductive, as the glenohumeral joint is deep-set and protected by muscle. Only rarely are intra-articular effusions or effusions from the bursae visible as an area of fullness on the anterior face of the shoulder. For the same reason, redness is unusual, even in cases of intense synovitis. Swelling of the acromioclavicular joint is easily visible and palpable.

Rupture of the supraspinatus tendon, severe lesions of the cervical roots or the brachial plexus and prolonged disuse can cause atrophy of the shoulder muscles, which is easy to see when it involves the supraspinatus or infraspinatus.

### Mobilization

This is the fundamental part of a clinical examination of the shoulder and should involve three different aspects:

a. *Active mobilization* – the patient carries out the movement unaided.

b. *Passive mobilization* – the examiner carries out the movement while the patient remains as relaxed as possible.

c. *Resisted mobilization* – the patient is asked to carry out the movement while the examiner offers resistance.

If active mobilization is free, full-range and painless, it is unlikely to be any significant pathology of the shoulder, as all the articular and periarticular structures take part in the movement.

If active mobilization is painful or limited in range, assessment of passive mobilization should follow. When the patient is relaxed, passive mobilization involves the joints and capsules, but leaves the tendons at rest. If passive mobilization is much less painful or less limited in range than active mobilization, the problem is much more likely to be periarticular and not articular. The opposite is the case if the pain and range restriction are similar during active and passive mobilization.

Resisted mobilization places tendons and bursae under tension, which causes intense pain if these structures have lesions. The appropriate maneuvers are well defined so that each one assesses specific structures. They must be carried out properly because if not interpretation will be erroneous.

---

### MAIN POINTS

In periarticular lesions, there is pain in selected active and resisted movements. Movement range can be reduced by pain. Passive mobilization is more ample and less painful than active mobilization.

In adhesive capsulitis and diseases of the glenohumeral joint, all active and passive movements are painful and frequently limited in range. The range of passive movements is also reduced. Resisted movements cause little or no exacerbation of pain.

---

The shoulder is already assessed to a reasonable extent in the general examination described in Chapter 6. If the patient complains of shoulder pain, either spontaneously or during the examination, or if mobility is significantly limited, a more detailed examination is necessary.

The method we suggest is as follows:

---

a. The patient is asked to repeat total abduction of the arm to 180°, if possible, telling us as soon as he feels pain and whether it goes away as he continues the movement. We suggest that you show the patient the movement and ask him to repeat it.

---

Normally, in supraspinatus tendonitis or subacromial bursitis, this maneuver causes pain in an arc between 30 and 120°, subsiding above this angle. In more severe cases, the pain may force the patient to interrupt the movement. If the patient is unable to maintain his shoulder at 90° after passive abduction, a rupture of the supraspinatus is highly probable. Pain that only appears above 120° abduction suggests osteoarthritis of the acromioclavicular joint (Figure 8.8.).

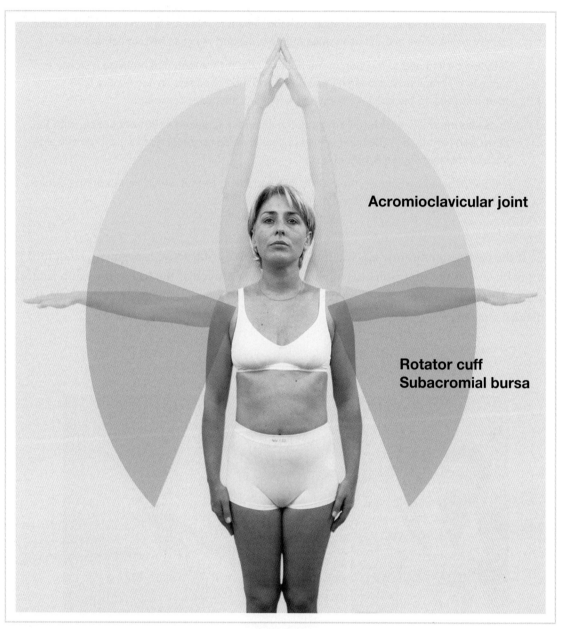

**Acromioclavicular joint**

**Rotator cuff
Subacromial bursa**

**Figure 8.8.** Clinical examination of the shoulder region: active abduction. Typical painful arcs.

b. We then ask the patient to raise his arms in front of his body, keeping the elbows extended.

Pain while performing this movement suggests a lesion of the biceps. In this case, the pain is located to the anterior aspect of the shoulder and upper arm. Note, however, that pain with this movement may also be caused by tendonitis of the supraspinatus or subacromial bursitis.

c. We now go on to passive mobilization. Ask the patient to relax his arm in your hand. Gentle passive movements and the assurance that this will hurt less can help to achieve this.

Standing behind and to the side of the patient, hold his forearm and mobilize it slowly and carefully to complete abduction (Figure 8.9A.) and then complete flexion (Figure 8.9B.). Your other hand lies on the patient's shoulder to feel any snapping or crepitus.

To assess internal and external rotation, the shoulder is placed in 90° abduction, with the elbow also bent to 90°. The hand is then pulled upwards (external rotation) and downwards (internal rotation) (Figure 8.10A. and B.)

Ask the patient how intense the pain is in comparison to that which he felt during active mobilization and assess the range of movement.

If the pain is significantly less intense than that felt during active movement, tendonitis is more likely – of the supraspinatus, if abduction is painful or of the biceps if flexion is most affected. In these cases, we can expect passive movements to show a full range, even though there may be some pain.

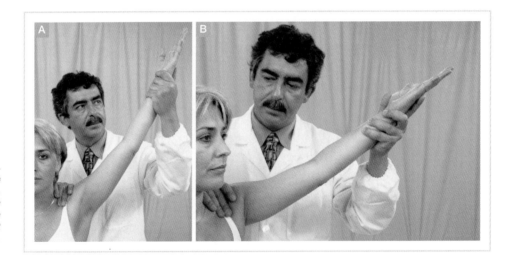

**Figure 8.9.**
Passive mobilization of the shoulder. **A.** Abduction. **B.** Flexion. *Please note: the correct interpretation of passive motion demands that the patient is relaxed.*

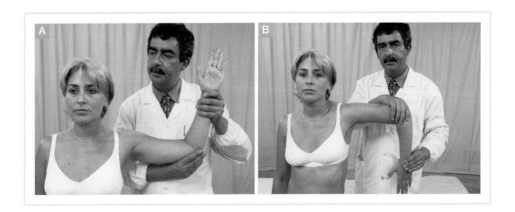

**Figure 8.10.**
Passive mobilization of the shoulder. **A.** External rotation. **B.** Internal rotation.

If, on the other hand, mobility is limited mechanically and not just by the pain, we should suspect an intrinsic lesion of the gleno-humeral joint and/or its capsule. In this case, we can sometimes detect crepitus or snapping in the joint. In glenohumeral synovitis, all movements are generally painful.

In the presence of limited abduction, it is useful to assess the glenohumeral separately from the scapulothoracic component. To do this, stand behind the patient and hold the lower vertex of the scapula, following its movement while inducing abduction of the arm (Figure 8.11.). With the shoulder blade immobilized, a normal glenohumeral joint allows about 90° abduction.

Significant limitation of all movements is highly suggestive of adhesive capsulitis, especially if external rotation is limited. Most arthropathies limit abduction earlier, leaving rotation, and especially internal rotation, relatively free.

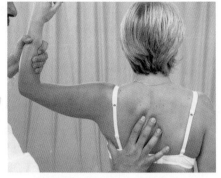

**Figure 8.11.** Precise evaluation of shoulder abduction due to the gleno-humeral joint. Immobilization of the scapula precludes the scapulo-thoracic component.

> d. Resisted mobilization also requires an appropriate technique.
>
> i) The patient's arms are placed at 90° abduction and about 30° ahead of the frontal plane, with the thumbs turned down. (The greater tuberosity is under the acromion.) Ask the patient to hold this position while you push his forearms down (Figure 8.12.).
>
> ii) The patient puts his hand on the opposite shoulder and raises his elbow until his arm is horizontal. He holds the position while you push his elbow down (Figure 8.13.).
>
> iii) With the patient's shoulder at 90° abduction and 30° anterior flexion, the elbows are bent to 90°. You push the shoulder down while raising and internally rotating the arm with the other hand (Figure 8.14. Subacromial conflict test).

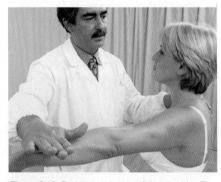

**Figure 8.12.** Resisted abduction of the shoulder. The rotator cuff (supra- and infraspinatus) is put under tension and the subacromial bursa is compressed.

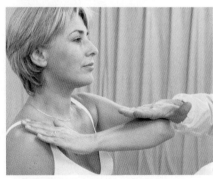

**Figure 8.13.** Subacromial impingement test. The rotator cuff (supra- and infraspinatus) is put under tension and the subacromial bursa is compressed.

The first two maneuvers require contraction of the supraspinatus, placing its tendon under tension. In addition, this contraction pulls the head of the humerus up towards the acromion, compressing the rotator cuff and the subacromial bursa against it. In the third maneuver, the observer induces the movement. If there is any inflammation of the supraspinatus tendon or bursa, the patient will complain of pain in the shoulder region – a positive maneuver. When these maneuvers cause pain in locations other than the shoulder, we should suspect hyperreactivity to pain, as in fibromyalgia for example.

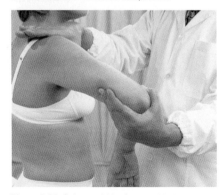

**Figure 8.14.** Subacromial impingement test.

In practice, it is very difficult in a clinical examination to distinguish between tendonitis of the supraspinatus and subacromial bursitis. This is not particularly important as the treatment is very similar.

e. We then test the biceps.

i. The patient raises his arms anteriorly to 30–45° flexion, with his elbows and wrists in extension and supination (Palms up test or Speed's test). He holds this position while you force his forearms down (Figure 8.15.).

ii. The patient places his arm along his body, the elbow bent to 90° and the hand semi-supine. He holds this position, while resisting your efforts to extend his elbow and pronate the hand (Yergason's maneuver – Figure 8.16.).

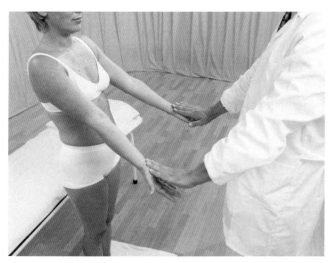

**Figure 8.15.** Palms up test (Speed's test). Pain in the shoulder suggests tenosynovitis of the long head of the biceps.

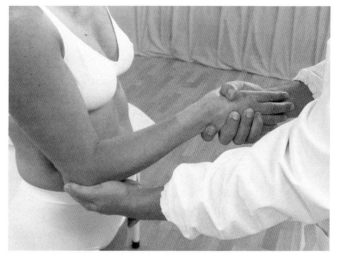

**Figure 8.16.** Yergason's test. The examiner tries to pronate and extend the forearm, while the patient resists. Pain in the shoulder suggests tenosynovitis of the long head of the biceps.

The maneuvers are positive if they cause pain in the anterior aspect of the shoulder and proximal third of the upper arm, suggesting tenosynovitis of the long head of the biceps.

### Palpation

As the shoulder is a deep joint, it is not possible to palpate the joint space or look for effusion. There are, however, two sites where palpation is particularly productive:

### Supraspinatus and infraspinatus tendon/subacromial bursa

With the arm at rest, they are the soft structures that you feel between the external border of the acromion, above, and the bony prominence of the greater tuberosity below (Figure 8.17A.). Alternatively, ask the patient to put his hand behind his back. This makes the greater tuberosity rotate forward to a position below and in front of the anterior vertex of the acromion (Figure 8.17B.).[2] Pain on deep palpation of these areas suggests a lesion of the supraspinatus or subacromial bursitis. If in doubt, compare with the other side.

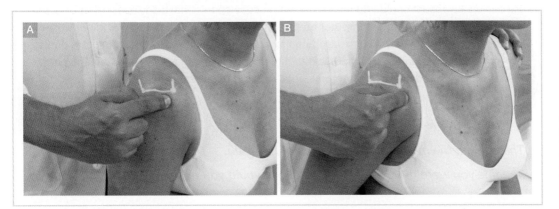

**Figure 8.17.**
Palpation of the insertion of the rotator cuff in the greater tuberosity of the humerus, with the shoulder in neutral position (**A**) or in internal rotation (**B**).

### Tendon of the long head of the biceps

To examine the tendon on the right side, stand behind and to the right of the patient and hold his forearm in your left hand. Run the fingertips of your right hand deeply across the head of the humerus. You will feel the greater and lesser tuberosities and the bicipital groove between them. If necessary, rotate the patient's shoulder inwards and outwards while you palpate. The tendon of the long head of the biceps and its sheath feel like a sinewy roll running along the groove and extending downwards. Local pain on palpation suggests tenosynovitis (Figure 8.18.).

Please note: As the glenohumeral joint is deeply located, it is difficult to absolutely confirm or exclude the existence of arthritis. We have to base our assessment on the rhythm of the pain, on the clinical context (monoarthritis of the shoulder is rare) and on passive mobilization: restriction of movements indicates a compromised joint. If the patient experiences pain during passive mobilization of the shoulder, rotating the arm to an angle of about 50°, there is probably inflammation of the synovium or capsule.

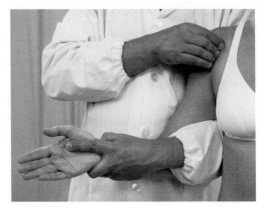

**Figure 8.18.** Palpation of tendon of the long head of the biceps. The tendon, surrounded by its synovial sheath, lies in the bicipital grove, on the anterior aspect of the humerus. It is easier to palpate while the shoulder is rotated internally and externally.

[2]Try it on yourself. Place your right hand at rest along your body. Press the head of the humerus with your left index finger just below the anterior vertex of the right acromion. Now rotate your hand inwards and outwards – the bony prominence that you can feel deep down gliding under your finger is the greater tuberosity.

## TYPICAL CASES
## 8.A. SHOULDER PAIN (I)

Mr. Figueiredo was a 48-year old draftsman. He was sent to us by his family doctor because of pain involving his right shoulder, which he had had for about 3 months. The pain troubled him particularly at night, stopping him lying on the right, his usual position. He felt no pain at rest, but movements caused intense pain, especially when putting on his jacket, washing his back, combing his hair or changing gear in the car. There was no significant morning stiffness.

He denied any recent or old trauma. He did not practice sport or have any special hobbies, but he spent a long time at the computer as part of his job. He mentioned sporadic, transient lumbar and cervical pain which he attributed to long hours sitting at the computer. He denied recent neck pain or paresthesia and said that moving his neck did not exacerbate the pain in his shoulder. He had no other symptoms or associated disease.

*Think about the most probable causes of this pain.*

*Imagine you were the patient's doctor. How would you examine him?*

A comparative inspection of the shoulders did not show any asymmetry. During the general rheumatologic examination, the patient complained of intense pain in his right shoulder during abduction, beginning at about 60° and with no relief on complete abduction. Anterior flexion of the arms caused some discomfort in the same area, though it was less intense. Passive mobilization of the shoulder in abduction caused pain, though it was much less severe than during active mobilization. The patient was anxious and unable to relax completely. Passive flexion of the shoulder was painless. The maneuvers of resisted abduction and resisted elevation of the arm with the hand on the opposite shoulder were painful. There was no significant pain in the palms up test or Yergason's maneuver. Palpation over the greater tuberosity of the humerus was very painful compared to the other side, particularly with the arm in internal rotation. The examination of the cervical spine and elbow was normal.

*Summarize this condition.[3]*

*What is your diagnosis?*

*Do we need diagnostic tests? Which ones?*

*What treatment would you choose?*

In view of the ineffectiveness of previous measures, we injected a mixture of local anesthetic and methylprednisolone around the supraspinatus tendon and the subacromial space (for technical

[3]A young patient with selective shoulder pain – pain worse during active than passive mobilization, without range limitations. Rotator cuff maneuvers positive.

guidance, see Chapter 30). The patient experienced considerable relief when we repeated active mobilization a few minutes later, which confirmed our diagnosis: supraspinatus tendonitis/sub-acromial bursitis.

We explained to the patient the cause of his pain and his anatomical condition. We said that the situation was highly likely to recur as, in most cases, it is related to a constitutional subacromial space conflict. We advised him to avoid repeated work with his arms raised above his shoulders and suggested that it would be a very good idea to use supports for his forearms when working at the computer. We told him to come back if the pain persisted. After 6 months we still had not seen him, but we would not be surprised if he came back with similar problems.

## SUPRASPINATUS TENDONITIS AND SUBACROMIAL BURSITIS
### *MAIN POINTS*

This is a very common condition in adults and the elderly.

When it appears in young people we should suspect glenohumeral instability.

The pain is usually unilateral and limited to the shoulder, rarely radiating to the arm. It is highly incapacitating.

As a rule, the pain is more intense during abduction than during flexion of the shoulder. It may be worse at night, especially lying on the same side.

Although it is usually an isolated problem, it may be associated with arthritis of the shoulder or other soft tissue lesions, especially tenosynovitis of the biceps.

A careful clinical examination usually provides the diagnosis.

Diagnostic tests are not necessary in typical cases, as they have nothing to add to the diagnosis or the choice of treatment.

Initial treatment is conservative, with topical and systemic anti-inflammatories and local protection.

In persistent or highly incapacitating cases, a local injection of glucocorticoids by an experienced professional is justified and usually solves the problem.

It is highly likely to recur and in exceptional cases may warrant surgery.

## *TYPICAL CASES*
## 8.B. FROZEN SHOULDER

Isabel dos Santos was a 62-year old farm worker. She came to our clinic because of pain and lack of mobility in the right shoulder, for which she had been on sick leave for the last 7 weeks. The pain was constant day and night and worsened with any attempt at movement. It was partially relieved by anti-inflammatories, but they did nothing for the limited mobility. When she first experienced these symptoms, she was sent for physiotherapy. The pain was exacerbated by mobilization, even when passive, however, and she refused any more treatment after a few sessions. She had been given an injection in the upper aspect of the shoulder. She had noticed no improvement.

When asked about trauma, she said that she had had a fall at work a few days before the shoulder pain appeared but that she had recovered immediately. She was being treated regularly for hypertension and diabetes, both of which were under control, and denied any other symptoms. She had undergone the menopause, spontaneously at 42. Her mother had been healthy and had died at the age of 82 as a result of a hip fracture.

Her clinical examination was normal. She was 1.48 m tall and weighed 45 kg.

Our general rheumatologic examination showed atrophy of the right shoulder muscles. The joint was almost completely immobilized and extremely painful. When asked to abduct her shoulder, the patient leaned her body to the left and only managed to raise her shoulder to about 40° abduction. Passive mobilization was extremely painful and highly limited in all directions, including internal and external rotation. On immobilizing the scapula, we found that almost all abduction was due to swinging the scapula. There were no anomalies in the cervical spine or the rest of the rheumatologic examination, apart from moderate dorsal kyphosis.

## FROZEN SHOULDER, ADHESIVE CAPSULITIS OF THE SHOULDER
## MAIN POINTS

This is a relatively uncommon, but highly incapacitating condition that can leave important sequelae if not treated properly.

It is an inflammatory, fibrosing process that affects the articular capsule and causes it to contract over the joint, thus limiting its mobility. Loss of external rotation is particularly suggestive of this condition.

The pain tends to be intense and constant, especially in the early stages of the disease, getting worse at night and with movement. It may subside spontaneously after a few weeks or months.

Limited active and passive mobility in all directions is an essential clinical clue. It may be the only manifestation in the late stages.

It may appear spontaneously, but there is often a history of trauma (even very small). Repeated tendonitis of the cuff, previous stroke and diabetes mellitus are predisposing factors.

Diagnostic tests serve essentially to rule out other pathologies like septic arthritis, intra-articular fracture, or aseptic necrosis of the humerus. In adhesive capsulitis, the standard x-ray of the shoulder is normal. Arthrography, CT scans and ultrasound can be used to confirm the diagnosis.

Although intra-articular injection of corticosteroids may be difficult, it helps to relieve the pain if administered in the initial stages of the condition.

Physiotherapy and regular exercise at home, together with analgesics and anti-inflammatories, play an essential role in restoring mobility, which may take up to 2 years.

In rare cases, recovery may require manipulation of the shoulder under anesthetic to break down the fibrosis, followed by physiotherapy.

*What do you think are the most likely diagnoses?*

*Would you ask for any diagnostic tests?*

*What treatment would you suggest in each case?*

In view of the symptoms, we thought the most probable diagnosis was adhesive capsulitis. We asked for a full blood count, sedimentation rate and anteroposterior x-rays in a neutral position and arranged to see her again soon. All these tests were normal. There were no signs of fracture or changes in the bone structure of the humeral head or articular space of the right glenohumeral joint, when compared to the left.

We gave her an intra-articular injection of a long-acting corticosteroid, using an anterior approach to the joint.[4] We noted considerable resistance to the pressure of the injection. We told the patient that we expected her pain to be greatly relieved and stressed the need for intense, prolonged physiotherapy. She would have to do regular exercises at home to increase the range of movement. We pointed out that complete recovery of mobility could take up to 2 years. We prescribed an anti-inflammatory for which she had already shown good tolerance, to take when necessary for the pain. We scheduled follow-up visits to assess mobility, which we recorded with a goniometer, for future reference.

*Reconsider the case. Have we forgotten anything, like additional tests?[5]*

*Consider the possible causes and their likelihood.*

*List the maneuvers that you think are necessary and their interpretation.*

---

[4]See Chapter 30 for guidance on the technique.

[5]In fact, we also looked for osteoporosis. This is a typical situation in which we should consider this condition as there are a number of risk factors: post-menopausal woman with an early menopause, underweight and a family history suggesting the disease.

*TYPICAL CASES*
## 8.C. SHOULDER PAIN (II)

António Rodrigues, a 43-year old stonemason, complained of pain in his left shoulder that had started 2 months before, after a particularly strenuous job. The pain was diffuse, but was more marked on the anterior aspect of the shoulder. He said that he had trouble picking up heavy weights and often dropped them because of the pain. Other movements were fairly easy. He denied any pain at night or at rest.

He was otherwise healthy with no other musculoskeletal or systemic complaints.

Our general examination did not find any anomalies. Active mobilization of the shoulder was complete and painless. The maneuvers for the rotator cuff were only slightly uncomfortable. The palms-up-test caused typical pain, however. Yergason's maneuver was also painful. Palpation of the left bicipital groove was much more painful than the right.

*What is your diagnosis?*

*How would you treat it?*

We diagnosed tenosynovitis of the long head of the right biceps.

We explained the situation to the patient, and suggested a period of rest, if possible with his arm in a sling. We prescribed anti-inflammatories, and scheduled a new appointment for a local injection if the situation did not clear up completely in 3 or 4 weeks.

*Imagine you are a general practitioner. What possible diagnoses do you think are likely? Why?*

*Would you request any diagnostic tests?*

## TENOSYNOVITIS OF THE LONG HEAD OF THE BICEPS
*MAIN POINTS*

This is a common condition in adults and the elderly.

The pain is usually unilateral and confined to the anterior face of the shoulder. It may be highly incapacitating.

As a rule, the pain is more intense on flexion of the shoulder. There may be nocturnal pain.

Although it is usually isolated, it can be associated with arthritis of the shoulder or other soft tissue lesions, especially supraspinatus tendonitis.

A careful clinical examination usually provides the diagnosis.

Diagnostic tests are not necessary in typical cases, as they have nothing to add to the diagnosis or the choice of treatment.

Initial treatment is conservative, with topical and systemic anti-inflammatories and local protection.

In persistent or highly incapacitating cases, local injection by an experienced physician is indicated.[6]

[6]See Chapter 30 for guidance on the technique.

*TYPICAL CASES*
## 8.D. SHOULDER PAIN (III)

António Sarmento was a 46-year old salesman. He came to us because of a deep, "dull" ache in his left shoulder, which was difficult to pinpoint and had started about 8 months before. The pain came in episodes and went away by itself after several minutes to 1 hour. He did not recognize a clear trigger for the pain, but he noticed it was related to more demanding physical activities, particularly climbing stairs. He attributed a curiously distressing character to it. It was sometimes associated with discomfort over the lower part of the sternum. He had been treated with anti-inflammatories to no avail.

Our systematic enquiry revealed no other alterations. He smoked about 30 cigarettes a day and was not taking any regular medication.

The patient was obese and good-humored. Our clinical and general rheumatologic examinations showed no alterations except hypertension (160/95 mmHg). Movements of both shoulders were free and painless, both on passive and active mobilization. Periarticular palpation was painless. The examination of the cervical spine was also normal, causing no pain in the shoulder. Auscultation of the heart and lungs showed no anomalies

On the basis of this information, we requested routine tests with an evaluation of serum lipids. His ECG showed slight elevation of the ST segment in the left precordial leads. After this finding the patient did an exercise test, which was positive, with clear signs of coronary ischemia coinciding with the pain in his shoulder, similar to that described spontaneously. The patient was referred to a cardiologist for a possible coronary angiography. When we saw him again about 3 months later he was asymptomatic following introduction of nitrates.

*He's your patient! What other questions would you ask him?*

## REFERRED SHOULDER PAIN
*MAIN POINTS*

Pain of cervical, coronary, pleural and subdiaphragmatic origin can radiate to the shoulder.

This pain is ill-defined and variable, depending on the cause.

A careful systematic enquiry can produce suggestive clues.

Regional clinical examination is normal.

An examination of the neck may show alterations and reproduce the pain, suggesting a cervical origin.

The treatment is oriented by the underlying cause.

*TYPICAL CASES*
## 8.E. SHOULDER PAIN (IV)

Carlos Soares, a 52-year old carpenter, decided to go to the doctor after many years of pain in both shoulders, because the symptoms were worsening and his functional disability was progressive. The pain had begun 10–12 years previously, and had continued since then with exacerbations and partial remissions. A workaholic, he attributed the pain to his occupation and continued to work in spite of everything, taking anti-inflammatories when it got worse. Now this was no longer possible. The pain in his right shoulder was incapacitating and its mobility was greatly reduced.

When asked, he also described a history of low back pain that had begun at the same time, with similar progression and characteristics: more intense when the work was harder. However, he also had pain at night and mentioned morning stiffness of the shoulder and lumbar region lasting about an hour.

He denied any systemic manifestations and his past medical history was not relevant.

*Plan the main points of a clinical examination of this patient.*

In the general clinical examination, we found obvious scaly erythematous lesions dispersed over the torso and scalp (Figure 8.19.), which the patient said he had had for years though it did not bother him.

Mobility of the lumbar spine seemed reduced and Schober's test (see Chapter 11) showed an elongation of 10–12.5 cm.

Mobility in his right shoulder was considerably reduced, limited to 120° abduction and 90° anterior flexion. Internal and external rotation were also reduced. Passive mobilization did not increase these ranges and was accompanied by moderate pain in all directions. The maneuvers for periarticular lesions were negative. There were no other alterations in the rest of the examination.

*Summarize this clinical case.[7]*

*What are the most probable diagnoses?*

*Would you ask for any diagnostic tests?*

*What treatment would you prescribe?*

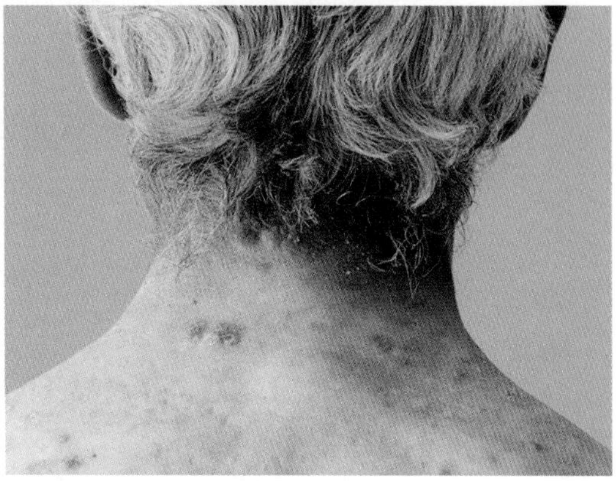

We requested lab tests, including a full blood count, sedimentation rate, liver and kidney tests, and x-rays of the shoulders (anteroposterior in neutral position and with external rotation), pelvis (anteroposterior) and lumbar spine (anteroposterior and profile). The tests showed a discreet elevation of the sedimentation rate to 32 mm in the first hour with no other alterations. The

**Figure 8.19.** Erythematous and scaling lesions – psoriasis.

[7]Inflammatory shoulder and back pain in a patient with psoriasis. Limited active and passive mobility in the painful areas.

radiograph of the shoulders showed diffuse osteopenia on the right, reduction of the joint space with some sclerosis of the articular surfaces and osteophyte formations (Figure 8.20A.). The x-ray of the pelvis showed sclerosis and partial blurring of the right sacroiliac joint (second degree sacroiliitis – Figure 8.20B.).

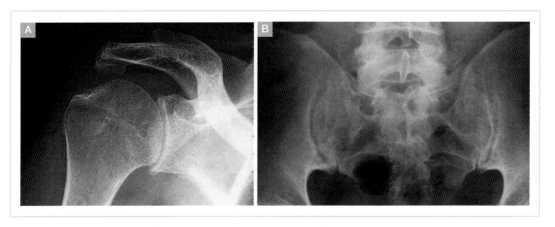

**Figure 8.20.**
**A.** Radiology of the shoulder – advanced arthritis. Note the joint space loss, diffuse osteopenia, displacement superiorly of the humeral head and osteophytes in the periphery of the glenoid surface. **B.** The X-rays of the pelvis revealed subchondral sclerosis, erosions and partial blurring of the right sacro-iliac joint.

## INFLAMMATORY SHOULDER PAIN
### MAIN POINTS

The shoulder can be involved in practically all types of polyarthritis.

Even when the complaints are focused in one area, it is essential to ask about other joints.

The inflammatory rhythm of the pain, an important clue to diagnosis, may be difficult to pinpoint, especially in manual workers.

Clinical examination is fundamental to the diagnosis. Pain on passive mobilization in several directions and limited active and passive mobility indicate joint disease.

Without proper treatment, arthritis can leave irreversible sequelae.

Treatment should begin early and be suited to the nature of the disease.

We considered that this confirmed the diagnosis of psoriatic arthritis, with involvement of the sacroiliac joints and the right shoulder, with secondary osteoarthritis of this joint and persistent inflammatory activity. It was unfortunate that the patient's joint disease was so advanced when he came to us.

The patient was advised to try to spare his shoulder as much as possible. We prescribed a long-lasting anti-inflammatory, to be taken with the evening meal, supplemented during the day, if necessary. We suggested regular exercises for both the affected regions. We recommended an intra-articular injection of the shoulder, which was highly effective. The patient was kept under clinical observation, saving further therapy for the involvement of any other articular areas.

## SPECIAL SITUATIONS

### Joint disease and instability of the acromioclavicular joint
Instability of the acromioclavicular joint is usually the result of trauma, such as a fall onto the outstretched arm. This joint can be involved in inflammatory arthropathies of several types.

Osteoarthritis may appear as a result of repeated trauma, usually from heavy manual labor. The pain is usually felt on the upper surface of the shoulder. Active mobilization causes pain in extreme movements in all directions and pain arising above 90° abduction is especially typical. The joint is accessible to local palpation, which may detect inflammatory or bony swelling and instability.

The most specific maneuver for examining this joint involves asking the patient to put one hand behind his back, with his elbow in extension. We then force adduction to the limit. The presence of acromioclavicular lesion is suggested by pain over the joint.

### Instability and subluxation of the gleno-humeral joint

This usually appears in young people, especially athletes, after violent movements like throwing a ball. It presents acutely with a "dead-arm" sensation, with intense pain, numbness and tingling in the arm, followed by a deeper pain. It is often followed by rotator cuff tendonitis for a few days or weeks. It has a marked tendency to recur, which is accentuated by repeated episodes of dislocation, even if each episode often resolves spontaneously.

In the presence of dislocation, there is a clear asymmetry of the shoulders on observation. To test stability, ask the patient to lie down with his upper limb hanging beside the examining table. Then immobilize the shoulder with one hand and hold the arm with the other. With the patient relaxed, try to induce anterior and posterior movements of the head of the humerus, noting the degree of instability and comparing it to the opposite side if necessary (Figure 8.21A.). Another way of testing stability consists of forcing external rotation and anterior projection of the humerus, while the arm is abducted to 90° (Figure 8.21B.). This maneuver assesses anterior instability and is positive if there is pain or a sensation of anterior dislocation of the head of the humerus. If posterior compression of the shoulder relieves this pain, this reinforces the suggestion of instability.

This suspicion justifies referring the patient to a special rehabilitation program.

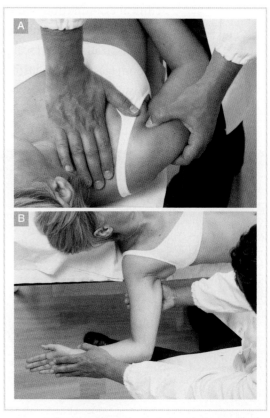

**Figure 8.21.** Shoulder stability test. **A.** The hand holding the upper arm tests the antero-posterior mobility at the joint level. The other stabilizes the collar bone and the acromion. **B.** The external rotation with anterior projection of the humerus causes pain. The diagnosis is reinforced if the pain subsides with posterior projection of the head of the humerus.

### Acute shoulder

Acute shoulder pain, sometimes accompanied by swelling, suggests trauma, infection or microcrystalline joint disease. Septic arthritis of the shoulder is rare but highly destructive and requires early treatment. Chondrocalcinosis and the deposit of hydroxyapatite crystals may result in acute, sometimes rapidly destructive arthritis.

These situations require urgent referral for diagnostic tests (joint aspirate, for example) and treatment. Stabilizing surgical procedures, preferably arthroscopic, are sometimes necessary.

## DIAGNOSTIC TESTS

Diagnostic tests are dispensable in most patients with regional shoulder pain. The enquiry and clinical examination will reveal diagnostic characteristics of soft tissue lesion: selectivity of painful movements, unlimited passive mobility that is less painful than active movement, resisted mobilization, and local palpation.

Some tests may be justified in cases of signs or symptoms suggesting joint disease or unclear, persistent clinical conditions.

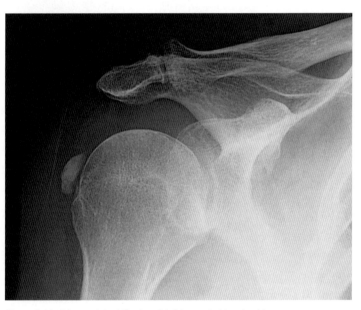

**Figure 8.22.** Subacromial calcification. Calcifying tendonitis or bursitis.

### Imaging

A *standard x-ray* of the shoulder is more productive in cases of joint disease and can show the typical characteristics of inflammatory or degenerative disease (Figure 8.20A.). It sometimes shows the presence of calcifications of the supraspinatus tendon or the subacromial bursa – calcifying tendonitis (Figure 8.22.). Although this finding will not alter the treatment, it indicates a chronic, recurring lesion, which is more resistant to conservative treatment. In some cases, we can see sclerosis and irregularity of the greater tuberosity, which indicates a similar pathology. X-rays can also show fractures and lytic lesions.

*Ultrasound scans* are more useful in soft tissue lesions and in experienced hands can detect inflammatory lesions or tears and pinpoint their exact location.

CT and MRI scans can make a valuable contribution to clearing up complex cases in specialized investigations.

### Other tests

Lab tests are indicated if there is reason to suspect inflammatory joint disease and are selected according to the nature of the joint disease suggested by the clinical evaluation. Changes in the full blood count and sedimentation rate are non-specific clues to inflammatory joint disease. Liver and kidney tests may be justified especially in preparation for possible disease-modifying treatment. Tests for rheumatoid factor are justified if the clinical assessment suggests rheumatoid arthritis. Suspected septic arthritis (acute/subacute monoarthritis, fever and leukocytosis) justifies referring the patient immediately to a specialized centre.

## TREATMENT

Most cases of regional shoulder pain correspond to soft tissue lesions and simple measures should be taken, as described above.

In the case of joint disease, which is potentially highly incapacitating, the patient should be sent to a specialist.

**1. Educating the patient.** Periarthritis of the shoulder is often related to an anatomical predisposition and repetitive work or leisure-related movements. As a result, they are highly likely to recur. Patients should be told this and taught how to avoid high-risk activities. They should be encouraged to take progressive, regular exercise as soon as the acute pain phase passes.

**2. Medication.** Anti-inflammatories, chosen according to the patient's particular condition (see Chapter 30), generally achieve marked relief of the pain. They can be aided by topical anti-inflammatories applied as a cream or patch several times a day in association with local heat.

In highly incapacitating cases or those that have resisted prior treatment, local (intra- or peri-articular) injection of an anesthetic and corticosteroid may be useful. These measures serve not only to confirm the diagnosis, but are also often effective in treating the condition itself. This kind of injection requires experience and a precise technique. In very advanced joint disease or ruptured tendons, performing a nerve block around the suprascapular nerve as it runs along the suprascapular groove may relieve the symptoms and improve mobility.

**3. Physiotherapy.** This is particularly useful in cases of persistent limitation of mobility, if the x-ray shows no signs of advanced, irreversible destruction of the joint structure. It is indispensable in cases of adhesive capsulitis.

The use of physical agents like deep heat and microwaves can be beneficial in cases of soft tissue lesions that are resistant to simpler measures.

**4. Surgery.** This is limited to situations that have resisted the above treatments. In cases of recurring subacromial lesion with a conflict of space, the surgeon may use subacromial decompression with acromioplasty and removal of the coracoacromial ligament, which can be done arthroscopically. A shoulder prosthesis may be necessary in cases of great functional disability with irreversible structural damage of the glenohumeral joint. The results are better when surgery is carried out at specialized centers.

## WHEN SHOULD THE PATIENT BE REFERRED TO A SPECIALIST?

Whenever passive mobility of the joint is significantly limited.

When x-rays show obvious alterations in the joint or bone.

Whenever shoulder pain is associated with confirmed or suspected arthritis (mono-, oligo- or polyarthritis). Suspected septic arthritis requires urgent referral.

When conservative measures prove ineffective, with continued significant suffering and disability.

## ADDITIONAL PRACTICE
### REGIONAL SYNDROMES. THE PAINFUL SHOULDER

22.A. PAIN AND STIFFNESS OF THE GIRDLES                    PAGE 22.2

# REGIONAL SYNDROMES
## THE ELBOW AND FOREARM

9.

J.A.P. da Silva, A.D. Woolf, *Rheumatology in Practice*, DOI 10.1007/978-1-84882-581-9_9,
© Springer-Verlag London Limited 2010

# 9. REGIONAL SYNDROMES THE ELBOW AND FOREARM

The elbow is a complex joint. Its great functional importance derives from its involvement in the positioning and optimizing use of the hand. Elbow pain is usually superficial and localized, often radiating to the forearm. It is exacerbated by exercise such as carrying heavy items or making a fist. Periarticular lesions are much more common than joint disease. The elbow may be involved in polyarthritis, but it rarely starts there. Osteoarthritis of the elbow is very rare.

Differential diagnosis is essentially clinical.

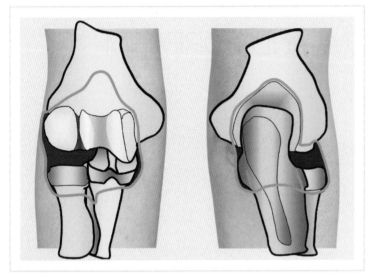

**Figure 9.1.** The elbow joints. The *green line* indicates the capsule insertion.

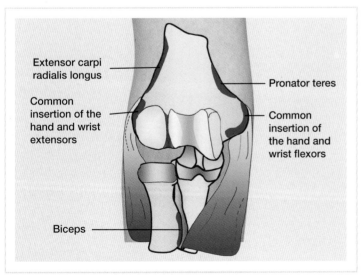

**Figure 9.2.** Muscle insertions around the elbow joint.

## FUNCTIONAL ANATOMY

The elbow combines three bones in three joints: the humeroradial, laterally, the humeroulnar, medially, and the proximal radioulnar joint. The humeroulnar joint conducts and limits flexion and extension. The other two joints are involved mainly in supination and pronation of the forearm and hand. When fully extended, the axis of the forearm and arm form a lateral angle (in valgus) of 5° (in men) to 15° (in women), which is lost when the elbow is in complete flexion.

A single capsule surrounds these three joints forming a voluminous recess at the extensor surface (Figure 9.1.). If there is accumulation of articular fluid or synovitis this is expelled during full extension, causing a palpable bulge around the olecranon, particularly on the medial side.

Immediately above the articular surfaces of the humerus are two bony protrusions whose identification is of the greatest clinical importance: the lateral and medial epicondyles.[1]

Tendons are inserted at the lower border of these protrusions. These tendons are the most common sites of pathology in the elbow: lateral (tennis elbow) and medial epicondylitis (golfer's elbow). The extensors of the forearm and wrist insert into the lateral epicondyle and the flexors insert into the medial epicondyle (Figure 9.2.).

[1]Find these references in your own elbow. With your arm slightly bent, palpate the external border of the distal end of the humerus. You will feel the protrusion of the epicondyle and, under it, a rounded structure – the radial head. The epitrochlea is in the same location on the inside, but is more prominent. The tendons of flexor and extensor muscles of the hand are inserted along the lower surface of these protrusions.

The elbow joint is served by a highly complex set of muscles. Extension is mediated by the triceps brachialis muscle, which joins the scapula and proximal humerus to the proximal end of the ulna (olecranon process). Elbow flexion is the result of the contraction of the biceps, (which joins the scapula to the radial tuberosity), the brachialis and the brachioradialis. Supination and pronation depend on specific muscles: the pronator teres, pronator quadratus, biceps and supinator.

The olecranon bursa covers the olecranon. It does not communicate with the joint, but is often the site of inflammation and effusion.

There are three other important points of reference.

- The ulnar nerve lies on the medial aspect, behind the medial epicondyle, in a tunnel consisting of branches of the humeroulnar ligament and the flexor carpi ulnaris. The ulnar nerve is easily entrapped along this route causing *ulnar nerve syndrome.*

- The anterior interosseous nerve, a branch of the median nerve, emerges between the two parts of the pronator teres, at the mid-point of the union between the upper and middle third of the anterior aspect of the forearm (Figure 9.3.). Compression of this nerve branch can cause pain in the forearm (*pronator syndrome*).

- In about 30% of people, the posterior interosseous nerve, a branch of the radial nerve, passes between the two parts of the supinator on the posterolateral surface of the forearm (about 5 cm below the epicondyle – Figure 9.4.). Local compression of this nerve can cause *radial tunnel syndrome.*

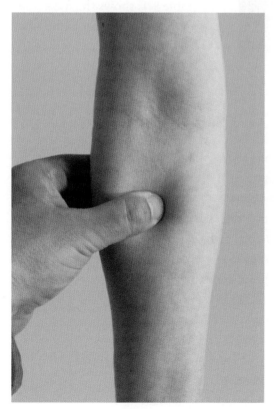

**Figure 9.3.** Tender point in the pronator syndrome.

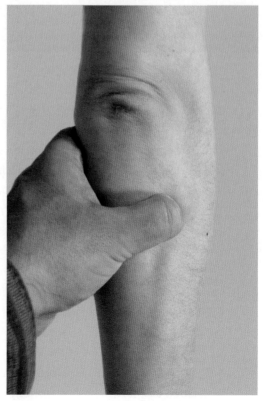

**Figure 9.4.** Tender point in the radial tunnel syndrome.

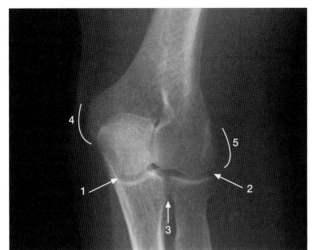

**Figure 9.5.**
Normal radiology of the elbow. Left side antero-posterior view in extension.
**1.** Humeroulnar joint.
**2.** Humeroradial joint.
**3.** Superior radioulnar joint.
**4.** Medial epicondyle.
**5.** Lateral epicondyle.

### Radiological anatomy

From an anteroposterior view (Figure 9.5.) note the size and regularity of the humeroradial, humeroulnar and radioulnar articular space and the regularity and density of the articular surfaces. The epicondyles may show erosion or calcification. The lateral view (Figure 9.6.) is not so clear. Look at the humeroradial joint and the regularity of the olecranon.

**Figure 9.6.**
Radiology of the elbow. Lateral view. Note the radio-humeral joint space and the regularity of the olecranon.

## COMMON CAUSES OF PAIN IN THE ELBOW AND FOREARM

Table 9.1. shows the most common causes of pain in the elbow and forearm.

| Etiology | Clinical clues |
|---|---|
| Lateral epicondylitis (Tennis elbow) | Pain at the lateral aspect of the elbow and forearm |
| | Worsens with extension of the wrist |
| | Pain on local palpation |
| Medial epicondylitis (Golfer's elbow) | Pain at the medial aspect of the elbow and forearm |
| | Worsens with flexion of the wrist |
| | Pain on local palpation |
| Olecranon bursitis | Pain at the vertex of the elbow |
| | Local swelling and tenderness |
| Trauma | History of trauma |
| Arthritis | Inflammatory pain |
| | Painful limitation of active and passive movements |
| | Posteromedial swelling |
| Referred pain | Pathology of the shoulder, neck, heart |
| | Local examination normal |

**Table 9.1.**
Common causes of pain in the elbow and forearm.

## THE ENQUIRY

The first thing we should do is to check that the problem is actually limited to this area and does not affect any other joints or areas, suggesting polyarthropathy or generalized pain.

In cases of tendonitis, the patient usually pinpoints the maximum pain on the medial or lateral aspect of the elbow. This pain often involves the same aspect of the forearm, sometimes as far as the distal third. Pain in tendonitis is usually exacerbated by exercise using the arm and forearm, such as carrying heavy items in the hands, or work involving flexion or extension of the wrist and fingers. The patient's work and leisure activities should be considered, as repetitive use is one of the main causes of these lesions.

Olecranon bursitis is normally obvious on local examination. It may be caused by repeated trauma (e.g. office workers), crystals (e.g. urate in gout) or infection. In other cases it is part of polyarthritis (e.g. rheumatoid arthritis).

Isolated arthritis of the elbow is rare and usually due to trauma or infection, but this joint is often involved in all types of polyarthritis. Osteoarthritis of the elbow is also rare. The type of pain, the clinical context and the physical examination are the basis of the diagnosis.

The presence of dysesthetic characteristics – burning sensation, electric shock, or tingling – should raise the possibility of radiculopathy or peripheral nerve compression – ulnar nerve syndrome. Sometimes, the symptoms caused by compression of the median nerve in the carpal tunnel radiate proximally, to the forearm.

Entrapment of the anterior or posterior interosseous nerves is relatively rare. It causes deep, undefined, persistent pain relatively unrelated to exercise, located respectively on the anterior and posterior aspect of the forearm. Curiously, the usual dysesthetic characteristics are often absent, although there may be paresthesia in the area of the median or radial nerve. When confronted with deep pain in the forearm, we should consider this possibility and conduct our physical examination accordingly (see below).

The forearm may be affected by pain radiating proximally from carpal tunnel syndrome, de Quervain's tenosynovitis or wrist arthropathy, though the symptoms are predominantly in the wrist and hand.

## REGIONAL CLINICAL EXAMINATION

### Observation

The first thing to look for is swelling around the elbow, which is common in cases of bursitis. The posterior aspect of the forearm and elbow is often the site of psoriatic plaques and rheumatoid nodules, which present as hard, painless subcutaneous lumps adhering to the deep planes. As a rule, there will be other signs of rheumatoid arthritis. There may also be gouty tophi, nodular accumulations of urate crystals with typical crepitus on compression. The clinical context will usually suggest gout (Figure 9.7.).

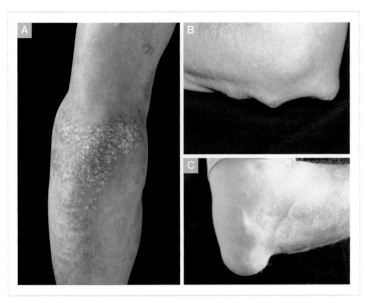

**Figure 9.7.** Common lesions in the posterior aspect of the forearm. **A.** Psoriatic plaque. **B.** Rheumatoid nodules. **C.** Gouty tophy (inspection could suggest olecranon bursitis but the lesion was firm on palpation).

Joint synovitis and effusion may cause visible swelling or other signs of inflammation, but they are better identified by palpation.

## Palpation

Palpation should focus on four main points:

1. Immediately below the lateral epicondyle, at the insertion of the common tendon insertion of the extensors of the wrist and fingers, the site of lateral epicondylitis (tennis elbow – Figure 9.8.)

2. Immediately below the medial epicondyle, in the common tendon of the flexors, the site of medial epicondylitis (golfer's elbow – Figure 9.9.)

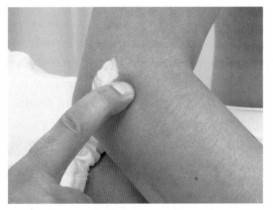

**Figure 9.8.** Palpating the insertion of the extensors of the wrist and hand, just below the lateral epicondyle.

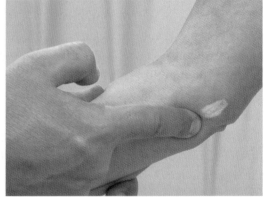

**Figure 9.9.** Palpating the insertion of the flexors of the wrist and hand, just below the medial epicondyle.

In either case, the exact point of maximum pain varies and we should palpate the whole tendinous part from the posterior to the anterior face, exerting adequate pressure.

3. The olecranon bursa and nodules should be palpated to ascertain their texture, tenderness, effusion or local warmth.

4. Palpation of the joint is not easy, as the anterior aspect is covered by muscle and there are no clear bone references on the posterior face. The examination for effusion or swelling is more effective if you insert the tips of your thumb and medial finger into the grooves on each side of the olecranon. The elbow is then fully flexed and extended (Figure 9.10.). Any effusion or voluminous synovial swelling will be expelled by the

olecranon in extension, as it occupies the olecranon fossa of the humerus. This is felt by the palpating fingers as a protrusion occurring with extension and disappearing with flexion of the elbow. There may be perceptible crepitus, if the cartilage is damaged.

Swelling and tenderness caused by synovitis may also be detected by palpating over the head of the radius. It is perceptible as a rounded bony structure on the posterolateral aspect of the elbow, below the epicondyle.

Slide the back of your hand along the posterior and anterior face of the elbow to look for a local increase in temperature.

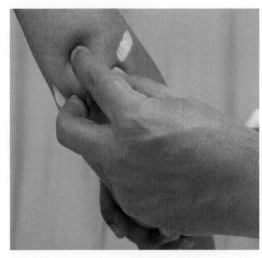

**Figure 9.10.** Examining for swelling or effusion of the elbow joints: during extension fingertips placed either side of the olecranon may sense the expulsion of excess joint fluid.

### Mobilization

The normal elbow is capable of about 145° flexion. Extension goes as far as 0°, and there may be hyperextension of up to −10° in many normal women. More pronounced hyperextension may be part of a *hypermobility syndrome* and may be associated with pain caused by subluxation and distension of the ligaments.

Active and passive movements of the elbow are not affected in lateral or medial epicondylitis. Joint diseases frequently result in early joint limitation, particularly extension, which the patient may fail to mention and may not have noticed. Occasionally, there is noticeable crepitus. Limitation of passive supination and pronation points to disease of the proximal or (especially) distal radioulnar joints.

Pain in epicondylitis can be exacerbated by resisted extension of the wrist. The same is the case with flexion in medial epicondylitis (Figure 9.11A. and B.).

If the local examination is normal, the possibility of referred pain from the wrist, shoulder or cervical spine should be considered. In these cases, pain is exacerbated by movements or palpation of these structures.

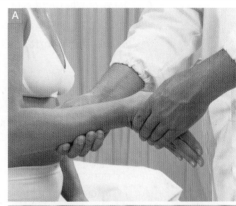
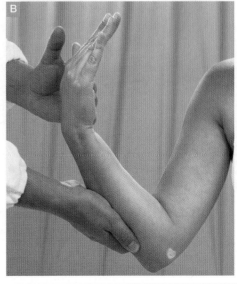

**Figure 9.11.** In lateral epicondylitis, the resisted extension of the wrist may induce pain in the lateral aspect of the elbow (**A.**). In medial epicondylitis, resisted flexion of the wrist will cause pain in the medial aspect of the elbow (**B.**).

### Neurological examination

In cases of suspected nerve root lesion, we must conduct a local neurological examination. The elbow receives sensitive innervation from C5 and C6 on the radial aspect and from T1 on the ulnar side. Both should be examined for sensitivity to pin-prick and touch (Figure 7.5.).

To assess muscle strength, test the following movements:

1. Resisted extension – triceps (radial nerve, C7)

2. Resisted flexion – biceps and brachialis (musculocutaneous nerve, C5/6)

3. Supination against resistance – biceps (musculocutaneous nerve, C5/6) and supinator (radial nerve, C6)

4. Pronation against resistance – pronator teres (median nerve, C6) and pronator quadratus (anterior interosseous branch, C8/T1)

Assess the reflexes of the biceps (musculocutaneous nerve, C5/6) and triceps (radial nerve, C7).

To test for ulnar nerve compression, suggested by paresthesia along the medial aspect of the forearm and hand, percuss over the ulnar tunnel (Tinel's test). If this reproduces the symptoms, ulnar nerve entrapment is likely, though false positives are common. Deep palpation or percussion of the exit points of the anterior and posterior interosseous nerves can trigger typical symptoms, suggesting nerve entrapment (pronator syndrome and radial tunnel syndrome, respectively).

---

### TYPICAL CASES
### 9.A. ELBOW PAIN (I)

Mário Alberto, a 38-year old computer operator, came to the surgery because of pain in his right elbow and forearm, which had started 3 months earlier and become progressively more intense and troublesome. The pain appeared only with movement and got worse when he picked up any objects, even light ones. When asked, he located the pain on the lateral aspect of the elbow and proximal forearm.

He denied any other joint problems, including his shoulder or cervical region. He had generally enjoyed good health until then.

The general rheumatologic examination revealed no pain or limited mobility. Active and passive movements of the elbow were easy and painless. There was no swelling, crepitus or local increase in temperature.

*Was our clinical examination complete?*

Compression of the common tendon of the extensors, below the epicondyle, caused intense pain, similar to the spontaneous pain and this was reproduced by resisted extension of the right wrist.

*What is your diagnosis?*

*Would you require any tests?*

*What treatment would you suggest for this patient?*

The observations above established a diagnosis of tennis elbow, with no need for additional tests. We suggested local application of a topical non-steroidal anti-inflammatory and a splint. We also recommended that he used supports for his forearms when working. Two weeks later, the patient had not improved. We gave him a local injection of 0.5 cc methylprednisolone (20 mg) around the tendon and recommended absolute rest of his right arm for 24 hours. We repeated our earlier suggestions in order to avoid any recurrences.

Please note: the symptoms of medial epicondylitis are much the same, but are located in the medial aspect of the elbow. Resisted flexion of the wrist exacerbates the pain. Work or leisure activities involving repeated forced flexion of the fingers (e.g. tennis, golf,… or an electoral campaign…) are predisposing factors. The treatment is very similar.

## LATERAL AND MEDIAL EPICONDYLITIS
### *MAIN POINTS*

These syndromes are very common in clinical practice, and are the most frequent causes of isolated pain in the elbow.

They appear most often in young and middle-aged adults, and are related to work or leisure activities requiring repeated flexion and extension of the wrists and fingers.

The pain has a mechanical rhythm and is located on the lateral aspect of the elbow and forearm in lateral epicondylitis and in the medial aspect in medial epicondylitis.

Active and passive mobility of the elbow is not affected.

Palpation of the corresponding muscle insertions causes intense pain.

Treatment is conservative: topical non-steroidal anti-inflammatories and splints or an elastic bandage in the initial stages and corticosteroid injections in persistent cases.[2]

Physical therapy may be important if the symptoms persist. Tendon decompression may be necessary in stubborn, incapacitating cases.

The patient should be advised about high-risk activities and ways of avoiding lesions such as suggesting palm-upwards method of lifting in lateral epicondylitis.

**NB:** Symptoms suggesting epicondylitis or medial epicondylitis may only be the most visible face of generalized pain or fibromyalgia. You must explore all the clinical symptoms.

[2]See Chapter 30 for guidance on this technique.

## 9.B. ELBOW PAIN (II)

José Silvares had been going to the same health centre for many years and suffered from tophaceous gouty arthritis that was resistant to treatment. He had had multiple episodes of migratory, recurring monoarthritis mainly affecting joints in his lower limbs. Over the years, he had developed progressive deformities in his hands and feet.

He went to emergency because of continuous, incapacitating pain in his left elbow. It had all started a few days earlier after a small local trauma which broke the skin and burst one of the nodules that he had had there for a long time. A whitish liquid came out, like liquid plaster. Inflammation had begun 2 days later…

On examination, we found that José had multiple nodules in his hands and elbows. The posterior aspect of his left elbow was very swollen and red, with fluctuation and pain on palpation. Attempts at mobilizing the joint caused intense local pain.

His family doctor decided to send him to hospital immediately because of suspected infection. The diagnosis of septic bursitis (*Staphylococcus aureus*) on top of tophaceous gout was confirmed. It required prolonged, systemic antibiotic treatment and local surgical debridement.

## OLECRANON BURSITIS
*MAIN POINTS*

This is reflected by swelling and pain over the olecranon. Palpation shows the presence of a fluctuant mass confirming presence of fluid.

Chronic bursitis caused by repeated trauma may develop without pain or signs of inflammation.

Intense pain, redness and local warmth suggest septic or microcrystalline bursitis. Olecranon bursitis may represent local involvement by polyarthritis (e.g. rheumatoid arthritis), in which case the signs of inflammation are moderate and the clinical context is suggestive.

Acute bursitis requires urgent treatment and should be referred to a specialized clinic. In other cases, the treatment depends on the underlying condition.

## TYPICAL CASES
## 9.C. ELBOW PAIN (III)

The patient, a 42-year old woman, was followed up by us and her family doctor for typical rheumatoid arthritis: chronic, symmetrical, additive polyarthritis, involving the small joints in the hands, wrists, elbows and ankles. The disease was well controlled on stable doses of immunosuppressant treatment, with no significant signs of inflammatory activity for the previous 2 years. We observed the patient every 6 months and her family doctor saw her in between.

At one of these visits, she complained to her doctor of growing inflammatory pain in her right elbow, which she attributed to hard farm work. Her doctor suspected reactivation of the arthritis in this location and asked us to examine her as soon as possible.

### What would you expect to find on examination?

We confirmed the diagnosis. Although the joint was normal on inspection, extension was reduced (with fixed flexion deformity of ~15°), and we were unable to increase the range with passive mobilization. Palpation of the peri-olecranon grooves during flexion/extension of the elbow showed swelling and slight pain. Palpation of the radial head was also painful. There was no obvious local warmth or redness over the elbow. Examination of the other joints revealed only moderate synovitis of a few MCP joints.

### What tests and/or treatment would you recommend?

There were no signs or symptoms suggesting general reactivation of the rheumatoid arthritis. We aspirated synovial fluid, which showed a high neutrophil count (8500/mm$^3$). Tests for crystals and bacteria were negative, thus excluding the possibility of septic arthritis. We decided to administer an intra-articular injection of a long-acting corticosteroid and asked the patient to keep her arm in a sling for 2 days. She was advised to do progressive exercises to recover the range of movement of the joint, following the period of rest.

We saw the patient two weeks later. The problem had resolved and she was back to normal.

## ARTHRITIS OF THE ELBOW
## MAIN POINTS

The elbow is often involved in polyarthritis, but is rarely the site of the initial episode. Monoarthritis of the elbow should suggest the possibility of septic or microcrystalline arthritis.

Osteoarthritis of the elbow is rare and suggests an underlying metabolic cause.

The following signs and symptoms point to arthritis:

- Inflammatory pain;
- Restricted motion and pain on active and passive mobilization;
- Swelling and pain on palpation of the joint;
- Redness and local warmth (inconsistent).

It is essential to conduct a systematic enquiry and general examination to look for symptoms and signs of a more general disease.

The treatment depends on the underlying condition.

The elbow is highly sensitive to the inflammatory process. Irreversible damage to the joint can appear in a very short time, with limitations of extension and supination/pronation. This justifies the early use of intra-articular treatment.

Monoarthritis of the elbow should be addressed in the same way as other monoarthritides (see Chapter 18).

## SPECIAL SITUATIONS

Although they are relatively rare, two syndromes involving peripheral nerve entrapment can cause pain of the forearm and may not be detected in our suggested clinical examination.

### *Radial tunnel syndrome*

This syndrome should be suspected when the patient describes deep, diffuse pain on the lateral and posterior aspect of the forearm. In some cases it may involve the lateral face of the elbow, suggesting lateral epicondylitis. The predominance of symptoms in the forearm, the presence of (inconsistent) paresthesia and muscle weakness favor this diagnosis.

The radial nerve may be compressed by abnormal fibrous bands behind the radial head. The posterior interosseous nerve, a branch of the radial nerve, is more often affected when it passes through the supinator muscle on the posterior aspect of the forearm, immediately below the elbow (about 30% of people have a fibrous arc here).

The following findings in the clinical exam are particularly suggestive:

- Reproduction of the pain by forced passive flexion or resisted extension of the middle finger

- Reproduction of the pain by extreme pronation of the forearm with flexion of the wrist

- Pain when pressure is applied with a tourniquet or sphygmomanometer cuff on the proximal forearm

- Weakness of extension of the little finger (posterior interosseous nerve)

- Pain on deep palpation of the posterolateral face of the forearm about 5 cm below the epicondyle (Figure 9.4.)

- Positive Tinel's sign at this site (posterior interosseous nerve) or over the radial head (radial nerve)[3]

The electromyogram/nerve conduction study is normal, except in very advanced phases of nerve lesion.

The treatment involves rest and mild exercise to begin with, then local anesthetic and corticosteroid injections if the symptoms persist. The use of splints or elastic bandages may bring relief, but the results vary. Surgical decompression may be necessary.

### *Pronator syndrome*

The anterior interosseous nerve, a branch of the median nerve, is compressed by the pronator teres muscle, 5–7 cm below the elbow.

---

[3]Tinel's (or Hoffman-Tinel's) sign consists of percussion on the site of potential compression of a nerve, preferably with a reflex hammer. The sign is positive if it causes tingling or pain in the innervation area.

This condition causes deep, undefined pain in the anterior aspect of the forearm. It tends to be continuous, although it is exacerbated by the use of the hands and wrists. Paresthesia in the area of the median nerve is suggestive but unfortunately inconsistent.

Evidence of muscular weakness or reproduction of the pain on resisted pronation suggests this diagnosis. In severe, chronic cases, there may be hypesthesia in the median nerve area. Deep compression of the site for about 30 seconds reproduces or exacerbates the symptoms (Figure 9.3.). The tourniquet test described above may also be positive.

The treatment is similar to that indicated for radial tunnel syndrome.

Please note: In either situation, do not forget to explore the possibility of generalized pain or fibromyalgia.

## DIAGNOSTIC TESTS

Generally speaking, diagnostic tests are unproductive and rarely necessary in regional pain of the elbow. Signs of joint disease or a history of trauma justify standard x-rays.

The presence of arthritis or acute bursitis of unexplained origin warrants fluid aspiration and analysis to look for crystals and bacteria and determine the total cell count and predominant cell type. Arthrocentesis of the elbow requires technical experience and laboratory facilities for synovial fluid studies. Suspected nerve entrapment may warrant electromyographic/nerve conduction studies.

## TREATMENT

The treatment of the most common causes of pain in the elbow and forearm has already been described and is within the scope of general practitioners. Avoid administering local injections if you are not trained or experienced in this technique.

### WHEN SHOULD THE PATIENT BE REFERRED TO A SPECIALIST?

Clinical signs and/or imaging results indicating mechanical or inflammatory joint disease of unknown cause.[4] In the case of arthritis, the referral should be urgent.

Clinically significant tendonitis or bursitis that is resistant to the measures used in general practice.

Persistent, debilitating pain of unknown origin.

[4]Osteoarthritis of the elbow is very rare. If there is no relevant history of trauma or previous arthritis, it almost always signifies metabolic joint disease, which requires appropriate etiologic investigation. See Chapter 16.

# REGIONAL SYNDROMES
## THE WRIST AND HAND

10.

J.A.P. da Silva, A.D. Woolf, *Rheumatology in Practice*, DOI 10.1007/978-1-84882-581-9_10,
© Springer-Verlag London Limited 2010

# 10. REGIONAL SYNDROMES THE WRIST AND HAND

The wrist and hand are extremely valuable sources of medical information. They are often the site of regional pathologies. Even more important, however, the hands provide significant and often diagnostic evidence in a variety of systemic rheumatic diseases.

For these reasons, it is essential to master the clinical examination of this area. *"The hand is the rheumatology patient's calling card."*

## FUNCTIONAL ANATOMY

The wrist and the hand make up a complex structural unit. While it is not essential for the clinician to master all the details of the anatomy, it is important to understand some basic aspects.

The wrist is made up of several joints (Figure 10.1.):

1. The radiocarpal joint, which is used for flexion/extension and adduction/abduction;

2. The distal radioulnar joint, which is involved in the supination and pronation of the forearm;

3. The intercarpal and carpo-metacarpal joints, which are involved in wrist movements, especially during forced flexion. The synovial cavity of the distal radioulnar joint is independent of the radiocarpal joint. All the others interconnect (except for the first carpometacarpal joint) .

The carpus consists of eight bones arranged in two transverse rows. These bones have many articulations between them and are stabilized by intrinsic ligaments.

The carpus articulates proximally, via the radiocarpal joint, with the distal extremity of the radius laterally, and medially with an articular disc (the triangular ligament of the carpus), which separates the radius from the distal extremity of the ulna.

The bones in the second row of the carpus articulate with the proximal extremities of the metacarpals. The joints that surround the base of the second and third metacarpals are practically immobile and, although they can be the site of pathology (e.g. in rheumatoid arthritis), they are not amenable to individual clinical examination. The fourth and fifth carpometacarpal joints provide the adjacent metacarpals with a slight capacity for flexion. In most people, the radiocarpal, inter-

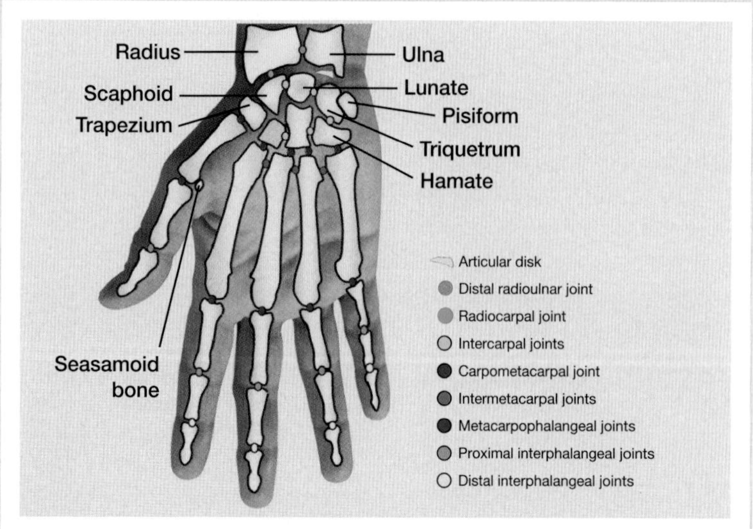

**Figure 10.1.** Bones and joints of the hand and wrist.

carpal and carpo-metacarpal joints (second to fifth) are connected by a common synovial cavity. This explains their combined involvement in arthritis when the wrist is affected.

The first carpometacarpal joint, which joins the trapezium to the base of the first metacarpal (first carpometacarpal joint or trapeziometacarpal joint), is particularly important. It has an independent capsule and synovial cavity. It is highly mobile (flexion/extension and adduction/abduction) and plays an extremely important role in the global function of the human hand, by allowing opposition of the thumb and fingers. It is often the site of osteoarthritis and deserves special attention during clinical examination of the hand.

The five metacarpophalangeal (MCP) joints are independent and are responsible essentially for flexion (about 90°) and extension (up to −10°), with slight adduction and abduction. The mobility of the first metacarpophalangeal joint (MCP1, of the thumb), with two sesamoid bones on the palmar face, is much more limited, not exceeding 30° flexion. The morphology of the proximal interphalangeal joints (PIPs) is similar to that of the metacarpophalangeals, permitting only flexion (90–100°) with 0° extension. The range of extension of the thumb interphalangeal joint (IFP1) is greater (45–60°), while flexion is more limited (80–90°).

There are four distal interphalangeal joints (DIPs, from the index to the little finger), with flexion of up to 90° and extension from 0 to −10°.

In normal circumstances, the segments of each finger are aligned along the same axis, in a slightly radial arrangement in relation to the axis of the wrist when at rest. In complete, forced flexion, the fingertips touch each other and press firmly into the palm.

Mobilization of the wrists and fingers depends on a large number of muscles joining the humerus and bones of the forearm to the fingers. Functionally, we can divide them into three groups. The flexors of the fingers are located along the palm face of the wrist and hand and the extensors along the dorsal face. The tendons of the long abductor and short extensor of the thumb run along the lateral aspect of the wrist.

These muscles insert in the phalanges by means of long tendons surrounded by synovial sheaths. As these structures often participate in the inflammatory processes, it is important to pay them particular attention. On the palm face, the tendon of the long flexor of the thumb on the radial side is covered by an independent sheath that extends from the distal forearm to the first interphalangeal joint. In most people, the other flexors are covered by a common tendon sheath that extends as far as the distal interphalangeal joint of the little finger, ending in the palm over the other tendons. The flexors of the index, middle and ring finger have independent synovial sheaths extending from the palm to the distal interphalangeal joint (Figure 10.2.). The tendon sheaths do not communicate with the cavity of the underlying joints.

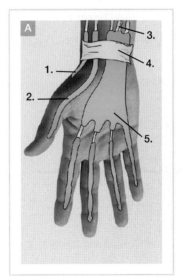 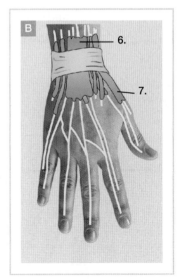

**Figure 10.2.** Tendon sheaths of the hand and wrist flexors.
**A.** Flexor tendons. 1. Flexor carpi radialis. 2. Flexor pollicis longus. 3. Flexor digitorum superficialis and profundus. 4. Flexor retinaculum. 5. Common sheath of flexor muscles. **B.** Tendon sheaths of the hand and wrist extensors. Common variant. 6. Extensor digitorum and extensor indicis. 7. Tendon sheath of abductor pollicis longus and extensor pollicis brevis muscles.

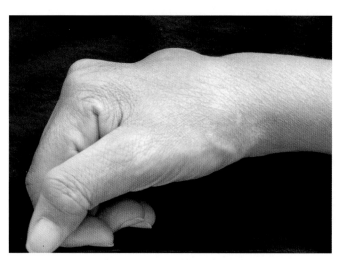

**Figure 10.3.** Tenosynovitis of the extensor tendons at the wrist may present as an hour-glass shaped swelling, due to the effect of the extensor retinaculum of the wrist.

The sheaths of the extensors are more numerous (usually six) and variable (Figure 10.2A.). It is worth remembering the one that envelops the tendons of the long abductor and short extensor of the thumb. It runs along the lateral aspect of the wrist, constituting the anterior border of the anatomical snuffbox. Inflammation of this synovial sheath is called De Quervain's tenosynovitis. The extensor retinaculum of the carpus forms a fibrous band over these synovial sheaths and cinches them, so that tenosynovitis of the extensors is frequently reflected by an hour-glass shaped swelling (Figure 10.3.).

Arranged between the metacarpals are the intrinsic muscles of the hand (the interosseous and lumbrical muscles), which reinforce the flexion of the metacarpophalangeal joints. Atrophy of these muscles is common in cases of chronic arthritis and neuropathic lesions, and is clinically detectable.

The hand is innervated by the radial, median and ulnar nerves. The radial nerve innervates the extensor muscles of the wrist and fingers and is responsible for the sensitivity in the lateral half of the dorsal aspect of the hand and most of the dorsal face of the thumb, and index and middle fingers (Figure 10.4.). The median and ulnar nerves innervate the flexor muscles of the wrist and fingers. The median nerve provides sensations for the palmar aspect of the thumb to the middle finger and the external half of the ring finger, together with the corresponding area of the palm. The area of sensation provided by the ulnar nerve includes the little finger, the medial half of the ring finger and the corresponding ulnar part of the hand, on the palmar and dorsal faces. It should be remembered, however, that there is considerable variation in these cutaneous distributions.

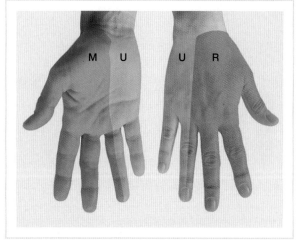

**Figure 10.4.** Sensory inervation of the hand. **M.** Median nerve. **U.** Ulnar nerve. **R.** Radial nerve.

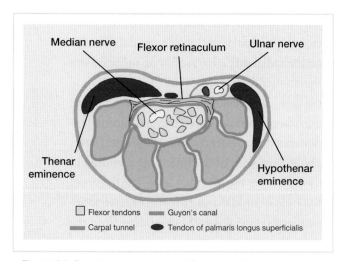

**Figure 10.5.** Carpal tunnel and ulnar tunnel (Guyon's canal).

The median nerve reaches the hand through the carpal tunnel, a non-distensible osteotendinous structure formed posteriorly by the bones and joints of the wrist and their capsule, in a concave form, and limited anteriorly by the flexor retinaculum. This channel houses all the flexor tendons and their sheaths, together with the median nerve, arteries and veins (Figure 10.5.). Understandably, inflammation in the synovium of the joints or tendon sheaths, fibrous alterations, bony deformities or fluid retention in this area can result in compression and subsequent dysfunction of the median nerve. This causes carpal tunnel syndrome. The ulnar nerve runs anteriorly to the retinaculum, and externally to the pisiform in its own canal (Guyon's canal) where it can also be compressed.

### Radiological anatomy

In x-rays of the wrists and hands (Figure 10.6.) examine all the joints from the wrist to the DIPs, running along each articular row. Note the size and regularity of the articular spaces and the presence of periarticular osteopenia or subchondral sclerosis. Examine any swelling or calcification of the soft tissue. If in doubt, compare with the other side.

In normal circumstances, the borders of the bones inside and on the periphery of the joints are regular, with a well-defined cortex. Note any calcification in the triangular ligament of the carpus and at the edge of the joints. Look for erosions (particularly of the styloid process of the ulna, MCPs and PIPs) and osteophytes (mainly in the first CMC, PIPs and DIPs). An oblique angle (Figure 10.7.) sometimes reveals erosions or osteophytes that are not detectable in an anteroposterior view.

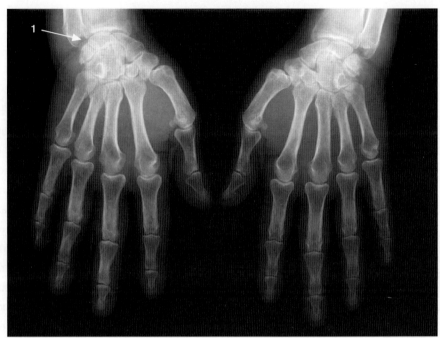

**Figure 10.6.** Normal radiography of the wrists and hand – antero-posterior view. **1.** Area of projection of the triangular ligament of the carpus.

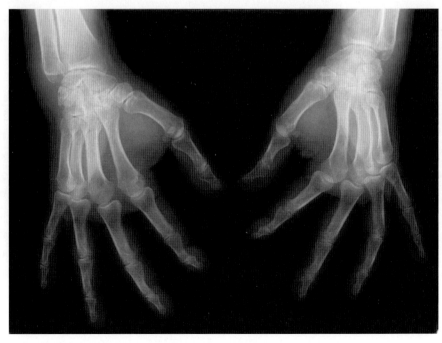

**Figure 10.7.** Normal radiography of the hand and wrist – oblique view.

## COMMON CAUSES OF PAIN IN THE WRIST AND HAND

The hand and wrist are common sites of pain, either limited to the region or as part of generalized rheumatic diseases (Table 10.1.).

Overall, carpal tunnel syndrome is the most common condition. De Quervain's tenosynovitis and osteoarthritis of the trapezo-metacarpal joint are also often found.

Both osteoarthritis and the different types of inflammatory arthritis frequently involve the hands, and the distribution of affected hand joints may be highly informative for reaching a correct diagnosis.

| Structure | Lesion | Clinical clues |
|---|---|---|
| Peripheral nerves | Carpal tunnel syndrome | Paresthesia of the hand confined to the area of the median nerve<br>Predominantly at night and in the morning<br>Tinel's and Phalen's signs |
|  | Ulnar nerve syndrome | Paresthesia of the ulnar aspect of the forearm and hand.<br>Tinel's sign of the ulnar tunnel in the elbow |
| Tendon sheaths and fascia | De Quervain's tenosynovitis | Pain in the lateral aspect of the wrist and thumb<br>Mechanical rhythm<br>Local pain on palpation<br>Finkelstein's maneuver |
|  | Tenosynovitis of the flexor tendons | Inflammatory or mechanical pain<br>Limited active flexion of the fingers<br>"Snapping" movement of the finger (trigger finger) |
|  | Dupuytren's contracture | Fibrosis and contraction of the palmar fascia in the palmar aspect of the 3rd, 4th or 5th finger |
| Joints | Osteoarthritis of the 1st carpometacarpal joint | Mechanical pain at the base of the thumb and radial aspect of the wrist |
|  | Nodal osteoarthritis | Mixed rhythm pain<br>Proximal and distal interphalangeal joints<br>Firm articular nodes |
|  | Arthritis | Inflammatory pain<br>Rubbery articular swelling |
| Referred | Cervical spine | Normal local examination<br>Associated manifestations |

**Table 10.1.** Most common causes of pain in the wrist and hand.

## THE ENQUIRY

A clinical enquiry with a patient whose complaints predominate in the wrists and hands will naturally aim to establish the clinical characteristics of each of the conditions mentioned above, with special attention to the aspects that distinguish them from each other.

It is important to take into account the relative prevalence of these different affections in general practice. Carpal tunnel syndrome, De Quervain's tenosynovitis, osteoarthritis of the 1st CMC and nodal osteoarthritis are much more common than inflammatory forms of arthritis. A thorough examination of the hands is mandatory in all patients, as it gives us a wealth of precise information that will help to narrow the differential diagnosis.

In this chapter we review the most important questions, assuming that the complaints are limited to the hands. However, a comprehensive, systemic enquiry is particularly important here, given that manifestations in the hands are frequently a sign of more disseminated diseases.

### *Where exactly does it hurt?*

In many cases, the patient indicates a reasonably precise area of pain, thus helping the doctor. As a rule, the pain due to osteoarthritis of the 1st CMC joint is limited to the base of the thumb and radial aspect of the wrist. The pain in De Quervain's tenosynovitis involves the same area, but may extend proximally to the forearm. In cases of mono- or oligoarthritis, the patient is usually able to identify the painful joints, which are often visibly swollen.

Patients sometimes say that the pain affects the "joints" of their hands. If several joints hurt, they will often say that they all hurt. We should not accept this at face value. It is hardly ever true! Ask the patient to place his hands on the desk and show you exactly which joints (or groups of joints) have been painful.

The exact distribution of the affected joints in the hand is invaluable in diagnosing a variety of joint diseases.

If the patient points to the palmar aspect of his hand or fingers, consider the possibility of tenosynovitis of the flexors, carpal tunnel syndrome or Dupuytren's contracture (the last of these is usually obvious on inspection and is usually painless). Many patients with carpal tunnel syndrome say that the pain or paresthesia affects the whole surface of the palm and not just the territory of the median nerve. Conversely, in ulnar nerve syndrome, the patient usually points to the ulnar border of the hand.

Patients with arthritis or osteoarthritis generally locate the pain on the dorsal face of the hand and fingers. Some patients describe typical trigger finger: one or more fingers hurt on flexion. If they are forcibly flexed, they "get stuck," and then spring free with a "snatching" or "triggering" movement when extended. Mobility is reasonable free, if forced flexion is avoided. This curious finding is diagnostic of stenosing tenosynovitis of the flexor tendons.

The patient very often has difficulty in pinpointing an exact location. The enquiry leaves an idea of imprecise, diffuse pain affecting most of the hand. This is an important clue to neurogenic or referred pain, which is extremely common in clinical practice. It is our cue to start asking more precise questions…

### Is there any paresthesia?

What we need to find out is whether the pain is paresthetic in nature: "*Do you feel pins and needles in your hand? Does it go numb?*" If the answer is yes or even ambiguous, this reinforces the suspicion of neurogenic pain caused by cervical root compression or, more often, a peripheral nerve lesion. The rhythm of the pain is a strong characteristic of this syndrome.

### Rhythm of the pain

"*Does your pain have a special timing? Is it worse in the morning, later in the day, at night, only with movement?…*"

In carpal tunnel syndrome the answer is usually clear cut. The discomfort occurs most at night and early in the morning and gets better with the use of the hands. Note that this is an inflammatory rhythm! It might suggest arthritis, but then pain would be focused in the joints and is not dysesthetic.

The pain in osteoarthritis of the 1st CMC joint and De Quervain's tenosynovitis is usually related to manual work and disappears at rest.

Arthritis of the hand is usually accompanied by typical inflammatory pain. Patients may be more precise about morning stiffness affecting the hands than any other area.

### How did the problem begin?

The onset of arthritis and tenosynovitis is usually much faster (from hours to weeks) than osteoarthritis or nerve entrapment (from weeks to months).

### Have there been any signs of inflammation?

> Patients often describe swelling of the hands and this can be misleading. Ask about its location and daily rhythm.

In most cases of joint disease, the swelling is not diffuse but localized around one or more joints. If there is synovitis of the interphalangeal joints, the swelling is usually fusiform as the inflamed synovium is limited by the capsule. Patients with swelling of the metacarpophalangeal joints usually point to the knuckles.

Many patients will mention diffuse edema all over the hand or on all the fingers, however. If you cannot see the edema, this symptom is difficult to interpret. In many cases, the patient will find that this edema fluctuates with the menstrual cycle, which suggests premenstrual fluid retention. The sensation of morning swelling of the hands is also common in patients with carpal tunnel syndrome, even without any clinical evidence.

Patients with fibromyalgia often mention diffuse and generally "accentuated" swelling in their hands. A variety of factors may contribute to the prevalence of this symptom in these patients, although it is not particularly important. It may be misleading, however, leading the physician to consider a variety of possibilities if the highly variable symptoms of fibromyalgia are not taken into account.

A description of redness, if consistent, deserves attention, as it is not found in many situations: infection, microcrystalline arthritis and psoriatic arthritis. It is rare in rheumatoid arthritis and very rare in osteoarthritis.

Ask the patient whether the color of his hands changes when they are exposed to cold. If it does, especially in three phases (pale → cynanotic → red), this indicates Raynaud's phenomenon, which is always significant. The way to approach this symptom is described in Chapter 25. Note that this phenomenon is often accompanied by paresthesia and pain, which may be the only cause for complaint.

Occasionally a patient says that a whole finger is red, swollen and painful. This can usually be verified by examination. If the examination confirms the presence of "dactylitis," this lends more weight to the possibility of infection, sarcoidosis or psoriatic arthritis.

### The general enquiry

It is always important to find out whether there is pain in any other locations. This is particularly important when the enquiry suggests arthropathy of the wrist or hand joints. For example, associated inflammatory back pain would suggest the possibility of seronegative spondylarthropathy. The symmetrical involvement of proximal metacarpophalangeal and interphalangeal joints indicates rheumatoid arthritis and other connective tissue diseases. Cervical pain or pain in the forearm may indicate referred pain.

The patient's general state of health and associated diseases are also important. A recent myocardial infarction may be responsible for Dressler's syndrome. Hypothyroidism can cause carpal tunnel syndrome. Raynaud's phenomenon is a clue to disease of the connective tissue, vasculitis or nerve compression upstream. Chronic obstructive pulmonary disease and lung cancer may account for clubbed fingers. Hepatitis or rubella infection may be the cause of reactive polyarthritis. Diabetes mellitus can have quite curious effects on the hands…

The presence of other manifestations, outside the hands, may lead you to consider a different "main syndrome."

## REGIONAL EXAMINATION

The clinical examination of the wrist and hand is extraordinarily informative about a wide variety of rheumatic diseases. Because it is easy to do, it should always be complete and thorough in all patients with local symptoms, regardless of the diagnosis you suspect after the initial enquiry. You will often be surprised…

### Observation

The palmar and dorsal aspects of the hand and wrist should be inspected carefully.

### Examine the skin

You may find signs here of such different diseases as psoriasis, systemic lupus erythematosus, scleroderma, dermatomyositis and vasculitis, among many others (Figure 10.8.). In cases of lupus, you occasionally find erythematous lesions on the dorsal aspect of the fingers, between the joints (Figure 10.8A.).

Reddish papules on the dorsal aspect of the finger joints (Gottron's papules) (Figure 10.8B.) are quite typical of dermatomyositis. They are sometimes associated with scaly erythematous lesions around the nails and ragged cuticles.

Stretched, wax-like skin on the fingers is a strong indication of scleroderma, which is typical of progressive systemic sclerosis (Figure 10.8C.). The skin is hard and inflexible on palpation.

In patients with connective tissue diseases (especially lupus and systemic sclerosis) the pads of the fingers may be affected by calcinosis, ulceration and focal necrosis, making their surface irregular and atrophic (Figure 10.8D.). Dark point-like lesions at the edge of the nails may correspond to micro-infarctions indicating small vessel vasculitis, which is relatively common in these patients.

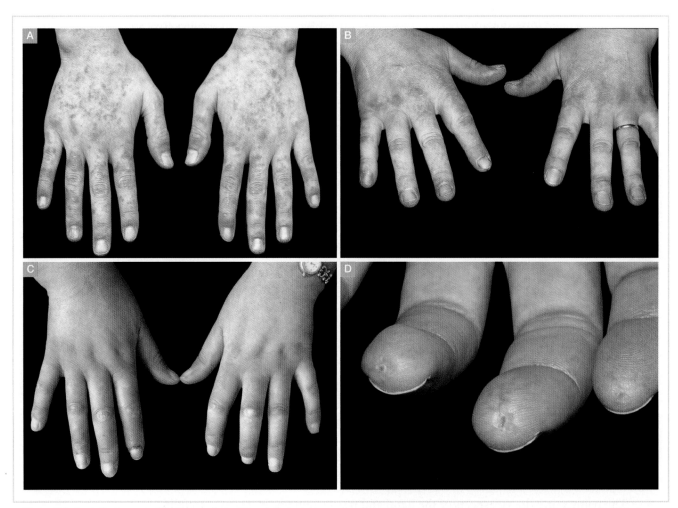

**Figure 10.8.** Hand skin changes in different rheumatic conditions. **A.** Systemic lupus erythematosus. **B.** Dermatomyositis. **C.** Systemic sclerosis. **D.** Subcutaneous infarcts.

Be sure to look at the nails. Mycotic infections are common, but the presence of coarse nail dystrophy or pitting (Figure 10.9.) may be the only manifestation of psoriasis.[1]

Long-lasting corticosteroid therapy can cause skin atrophy, making it friable and prone to bruising. This is often prominent on the dorsal aspect of the hands.

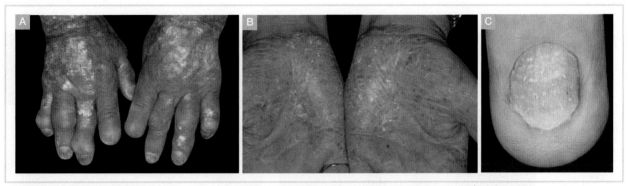

**Figure 10.9.** Psoriasis may present with typical patches in the hands (**A.**) or palmar keratosis (**B.**) Nail dystrophy and pitting (**C.**) are more common when the distal interphalangeal joints are involved.

## Look for signs of muscle atrophy

When carpal tunnel syndrome is chronic and severe it leads to atrophy of the muscles in the thenar eminence. Chronic lesions of the ulnar nerve lead to atrophy of the hypothenar eminence. Chronic arthritis of the wrist and hands often results in generalized atrophy of the intrinsic muscles of the hands, forming depressions between the tendons of the extensors (Figure 10.10.).

## Swelling

Visible swelling of the back of the wrist is usually due to tenosynovitis of the extensors. Bound by the posterior ligament of the carpus, these swollen structures assume the shape of an hourglass (Figure 10.3.).

Synovitis of the metacarpophalangeal joints may cause the recesses between the nodes of the fingers to fill up (Figure 10.10.). However, swelling of these joints should always be confirmed by palpation. The same is the case for the fusiform swelling around proximal interphalangeal

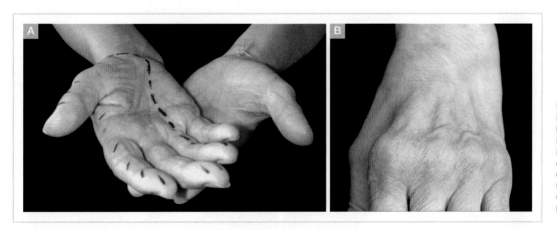

**Figure 10.10.** Muscle wasting in the hands. **A.** Thenar eminence wasting is typical of advanced carpal tunnel syndrome. **B.** Diffuse muscle wasting in chronic inflammatory polyarthritis.

[1]Pitting consists in the presence of pointlike depressions in the ungual bed. Some authors consider that a total of 50 or more of these depressions in the ten nails of the hands confirms a diagnosis of psoriasis, even if there are no skin lesions.

joints – they are strongly suggestive of arthritis but it is palpation that will confirm the suspicion (Figure 10.11.).

Synovial cysts in the wrist (extensions of the synovium of the wrist due to partial rupture of the capsule), also known as ganglia, are common and usually painless. They present as a soft, localized swelling (Figure 10.12.).

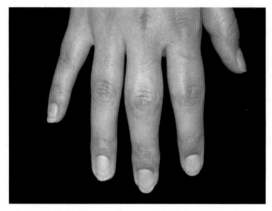

**Figure 10.11.** Fusiform swelling around the 2nd and 3rd proximal interphalangeal joints

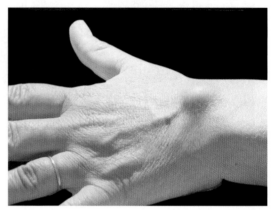

**Figure 10.12.** Synovial cyst of the wrist. The swelling is soft on palpation.

### Nodes

Nodes are relatively frequent in the hands. Rheumatoid nodules are usually found over the extension surface of the joints, and other areas subjected to friction. They are firm and painless, with no signs of inflammation, and adhere to the deep fascial planes (Figure 10.13A.).

Gouty tophi may form coarse swellings around the joints, if hyperuricaemia is not properly controlled. The superficial accumulation of urate crystals can give a suggestive whitish color (Figure 10.14B.). Firm palpation may elicit a typical crepitus.

Localized bony swellings on or near the dorsal aspect of the proximal (Bouchard's nodes) or distal (Heberden's nodes – Figure 10.14.) interphalangeal joints are highly suggestive of nodal osteoarthritis. This feature is quite different from the diffuse, spindle-shaped swelling observed in synovitis (Figure 10.11.).

**Figure 10.13.**
Nodules of the hands.
**A.** Rheumatoid nodules – usually small with a regular surface. **B.** Irregular nodules with white deposits – gouty tophy.

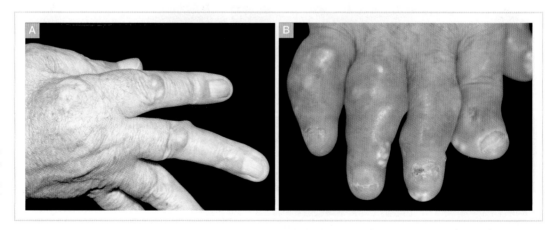

## *Malalignment*

Malalignment between the axis of adjacent bone segments is a sign of advanced joint disease. It is very common in the late stages of both rheumatoid arthritis and nodal osteoarthritis. The typical deformities of these diseases are, however, quite different.

In rheumatoid arthritis, malalignment occurs mainly along the anteroposterior plane, as shown in Figure 10.15A. The most frequent deformities are in flexion or extension of the MCP, PIP or DIP joints. Ulnar deviation of the fingers is common, but the deviation takes place at the MCP joint. In advanced nodal osteoarthritis, the hand may look disorganized and angular. There may be radial or ulnar deviation of one phalange over the other, which is accentuated by the nodules (Figure 10.15B.). An angular deformation at the base of the thumb suggests advanced osteoarthritis of the 1st CMC joint (Figure 10.16.).

The wrist is often deformed in arthritis. Synovial swelling is only visible when the disease is very active. In more advanced stages, however, the structural disorganization of the radiocarpal joint often leads to palmar subluxation of the carpus, making it look like the "back of a fork" (caput ulnae – Figure 10.17.).

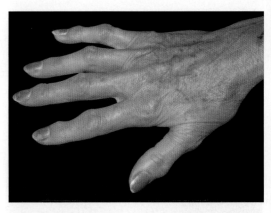

**Figure 10.14.** Nodal osteoarthritis of the hands. Discrete bony nodules around PIP (Bouchard nodes) and DIP joints (Heberden nodes).

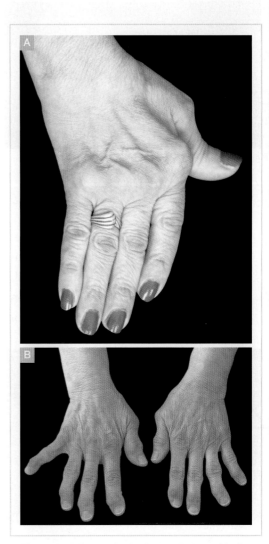

**Figure 10.15.** Finger deformity. **A.** Ulnar deviation of the fingers in rheumatoid arthritis. **B.** Nodular deformity of the finger, with deviations of one phalanx over the other in nodal osteoarthritis.

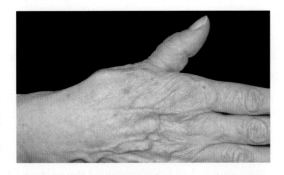

**Figure 10.16.** Osteoarthritis of the first CMC joint is frequently associated with squaring at the base of the thumb.

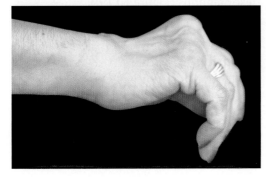

**Figure 10.17.** Palmar subluxation of the wrist in a patient with advanced rheumatoid arthritis.

### Mobilization

First ask the patient to completely flex and extend his wrists. Then ask him to close his hand tight and slowly stretch his fingers as far as possible. If the active movement is limited, check whether passive mobilization is more complete.

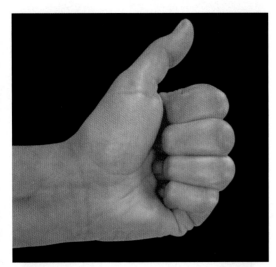

**Figure 10.18.** Active flexion of the fingers: fingertips should press firmly on the palmar aspect of the hand.

The wrist should flex about 80° and extend to approximately 70°. With the hand closed, the tips of the fingers should press hard into the palm of the hand (Figure 10.18.). Extension of the fingers should be smooth, with no "snatching," and reach 0° extension in all the joints (45–60°, in the thumb interphalangeal).

If mobility is at all limited, repeat the movements passively. There are two possibilities: (a) passive range of movement is no greater than active or (b) passive mobility is clearly wider than active.

What do these differences mean?

If the patient can carry out full active movements, we will be reassured that there is no major damage. Limitations in active as well as in passive movement indicate that the problem is structural, i.e. something is stopping the joints from moving completely: an articular lesion or fibrosis of the capsule. Passive mobility obviously does not require the patient's tendons, muscles, peripheral nerves or CNS. Lesions of these structures do not affect passive mobility, even if active movements are limited. Therefore, if passive mobility is more ample than active mobility, these structures should be assessed further.

The most common cause for this is tenosynovitis of the flexor tendons. In this very common condition, one or more fingers do not touch the palm of the hand, though we can make them do it easily. The presence of trigger movements of the finger suggests stenosing tenosynovitis.

In Dupuytren's contracture, the patient is unable to extend completely his ring finger (more rarely, the middle or little finger), due to hard thickening of the palmar fascia that holds the flexor tendons (Figure 10.19.).

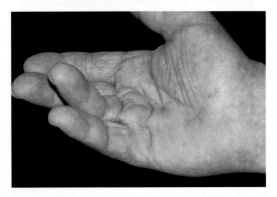

**Figure 10.19.** Dupuytren's contracture. Notice the thickening and contraction of the palmar fascia, proximal to the fourth finger. Active and passive extension of the fourth finger was limited.

### Palpation

**a) Palpate any visible nodules**

Feel their consistency, texture and location.

Rheumatoid nodes can affect the hands. They are firm, rubbery and painless and adhere to the deep fascial planes (Figure 10.13A.). The surface of gouty tophi (Figure 10.13B.) is irregular and sometimes whitish. They may deform slightly on pressure, with crepitus. Bouchard's and Heberden's nodes (on the proximal and distal interphalangeal joints, respectively, Figure 10.14.) are typical of nodal osteoarthritis of the hands. They have a bony consistency, (they comprise osteophytes) and are usually painless. Synovial cysts (ganglia), usually in the vicinity of the wrist, are soft and malleable.

Almost all of us have two small palpable nodes, one on either side of the palmar face of first metacarpophalangeal joint. What could they be?[2]

### b) Palpate the joints of the wrist

Use the back of your hand to check for local increase in temperature. Hold the patient's hand between yours and use your thumbs to explore the articular space between the radius and the carpus. Also palpate the processes of the radius and ulna on the lateral and medial face of the wrist, respectively (Figure 10.20.). If you find swelling on the back of the wrist, try to distinguish between tenosynovitis of the extensors and arthritis of the wrist, mobilizing the patient's fingers while palpating (in tenosynovitis, the swelling may move slightly with the mobilized tendon).

It is important to feel the bony contours under your fingers. The loss of typical definition indicates that there is something additional between your fingers and the bone – probably an

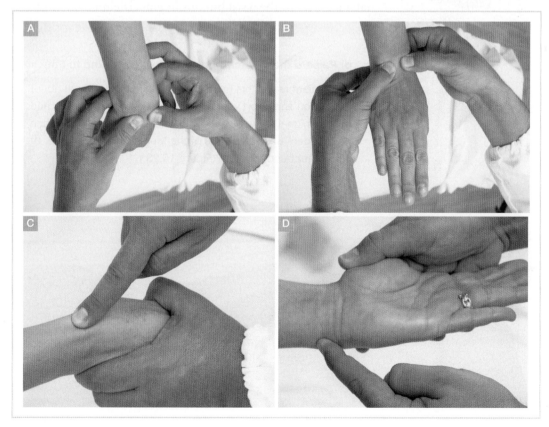

**Figure 10.20.**
Palpation of the wrist. **A**. and **B**. The index fingers of the examiner palpate the palmar aspect of the wrist. The thumbs explore the joint line for tenderness, swelling or crepitus, while the wrist is passively flexed and extended. Palpate also the radial **C**. and ulnar **D**. processes.

[2]Sesamoid bones.

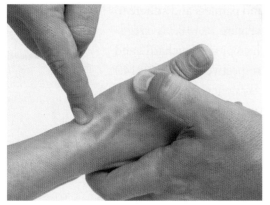

**Figure 10.21.** Palpation of the tendon sheath of the abductor pollicis longus and extensor pollicis brevis – De Quervain's tenosynovitis. Palpation during resisted abduction increases pain.

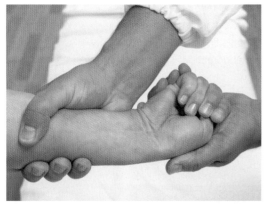

**Figure 10.22.** Finkelstein's maneuver. Positive in De Quervain's tenosynovitis.

inflamed synovium. The articular space of the radiocarpal joint is not easy to define as the edges of the articular surfaces are rounded and do not provide a clear, palpable reference. Experience acquired by repeating this assessment on all patients markedly increases the ability to detect small degrees of swelling. Pain on palpation along the articular space also suggests local inflammation.

### c) Explore the possibility of de Quervain's tenosynovitis

The tendons affected in this condition form the anterior (palmar) border of the so-called anatomical snuffbox. If there is inflammation, palpation is painful. This pain may be exacerbated if the thumb is placed in resisted abduction (Figure 10.21.).

**Finkelstein's maneuver** is very sensitive and specific to this condition. Ask the patient to hold his thumb between the clenched fingers of his hand. Hold the patient's hand and firmly induce passive adduction (Figure 10.22.). Pain in the outer edge of the wrist is typical of de Quervain's tenosynovitis. Osteoarthritis of the 1st CMC joint can also cause pain on the lateral aspect of the wrist but not in Finkelstein's maneuver.

### d) Palpate the metacarpophalangeal joints (2nd to 5th)

The patient leaves his hand at rest. Place the MCPs at about 45° flexion and insert your index finger behind these joints and pull them gently towards you. Now palpate the articular space and borders using the pads of the thumb and index finger of your other hand together (Figure 10.23.).

**Figure 10.23.**
Palpation of metacarpo-phalangeal joints. The index finger of the examiner palpates the palmar aspect of the MCP while the sharpness of the joint line is explored with the tips of the index and thumb of the other hand.

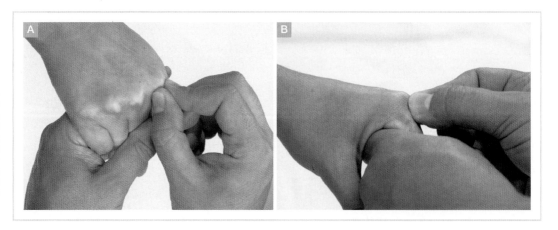

These spaces are clearly perceptible in normal hands. With experience, it is possible to identify even slight swelling of the synovium. The bony relief becomes ill-defined (increasing with higher degrees of inflammation). Note that the base of the first phalanx runs under the head of the metacarpal in flexion. The joint space is located 1.5–2 cm below the dorsal face of the metacarpal (Figure 10.23B.). An index finger placed under/behind the MCPs is very useful, as it makes the base of the phalanx more perceptible and pushes forward any articular effusion that there may be.

Repeat the operation for each joint of the four fingers (the MCP of the thumb is palpated differently). These joints are very often affected in rheumatoid arthritis, lupus, psoriatic arthritis, etc.

It is very rare to find bony (hard) swelling of the MCPs. This is typical of osteophytes and therefore osteoarthritis – which is unusual in this location.

### e) Palpate the first MCP and the proximal interphalangeals

Place the pulps of your index finger and thumb on each side of the joint. They will act as sensors only, without moving. Place the thumb and index finger of your other hand on the dorsal and palmar faces of the joint, exerting and relieving pressure repeatedly (Figure 10.24.).

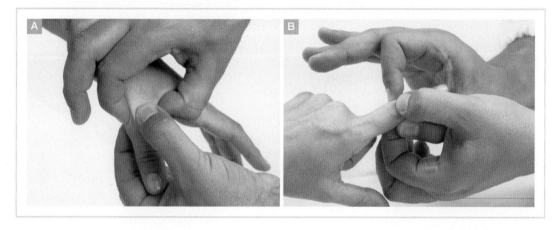

**Figure 10.24.**
Palpation of the first metacarpo-phalangeal and proximal interphalangeal joints: look for tenderness and fluctuance.

The synovium of these joints is strictly delimited by the capsule. If there is any swelling or articular effusion, the synovium acts like a small sac of water. When we palpate in an antero-posterior direction, there is transverse expansion that the sensor finger and thumb identify as fluctuation. The technique must be accurate to avoid mistakes.[3] Fluctuation suggests synovitis, i.e. arthritis. This interpretation is reinforced if palpation causes pain (there can be swelling without pain and pain without swelling).

These joints are often the site of inflammation in rheumatoid arthritis, psoriatic arthritis, lupus, etc.

[3]We all have fluctuation *between* the finger joints because the local soft tissue is enveloped by a fascia. Try to find fluctuation in someone else's phalanges. To avoid mistaking this sign for synovitis when assessing the interphalangeal joints, your fingers must only touch the patient's joint: use the tips of your fingers and not the whole of your distal phalange.

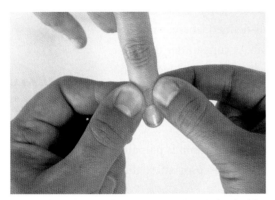

**Figure 10.25.** Palpation of the distal interphalangeal joints: look for tenderness, fluctuance and bony nodules.

### f) Palpate the distal interphalangeal joints

The method is similar to that used for the proximal interphalangeals (Figure 10.25.). Swelling is much rarer and fluctuation is not always perceptible because of the small volume of the joint. The most common alteration here is Heberden's nodes (bony nodules that are typical of nodal osteoarthritis of the hands).

Inflammation of the DIPs is very suggestive of psoriatic arthritis, particularly when it is found in combination with nail pitting. Rheumatoid arthritis and lupus usually spare these joints.

### g) Palpation of flexor tendons and their synovial sheaths

Place your thumb gently on the path of the flexor tendon of the index finger, on the palmar face of the hand, immediately above the metacarpophalangeal. Use it as a sensor while you passively flex and extend the patient's finger, holding it by the distal phalange (Figure 10.26.). Repeat the maneuver with the other fingers.

**Figure 10.26.**
Palpation of flexor tendon sheaths. The thumb feels for crepitus, swelling or nodules adherent to the tendon, while the finger is passively mobilized.

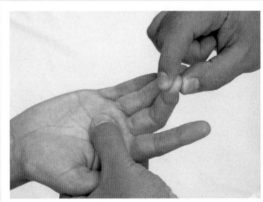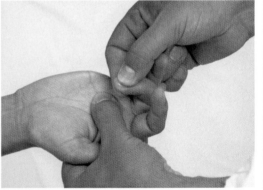

Assessment of the flexor tendons is especially important if there is limitation of active flexion of the fingers but not of passive mobilization. In tenosynovitis you will feel thickened tissue gliding under the palpating fingers, sometimes with crepitus and pain. This is an inflamed synovial sheath, which is dragged by the tendon to which it adheres. In the case of trigger finger, look for a nodule adhering to and moving with the tendon, which is almost always perceptible.[4]

---

[4]The nodule that we feel is a thickening of the tendon itself, located near the opening of the tendon sheath. When the patient flexes his fingers hard, the nodule is forced into the sheath. When extending them again, he has to make an effort for the nodule to overcome the resistance of the entrance to the sheath. This forced exit results in a trigger movement, though once it is out it moves freely.

**NOTE**

The distribution of the affected joints in the wrist and hand and the types of changes are very important for differential diagnosis of the most common joint diseases in this area (Figure 10.27.).

The accompanying alterations – manifestations on the skin or nails, nodules, malalignment, etc. – also help the diagnosis.

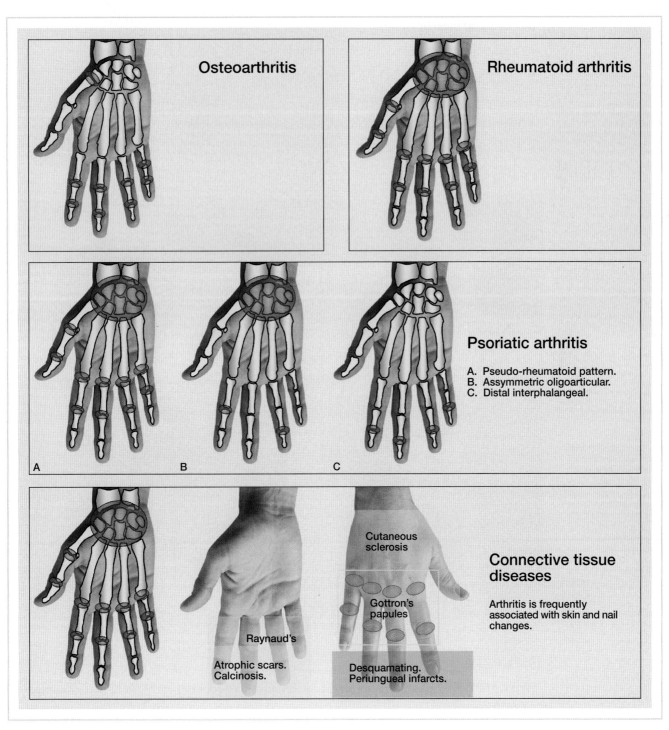

Osteoarthritis

Rheumatoid arthritis

Psoriatic arthritis

A. Pseudo-rheumatoid pattern.
B. Assymmetric oligoarticular.
C. Distal interphalangeal.

A   B   C

Cutaneous sclerosis

Gottron's papules

Raynaud's

Atrophic scars. Calcinosis.

Desquamating. Periungueal infarcts.

Connective tissue diseases

Arthritis is frequently associated with skin and nail changes.

**Figure 10.27.** Writs and hand joints typically involved in the different arthropathies.

### The neurological examination

A neurological examination is particularly indicated if the prior assessment suggests neurogenic pain: paresthetic pain, predominating at night, suggestive location, related to movements of the neck, weakness, etc.

Atrophy of the thenar and hypothenar eminences on the palmar face of the hand is also suggestive.

#### h) Assessing muscle strength

Successively test the patient's strength in the following movements (Figure 10.28.):

- Extension of the wrist (root C7, radial nerve)

- Opposition of thumb and index finger (root C7/8, median nerve)

- Resisted flexion of the fingers (root C6–C8, median nerve)

- Spreading the fingers (root C8/T1, ulnar nerve)

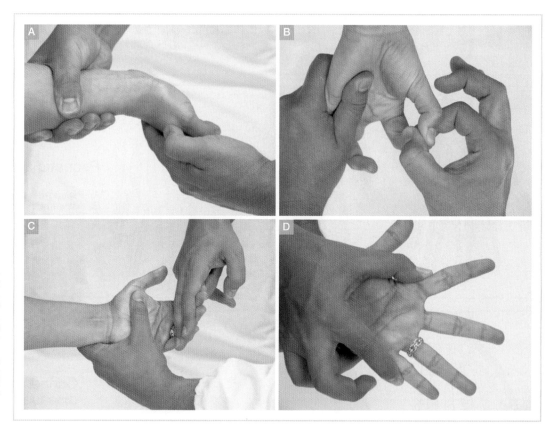

Figure 10.28.
Neurological examination of the hand and wrist.
**A.** Extension of the wrist (C7, radial nerve).
**B.** Opposition of the thumb and index finger (C7–C8, median nerve).
**C.** Resisted flexion of the fingers (C6–C8, median nerve). **D.** Spreading of the fingers (C8-T1, ulnar nerve).

#### i) Assessing sensitivity to pain

Hypoesthesia of the hand is only found in very advanced root or nerve lesions and is not necessary to prove a neurogenic lesion. Its assessment should take into account the sensory areas of the peripheral nerves (Figure 10.4.) and the radicular dermatomes (Figure 7.5.).

### j) Tinel's sign

Tinel's sign is checked by percussion on a point of the path of a nerve. It is positive if it results in dysesthesia radiating to the sensory area of the nerve (it sometimes radiates proximally). Depending on the area affected by the spontaneous "neurogenic" symptoms, you may perform:

- Tinel of the median nerve in the carpal tunnel (Figure 10.29A.);
- Tinel of the ulnar nerve in Guyon's canal (Figure 10.29B.);
- Tinel of the ulnar nerve in the elbow (Figure 10.30C.).

### k) Phalen's test

Place the patient's wrists in forced flexion so that the backs of his hands press against each other for about 60 seconds (Figure 10.30.). In carpal tunnel syndrome this test often reproduces symptoms: paresthesia in the territory of the median nerve.

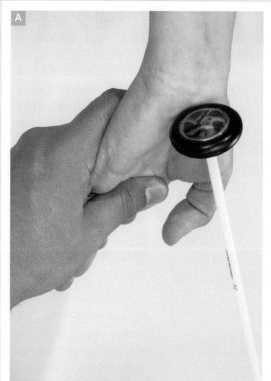
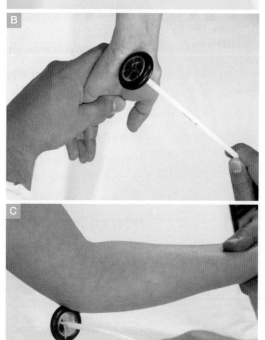
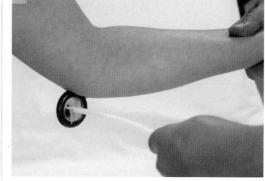

**Figure 10.29.** Tinel's sign. **A.** Tinel of the median nerve in the carpal tunnel. **B.** Tinel of ulnar nerve in the ulnar tunnel. **C.** Tinel of the ulnar nerve in the elbow.

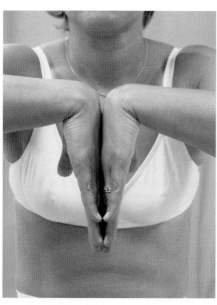

**Figure 10.30.** Phalen's test. This position is kept for about 1 minute: paresthesia in the median nerve distribution suggests carpal tunnel syndrome.

*TYPICAL CASES*
**10.A. PAIN IN THE HANDS (I)**

Maria de Jesus, a 54-year old cook, said that she was finding it increasingly difficult to do her job. She would wake up several times a night with pain in her hands, especially her right one, which prevented her from sleeping. The pain was relieved by moving her hands. She felt that her hands were "swollen" and "numb" in the morning. This usually got better with time, but she was "clumsy." She kept dropping things (she had broken more dishes in the last 3 months than in the rest of her life!). She denied pain in any other locations, except for the mechanical back pain that she had been having for about 10 years. During our systematic enquiry she said that she had been feeling tired and forgetful but that it was "probably lack of sleep." She had recently put on 6 kg.

*Imagine the essential steps of the clinical examination that you would give her.*

Our clinical examination revealed an obese patient (weight: 78 kg; height: 1.54 m) with no physical anomalies in the physical examination other than firm edema in her legs. The whole rheumatologic examination was normal, with no pain or limitation of movements. Her hands were also normal, with no swelling, muscular atrophy or alterations in the skin or nails. There were no limitations to active or passive mobility, and palpation was painless, with no signs of synovitis or tenosynovitis.

*How would you explain her symptoms?*

*Would you conduct any further clinical assessments?*

We asked the patient again about the pain. Yes, she had had some tingling. She said that her whole hand was affected but, when pushed, admitted that the little finger was not involved.

We tested for Tinel's sign in the median nerve and conducted Phalen's test, both of which were positive bilaterally. The examination of the cervical spine was normal.

*What are the possible diagnoses?*

*Would you request any diagnostic tests?*

We confirmed the diagnosis of carpal tunnel syndrome, without additional tests.

*Could the history of weight gain, edema and tiredness have some other significance?*

We advised Maria de Jesus to wear a splint on her wrist and we asked for a thyroid hormone test. Two weeks later, the results confirmed the diagnosis of hypothyroidism, and she was started on thyroxin. We discussed alternative treatments with the patient and decided to postpone a possible corticosteroid injection into the carpal tunnel until after a course of thyroid replacement.

After 6 weeks, Maria de Jesus was "a new woman...".

## CARPAL TUNNEL SYNDROME
### MAIN POINTS

This is a very common condition, especially in middle-aged women.

The main symptoms are pain and paresthesia of the median nerve area (or the whole hand...), mainly at night and in the morning, which improve with movement.

Patients often lose manual dexterity and describe diffuse, discreet swelling of the hands in the morning.

Clinical examination finds no signs of joint disease or limitation of movement.

Positive Tinel's and Phalen's tests reinforce the diagnosis.

Atrophy of the thenar eminence and loss of sensitivity in the median nerve territory are later manifestations.

Most cases have no identifiable underlying cause. Diabetes, hypothyroidism, pregnancy, work with vibrating machinery and intensive use of the hands are risk factors. It often accompanies synovitis or tenosynovitis of the wrist (e.g. in rheumatoid arthritis).

An electromyogram is justified in doubtful cases or if surgery is considered. Lab tests are only justified to look for the underlying cause and are oriented by clues collected in the general enquiry and examination.

Therapy consists basically of local protection (splints) and treatment of any identifiable underlying disease.

Corticosteroid injections can be administered in cases of intense or persistent symptoms.[5] Decompression surgery is sometimes indispensable.

### TYPICAL CASES
### 10.B. PAIN IN THE HANDS (II)

It all seemed to have started at the age of 50, after the menopause. The patient had aches and pains here and there that she considered normal for her age. At the age of 56, the pain in her hands became persistent and daily. It was this pain that brought her to us at the age of 62. The pain appeared mainly after prolonged use of the hands (e.g. after crocheting for a long time, one of her favorite occupations that she could no longer do...). She often woke up with pain and stiffness in her hands lasting up to about an hour in the worst phases. She had only noticed swelling once, two years previously. The second DIP of her right hand had been swollen and red with a blister that had burst and produced some fluid. She had noticed progressive deformation in several joints. But, "Doctor, this must run in the family. My mother's hands were all deformed when she died. That's what worries me most..."

We asked her to show us her hands (Figure 10.31.) and point to exactly where it hurt. She indicated the base of her thumbs and, diffusely, the proximal and distal interphalangeal joints. The metacarpophalangeal joints and wrists were not affected. She also had typical mechanical pain in her knees and lumbar region.

Palpation of the trapeziometacarpal joints was painful.[6] Palpation of the PIPs and DIPs was painless, but there were firm nodules located on either side of the dorsal face of several joints. Finkelstein's maneuver was negative.

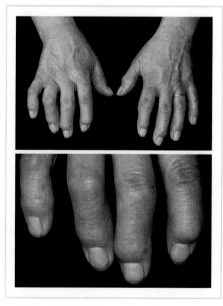

**Figure 10.31.** Clinical case "Pain in the hands (II)". Notice the nodular deformities around the PIPs and DIPs, as well as the deviations of some phalanges.

[5]For guidance on the technique, see Chapter 30.

[6]The 1st CMC (Trapeziometacrpal joint) can be palpated at the base of the thumb in the anatomical snuff box. The joint space is not perceptible but in osteoarthritis there is pain and osteophytes are occasionally perceptible.

*Give a brief description of this case.*[7]

*What is your diagnosis? Are there any alternative possibilities?*

*Would you ask for any diagnostic tests?*

*Would you like to consider the treatment?*

Our clinical examination left no doubt. The patient had nodal osteoarthritis of the hands and osteoarthritis of the 1st carpo-metacarpal joints.

We explained the nature of the condition to the patient and told her that, unfortunately, there was no way of stopping its progression to deformity. We stressed, however, that patients with nodal osteoarthritis maintain good mobility and function in spite of the deformities. We suggested local application of heat and topical anti-inflammatory creams. We recommended paracetamol to relieve the pain when necessary, reserving anti-inflammatories for use if this measure failed. This condition is described in more detail in Chapter 16.

*TYPICAL CASES*

**10.C. PAIN IN THE WRIST (I)**

Graça Oliveira, a 42-year old domestic employee, described increasingly intense pain in her left wrist and the distal part of her left forearm for about three weeks (she was left-handed). The pain worsened while she was working and continued to bother her somewhat even when at rest. There was no pain at night and no paresthesia. She denied any recent trauma and had noticed no signs of inflammation.

She had always been healthy and this was the first episode of such symptoms.

On examination, inspection and mobility of wrists and hands were normal. Palpation of the joints revealed no abnormalities, thus excluding the possibility of synovitis. Tinel's and Phalen's tests were negative.

*Find out for yourself. What else is there to explain her pain?...*

*What aspects of the clinical examination haven't we explored?*

That's right. Palpation of the tendons on the outer border of the wrist caused pain, which was more marked at the anterior edge of the anatomical snuffbox. We noted slight thickening in this tendon. Abduction or resisted flexion of the thumb caused pain similar to the spontaneous pain, exacerbated by simultaneous palpation of the tendon. Finkelstein's maneuver caused intense pain.

This allowed the diagnosis of De Quervain's tenosynovitis, without the need for additional diagnostic tests. We advised her to rest her left arm for about a week and recommended local friction with an anti-inflammatory cream after applying heat for 5–10 minutes. The patient came back 2 weeks later as she had not improved.

We then administered a careful injection of corticosteroid into the tendon sheath and recommended complete rest of the arm for 2 days. With the patient, we explored the possibility of

---

[7] A 62-year old woman with mixed-rhythm pain in the small joints of her hands and progressive deformation with stony nodes.

diminishing repeated use of the thumb with special splint. She said that this was incompatible with her work.

A couple of weeks later she told us on the phone that she no longer had any symptoms. The risk of recurrence is high, however.

## DE QUERVAIN'S TENOSYNOVITIS
### MAIN POINTS

This consists of the inflammation of the tendon sheath of the long abductor and short extensor of the thumb.

It appears particularly in middle-aged women and is associated with repetitive manual work.

The pain is predominantly mechanical and located in the radial edge of the wrist, with some proximal or distal radiation.

The diagnosis is based on pain on local palpation, resisted mobilization and Finkelstein's maneuver.

The initial treatment involves rest and topical anti-inflammatories.

Local corticosteroid injection may solve the problem, but it must be carefully administered[8].

Protecting the joint, with the use of appropriate splints (Figure 29.2.), is helpful in preventing recurrence.

### TYPICAL CASES
### 10.D. PAIN IN THE HANDS (III)

The symptoms had been going on for about 4 months when we saw the patient for the first time. She described pain and inflexibility in both hands, especially in the morning. The stiffness sometimes lasted up to 2 hours. By the afternoon she had practically no symptoms. Her family doctor had prescribed anti-inflammatories, which relieved the pain without eliminating it all together. She attributed epigastric pain to this medication.

She denied any other articular or extra-articular complaints during a thorough enquiry.

The general clinical examination showed no alterations other than reduced active flexion of the fingers. Careful palpation of the metacarpophalangeal and interphalangeal joints was painless with no signs of articular swelling.

### How would you continue investigating this case?

We tested passive mobility. It was quite easy to flex the fingers completely, much beyond active mobility. Palpation over the flexor tendons of the fingers, with simultaneous passive mobilization, was painful and showed clear thickening of the tissue adjacent to the flexor tendons of the index and middle fingers on the left and the index, middle and ring fingers on the right. There was discreet crepitus.

---

[8]Injection of corticosteroids into the tendon weakens it and may lead to a subsequent rupture. For guidance on the technique, see Chapter 30.

## ARTHRITIS OF THE WRIST AND HANDS
### MAIN POINTS

Practically all types of arthritis can involve the hands.

The diagnosis of arthritis requires demonstration of joint inflammation, i.e. synovial swelling, on clinical examination.

The clinical examination technique should be thorough.

Monoarthritis of the wrists and hands is relatively rare. After excluding septic or microcrystalline arthritis, we should consider the possibility of incipient polyarthropathy.

The systematic enquiry and general examination are essential to the differential diagnosis.

The distribution of the affected joints in the wrists and hands is highly suggestive of the type of arthritis (Figure 10.27.).

The lab tests and treatment indicated depend on the overall clinical context.

Tenosynovitis often accompanies arthritis of the hands, and can be the first sign of this condition.

A diagnosis of inflammatory arthritis of any kind justifies sending the patient to a specialist as soon as possible.

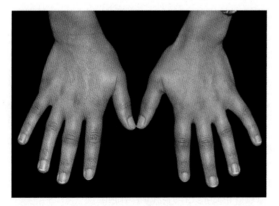

**Figure 10.32.** Clinical case "Pain in the hands (III)". Please note that although inspection suggests joint swelling, this can only be proved by palpation.

*What is your diagnosis?*

*Are any diagnostic tests necessary?*

*How would you interpret them?*

*What approach would you take?*

Our examination showed that the patient had **tenosynovitis of the finger flexors**.

This condition in a young woman (aged 38), who did not do hard manual work and had no other manifestations, strongly suggested incipient polyarthritis.

We therefore changed her anti-inflammatory treatment, opting for a long-acting agent to be taken at night in order to guarantee maximum efficacy in the morning, associated with some gastric protection. We requested several lab tests: full blood count, sedimentation rate in the first hour, liver enzymes, creatinine, glucose, urinalysis, rheumatoid factor and antinuclear antibodies.

For personal reasons, the patient was only able to see us again 3 months later. The pain had become worse and so had the stiffness, which now lasted the whole morning. The pain kept her awake at night and now involved her right wrist and her toes. She had noticed edema in her hands about 2 months before (Figure 10.32). She continued to deny any extra-articular manifestations of any kind. The epigastric pain had disappeared.

On examining her we now noticed a moderate reduction in flexion of the fingers, which could not be reduced passively. The signs of tenosynovitis persisted but were now accompanied by clear swelling, without redness, of the first, second and third MCPs on the left and the first and second on the right. There was fluctuation and pain on palpation of the right and left first, second and third PIPs and the third left PIP. Her right wrist was painful on palpation, with appreciable swelling and slight local heat. Transverse palpation of the metatarsal-phalangeal caused pain.

*Give a brief description of this clinical condition.*

*What is your interpretation now?*

There was now evidence of polyarthritis (inflammatory pain, with signs of inflammation in several joints), which was additive (as more joints were becoming involved), symmetrical (MCPs on each side, PIPs on each side) and predominantly peripheral (wrists and small joints of the hands), with no systemic manifestations. These characteristics are highly suggestive of rheumatoid arthritis. Psoriatic arthritis or another disease of the connective tissue was possible, even with no extra-articular manifestations.

When the lab tests came back, the blood count, creatinine and liver enzymes were normal. The sedimentation rate was high at 53 mm in the first hour. The rheumatoid factor and antinuclear antibodies were negative.[9]

We explained the situation to the patient and started her on appropriate treatment for rheumatoid arthritis (Chapter 19).

## TYPICAL CASES
## 10.E. PAIN IN THE HANDS (IV)

Alice, aged 32, was referred to us by her GP because of pain in her hands, which had been developing for several months and was "unresponsive to non-steroidal drugs." The pain mainly affected the small joints of her hands, particularly at night and in the morning, with morning stiffness lasting from 30 to 60 minutes. She described mild hand swelling, particularly in the morning.

The pain was not incapacitating, but was still troublesome and worrying. She described transient episodes of intense pain in which her hands turned purple. These episodes were especially triggered by cold and emotional stress. No other joints were involved.

*What possible diagnoses are you thinking of?*

*What additional information would you want?*

The systematic enquiry was particularly interesting. The episodes of acute pain were accompanied by a clear change in color of some fingers (especially the index and middle finger of each hand), which first went very pale and later cyanotic. This had been happening for several years, particularly in winter, but she had never thought much of it. When asked, she said that she often had long-lasting painful mouth ulcers but denied any vaginal ulcers. Her eyes were frequently itchy and red, especially in the evening. Her skin had become quite sensitive to the sun the previous summer and she had suffered an erythematous reaction on her face and hands, which had gone away after a few weeks.

Her medical history included hospitalization due to pleural effusion with fever. This was attributed to pulmonary tuberculosis and had responded to treatment. All these "little things" had begun 4 years previously during her first pregnancy and she had been perfectly healthy until then.

Our general examination did not reveal any changes in her skin or mucosae. The chest examination was normal. Inspection of the hands found slightly spindle-shaped PIPs which were painful on palpation, but with no clear synovitis. There were small, scaly erythematous lesions on the backs of her fingers. Tinel's and Phalen's tests were negative.

[9]NB: rheumatoid factor is only positive in about 75% of cases of rheumatoid arthritis and this percentage is lower in the first months of the disease. The diagnosis is based on the clinical assessment even with a negative rheumatoid factor (see Chapter 19).

## THE HANDS IN CONNECTIVE TISSUE DISEASES
### MAIN POINTS

All connective tissue diseases (CTDs) can cause joint pain or arthritis of the hands, which is often the first manifestation.

As a rule, synovitis is much more pronounced in rheumatoid arthritis than in other CTDs. There are often alterations of the skin and mucosae.

Always pay attention to inflammatory joint pain, especially in young people with no generalized pain.

A systematic enquiry and examination, focusing on the common extra-articular manifestations of CTDs, are the key to diagnosis.

Pay attention to the clinical information, even if none of it is conclusive, and consider the degree of probability of a systemic disease.

A clinically founded suspicion of CTD warrants requesting appropriate diagnostic tests and sending the patient to a specialist as soon as possible.

*Briefly summarize this patient's problems.*

- Peripheral, inflammatory polyarthralgia;

- Photosensitivity;

- Raynaud's phenomenon;

- Recurring mouth ulcers;

- Itchy eyes (xerophthalmia?);

- A history of pleurisy (tuberculosis?).

And all this in a young woman who we would expect to be healthy!

*Review your possible diagnoses...*

It's just as you think. We have sufficient information to suspect a systemic disease of the connective tissue. Note that, in practice, the difficulty of such cases lies in actively searching for and assessing relevant clinical data, which requires a systematic, focused enquiry and examination.

*What diagnostic tests do you think are important?*

The full blood count that we requested showed leucopenia, with normal red cell and platelet counts. Her liver enzymes and creatinine were normal. The urinalysis showed red cell castes with mild proteinuria and hematuria. Her sedimentation rate was high at 48 mm in the first hour, while reactive C protein was normal. Immunofluorescence for antinuclear antibodies was positive, at a titer of 1:320, with a homogeneous pattern.

The diagnosis of systemic lupus erythematosus was thus made. We set up some additional tests and prescribed the appropriate treatment.

## SPECIAL SITUATIONS

### Ulnar nerve syndrome

This is much less common than carpal tunnel syndrome. It causes paresthesia of the ulnar nerve territory, affecting only the medial border of the hand and fingers, if the compression is in Guyon's tunnel. The ulnar border of the forearm may also be involved if the compression is on the posteromedial aspect of the elbow joint. Positive Tinel's test at the sites of possible compression reinforces the diagnosis. There may be weakness in adduction of the little finger and hypoesthesia in the affected area. It requires differential diagnosis with C8 radiculopathy. An electromyogram may be necessary to confirm the diagnosis. Treatment involves avoiding local trauma by protecting the joints. If this is insufficient, it is worth administering a corticosteroid injection in the vicinity of the compression. Surgical decompression is necessary if the symptoms persist or if there are significant neurological signs.

### Dupuytren's contracture

This consists of fibrous thickening of the palmar fascia (i.e. not the tendons or tendon sheaths) thus preventing complete extension of the affected fingers, and leads to a fixed flexion deformity. The first and most commonly affected digit is the ring finger (Figure 10.20.). It is more common in men aged over 50. Palpation shows a hard, tense band. Diabetes mellitus, alcoholism and hard manual labor are predispositions, but most cases are idiopathic. There is a family predisposition.

Treatment is difficult and in the initial stages is aimed at protecting the area from repeated trauma and distending the tissues by means of local heat and extension exercises. Treatment of advanced, incapacitating forms usually requires surgery.

### Trigger finger

This is the result of stenosing tenosynovitis of the flexor tendon of one or more fingers. The patient describes pain in the palm while his finger often "gets stuck." In more advanced stages, the finger may remain fixed in flexion. It is released by active or passive extension of the finger, with pain and a triggering movement. Palpation of the flexor tendon and its sheath generally reveals a palpable node that moves with the tendon during passive mobilization. It can be improved by wearing splints and changes in the patient's daily activities. A corticosteroid injection may be highly effective. Surgery is occasionally needed.

### Diabetic hand syndrome

A hands in diabetes are often the site of rheumatic complaints. Carpal tunnel syndrome, ulnar syndrome and tenosynovitis are the most common conditions in these patients.

Diabetic hand syndrome consists of a diffuse thickening of the soft tissues of the hand and fingers (fascia, tendons, capsules and ligaments), which limit mobility, particularly extension, without concomitant joint disease. It is known as diabetic chiroarthropathy and is usually painless. A typical feature of the clinical examination is the so-called *prayer sign*. Ask the patient to put his hands together as if praying. Patients with this condition find it difficult to join the palms of their hands due to the inability to extend completely the different joints (Figure 10.33.). The onset and progression of this syndrome occur in parallel with diabetic microangiopathy.

Treatment involves general care, physical therapy to maintain the elasticity of the tissues and tighter control of the diabetes.

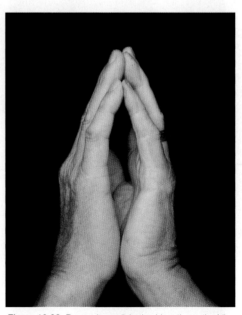

**Figure 10.33.** Prayer sign – diabetic chiroarthropathy (diabetic hand syndrome). The patient is unable to press both hands together.

### Finger clubbing: hypertrophic osteoarthropathy

Hypertrophic osteoarthropathy is a complex condition involving joint disease and generalized periostosis (periosteum inflammation and bone deposition). It usually appears in association with conditions such as lung diseases with chronic hypoxia, lung neoplasm, cyanotic heart disease, heavy smoking, liver cirrhosis, inflammatory gut disease, etc.

It is reflected by pain in a variety of locations. A burning sensation in the pads of the fingers is common. The lower limbs are often affected by deep, diffuse pain, which is typically worse when the legs are hanging.

Finger clubbing (or drumstick finger – Figure 10.34.) is one of its earliest, most common signs. The pads of the fingers thicken and swell and nails take on a convex shape. The perimeter of the finger at the base of the nail is larger than that of the DIP. Loss of space between the nails when we press two nail beds together is a particularly specific sign, reflecting loss of angle of nail bed (Figure 10.34C.).

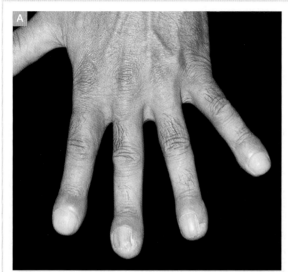

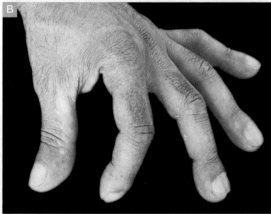

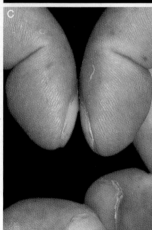

**Figure 10.34.**
Clubbing. Notice the deformity of the distal phalanxes (clubbed fingers). Loss of the nailbed angle is an early sign of this condition.

### Generalized edema of the hands

Occasionally a patient may describe generalized swelling of the hands, affecting not only the area around the joints but also the tissue of the back of the hand and wrist with pitting (boxer's hand).

This situation may rarely reflect acute or exacerbated arthritis, as in rheumatoid arthritis. The hand of a patient with scleroderma may suggest this condition as in its initial phases skin edema predominates before sclerosis.

Algodystrophy (or reflex sympathetic dystrophy) may cause diffuse edema of the hands with suggestive changes in color (mauve) and increased sweating. This condition is described in Chapter 14.

The most common symptom of the rare condition RS3PE (remitting seronegative symmetric synovitis with pitting edema) is accentuated diffuse edema of both hands. It may respond perfectly to corticosteroid treatment but often progresses into typical rheumatoid arthritis.

Before considering these possibilities, however, do not forget to exclude other conditions like venous or lymphatic compression, allergic reaction or hypothyroidism.

## DIAGNOSTIC TESTS

A wide variety of rheumatic conditions of the wrist and hand may be diagnosed clinically, without the need for additional diagnostic tests. This is so for De Quervain's tenosynovitis, nodal osteoarthritis, osteoarthritis of the 1st CMC, Dupuytren's contracture, diabetic hand syndrome, and, to a large extent, rheumatoid arthritis, etc.

Carpal tunnel and ulnar tunnel syndrome do not normally require tests. An electromyogram may be justified if clinical assessment is not conclusive, if motor symptoms suggest severe median nerve compression and/or if surgery is likely. The need for tests to detect a pathology underlying these syndromes (glycemia, thyroid hormones, etc.) depends on the clinical context. As with many investigations, they are not very useful if requested indiscriminately.

If we suspect arthritis, there is a clear need for acute phase reactant studies, full blood count, basic biochemistry and other tests applicable to the diagnosis and to prepare for subsequent treatment. Rheumatoid factor and antinuclear antibodies are important tests in suspected polyarthritis, but they should never replace clinical assessment.

**In rheumatology, no test can make the diagnosis in the absence of compatible clinical symptoms.**[10]

### *Imaging*

X-rays of the hands and wrists (anteroposterior and oblique angle) are justified whenever the clinical assessment suggests joint disease.

Reading these x-rays follows the same principles as for other joints:

> Look at the alignment of the bones.
>
> Assess the width and symmetry of the articular space.

Both arthritis and osteoarthritis involve loss of articular space. In arthritis, it tends to be homogeneous and uniform along the space. In osteoarthritis, the loss is often asymmetrical, depending on the lines of pressure exerted through the joint (Figure 10.35.).

> Look at the bone density around the joints.

**WHEN TO CONSIDER ARTHRITIS OF THE WRIST AND HANDS**
*MAIN POINTS*

Inflammatory pain

Rubbery swelling and/or pain in the joints on palpation

Signs of inflammation (inconstant)

Elevated acute phase reagents (usual)

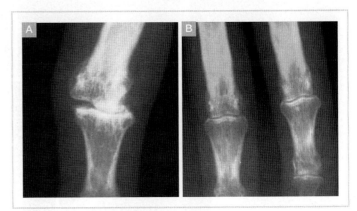

**Figure 10.35.** In osteoarthritis (**A.**) joint space loss is usually focal or asymmetrical, while in inflammatory arthritis (**B.**) it tends to be uniform and diffuse.

---

[10]A truth of La Palisse: for there to be rheumatoid arthritis, there must be … arthritis.

In rheumatoid arthritis, periarticular osteopenia is one of its most typical signs and occurs early in the course of the disease. Conversely, osteoarthritis is associated with thickening of the subchondral bone – subchondral sclerosis. Curiously, although psoriatic arthritis is inflammatory, it does not cause pronounced osteopenia (Figure 10.36.).

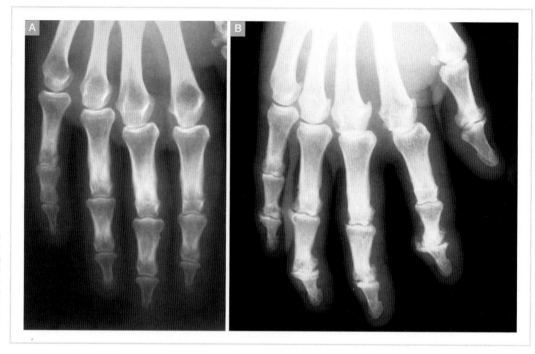

**Figure 10.36.** In rheumatoid arthritis (**A.**) periarticular osteopenia is an early radiological feature. In osteoarthritis (**B.**) subchondral bone sclerosis is a typical finding. Also notice the loss of joint space in both conditions.

Examine the edges of the joint for erosions or osteophytes.

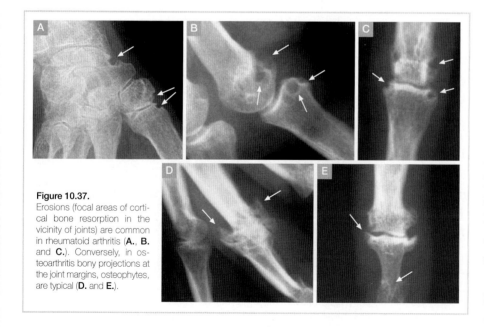

**Figure 10.37.**
Erosions (focal areas of cortical bone resorption in the vicinity of joints) are common in rheumatoid arthritis (**A.**, **B.** and **C.**). Conversely, in osteoarthritis bony projections at the joint margins, osteophytes, are typical (**D.** and **E.**).

Erosions look like small "bites" near the insertion points of the capsule and synovium. They are highly suggestive of rheumatoid arthritis and predominate in the joints usually affected by this type of arthritis: MCPs and PIPs. The styloid process of the ulna is also a common site of rheumatoid erosion. Lupus and other CTDs do not cause erosions, in spite of the articular inflammation.

In osteoarthritis, on the other hand, there are usually bony spurs (osteophytes) (Figure 10.37.).

Psoriatic arthritis is peculiar in this respect. It tends to cause erosions in the top of the proximal phalange and spurs in the base of the distal phalange, sometimes producing a "pencil in cup" appearance (Figure 10.38.).

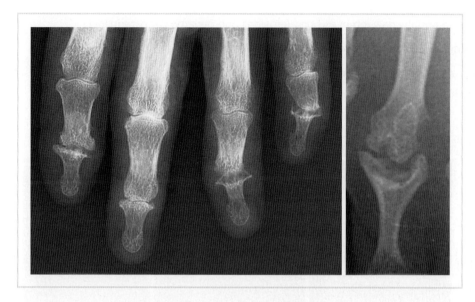

**Figure 10.38.** In advanced psoriatic arthritis, the association of erosions and exostoses may suggest so-called "pencil in cup" deformities.

Look for calcification of the cartilage or soft tissue – pay particular attention to the triangular ligament of the carpus (Figure 10.39.).

Assess the distribution of the affected joints and compare it with the typical pattern of each joint disease.

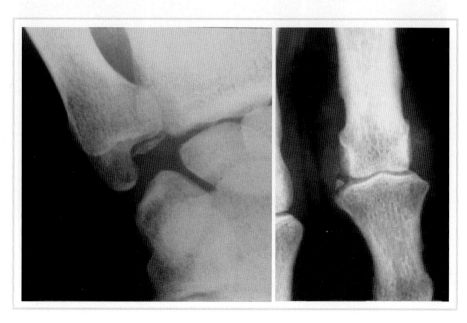

**Figure 10.39.** Chondrocalcinosis. Notice the calcification of the triangular ligament of the carpus and the interphalangeal joint.

## IMAGING OF THE HANDS
### *MAIN POINTS*

In simple terms, we can say that some radiological characteristics distinguish between the most common diseases of the wrist:

- Rheumatoid arthritis only removes bone (erosions and periarticular osteopenia)

- Osteoarthritis adds bone (osteophytes and subchondral sclerosis)

- Psoriatic arthritis does both (erosions and spurs, with no osteopenia or subchondral sclerosis) (Figure 10.40.)

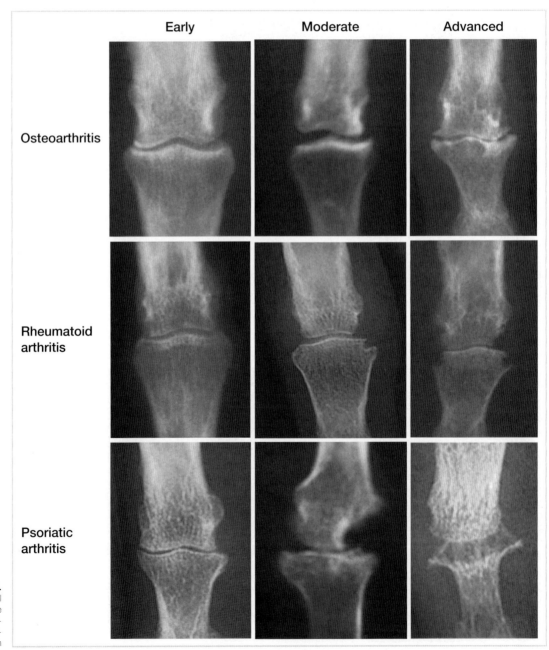

**Figure 10.40.**
Typical radiological features of the three arthropathies in different stages of progression

Bone scintigraphy is hardly ever justified to study the hands. Clinical assessment is highly informative and careful examination of the joints is usually more conclusive than scintigraphy.

## TREATMENT

We have already dealt with the principles of treating lesions of the soft tissue and osteoarthritis of the hands. If pain and disability do not respond to medication, splints on the thumb or wrist can relieve the symptoms and improve mobility (Figures 29.2. and 29.3.). Corticosteroid injections play an important part in treating some of these conditions, but should only be administered with a specific indication and by a trained physician.

When confronted with arthritis, a GP should refer the patient to a specialist as soon as possible. Even in chronic diseases like rheumatoid arthritis, the first few months are a crucial opportunity to avoid irreversible structural lesions, which is only possible with appropriate, timely treatment. Acute arthritis or suspected connective tissue disease warrant urgent referral.

If in doubt, GPs may request basic diagnostic tests such as acute phase reactants, rheumatoid factor or antinuclear antibodies, but should avoid wasting too much time using sophisticated tests, while awaiting an appointment with a consultant, you should resist the temptation to prescribe corticosteroids or immunosuppressants. Although they may provide rapid relief, it will be transient and there is a significant risk of side effects. Such hasty treatment may also blur the clinical features and influence results of diagnostic tests, making a definite diagnosis more difficult for the specialist. If you feel the need to resort to corticosteroids, consider whether your patient would not be better going to the ER at a hospital with a rheumatology department.

---

### WHEN SHOULD THE PATIENT BE REFERRED TO A SPECIALIST?

Whenever and as soon as your clinical assessment demonstrates arthritis.

Whenever there are reasonable indications of connective tissue disease.

Whenever an x-ray shows loss of articular space or erosions, even if the clinical examination is not very suggestive.

Whenever soft tissue lesions are resistant to conservative treatment.

## ADDITIONAL PRACTICE
### REGIONAL SYNDROMES. THE WRIST AND HAND

# REGIONAL SYNDROMES
## LOW BACK PAIN

11.

J.A.P. da Silva, A.D. Woolf, *Rheumatology in Practice*, DOI 10.1007/978-1-84882-581-9_11,
© Springer-Verlag London Limited 2010

# 11. REGIONAL SYNDROMES LOW BACK PAIN

ow back pain is the most common complaint after the common cold. Almost everyone has at least one episode of low back pain during their lives. In the USA, it accounts for around 3% of all visits to doctors.

Low back pain often takes the form of an acute episode which occurs most commonly between the ages of 30 and 50. About 90% of episodes of acute backache clear up in less than 8 weeks regardless of the treatment. A small minority of people will, however, have recurring acute attacks or their condition will become chronic, with considerable pain and disability. Chronic low back pain is an important public health problem with a significant social and economic impact involving substantial direct and indirect costs.

In most cases of chronic mechanical back pain, it is impossible to make a precise diagnosis because of the complexity of the structures in question and the multiplicity of potential factors. The course of chronic back pain is closely related to psychological and social factors that are difficult to assess. Even in these cases, however, we can arrive at an approximate diagnosis that enables us to help the patient.

Only a small percentage of cases involve a specific etiology requiring special diagnostic and therapeutic action, but it is precisely these cases that require our attention most. Low back pain may be the first manifestation of a potentially fatal disease.

> **The approach to patients with low back pain has three main goals:**
>
> 1. Preventing acute episodes from becoming chronic
>
> 2. Identifying cases requiring specific treatment (red flags)
>
> 3. Relieving the symptoms and, in particular, improving the patient's physical and social functions while avoiding unnecessary tests

## FUNCTIONAL ANATOMY

The functional anatomy of the lumbar spine is very similar to that already described for the cervical spine: a set of five vertebrae one on top of the other separated by intervertebral discs.

Posteriorly, pedicles project on either side of the vertebral body. The transverse processes extend laterally from them. The upper and lower joint surfaces that extend from the pedicles, form facet joints with the adjacent vertebrae. The alignment of the lumbar facet joints is almost anteroposterior, which is why they are capable only of flexion and extension. Rotation of the torso depends, therefore, on the thoracic spine.

The lumbar spinal canal contains and protects the end of the spinal cord (the medullary cone ends at approximately L1/L2) and the nerve roots forming the cauda equina. The first lumbar root emerges between L1 and L2 and so on (Figure 11.1.).

The vertebrae and their joints are stabilized by a large number of ligaments, which may be the site of back pain-causing lesions, but are impossible to evaluate separately either clinically or by imaging. These ligaments and their insertions are common targets of pathology in ankylosing spondylitis and the other seronegative spondyloarthropathies.

The lumbar spine is mobilized by muscles running along the vertebral grooves, which have multiple insertions along the posterior aspect of the spine. The nerve roots and regional nerve branches are located between these muscles. They may all be the site of disease but cannot be examined individually.

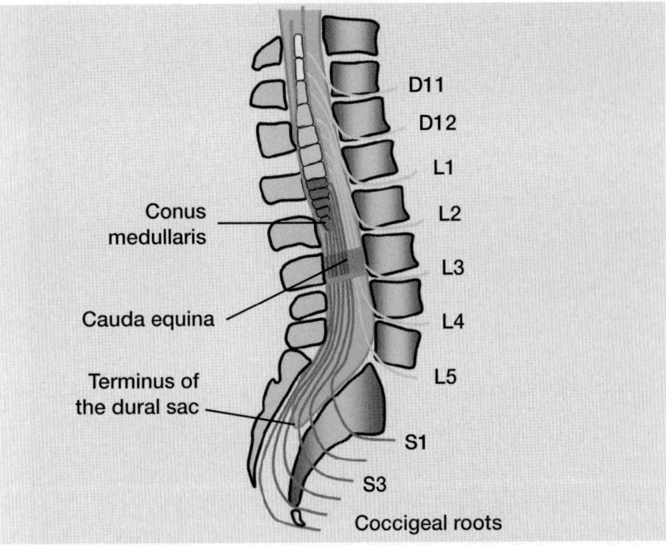

Some aspects require closer attention.

The intervertebral foramen through which the nerve roots emerge is limited anteriorly by the intervertebral disk, which may herniate, compressing the root and leading to neurogenic pain (e.g. sciatica) (Figure 11.2.). Posteriorly, the nerve roots are in contact with the facet joint. This is a synovial joint that is frequently affected by osteoarthritis, often with exuberant osteophytes. These osteophytes may cause compression of the root just like a herniated disk, and usually the symptoms are indistinguishable.

The lumbar spinal canal houses the roots that innervate the lower limbs and sacral region. In some people it can be constitutionally narrow. The canal may be reduced further by spondylolisthesis (when a vertebral body slides over the one below it), by prolapsed disks or by large osteophytes from the intervertebral joints. Neural tumors, such as neurofibroma or meningioma are less common causes. When the canal is markedly narrowed, the roots may be compressed to the point of dysfunction, causing pain and weakness in the area served by that root or diffuse exercise-dependent pain (claudication) and neurological deficit affecting the lower limbs (lumbar stenosis) or only the sacral roots (cauda equina syndrome).

![Figure 11.1]

**Figure 11.1.** Emergence of lumbar, sacral and coccigeal nerve roots.

Labels: Conus medullaris, Cauda equina, Terminus of the dural sac, D11, D12, L1, L2, L3, L4, L5, S1, S3, Coccigeal roots

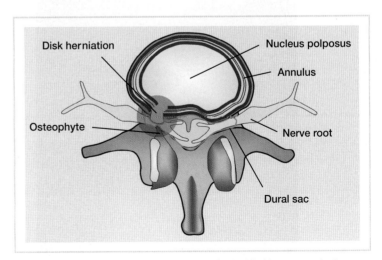

**Figure 11.2.** Emergence of lumbar nerve roots. On the *left side:* compression by extruded nucleus polposus (disk herniation) or by osteophytes from the facet joint.

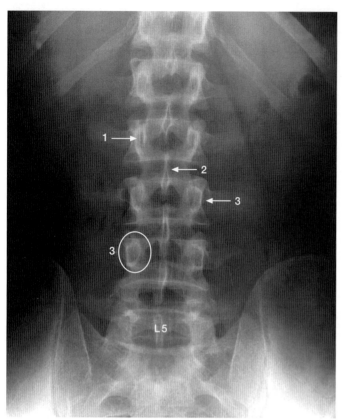

**Figure 11.3.** Lumbar spine radiograph: antero-posterior view. **1.** Facet joint. **2.** Projection of the spinous process. **3.** Projection of the pedicle.

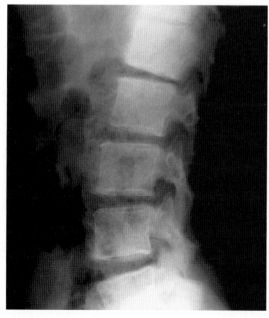

**Figure 11.4.** Lumbar spine radiograph: lateral view.

### *Radiological anatomy*

In an anteroposterior x-ray (Figure 11.3.) the alignment of the vertebrae may be seen. Malalignment is called scoliosis. Look for lytic lesions (the "disappearance" of a pedicle or a tranverse process may be the only sign of a metastasis). Note the regularity of the intervertebral spaces and the articular borders as well as the presence of osteophytes or syndesmophytes. The facet joints of the lower vertebrae can, at times, be seen in this projection.

On the lateral film (Figure 11.4.) we get a better idea of the morphology of the vertebral bodies (crush fractures, osteophytes, or squaring of the anterior border) and the size of the intervertebral spaces (i.e. the disc spaces): they increase slightly from L1 to L4 (L4–L5 is generally covered by the iliac bone). Look at the regularity and density of the vertebral platforms. Look for any accentuation or reduction of the normal lordosis.

Look for any calcification of the intervertebral disks or ligaments. Assess the contrast in density between the vertebral body and the neighboring tissue, as a reduction may indicate osteoporosis. Do not mistake the superimposition of intestinal gas for a lytic lesion. Spondylolisthesis is clearly seen in this projection (anterior dislocation of a vertebra over the one below).

## COMMON CAUSES OF LOW BACK PAIN

The most common causes of low back pain are shown in Table 11.1. Almost all cases will fall into one of the first three categories. Our main goal is to distinguish them from the others and treat them all as effectively as possible.

| Nature of the problem | Suggestive manifestations |
|---|---|
| Acute mechanical low back pain | Acute pain |
| | Paravertebral muscle spasm |
| | Young patient |
| Chronic mechanical low back pain | Chronic, recurring mechanical pain |
| | No systemic manifestations |
| | No neurological signs |
| Fibromyalgia | Generalized pain |
| | No limitations to mobility |
| | Diffuse tenderness on palpation of the |
| | paravertebral (and other) muscles |
| Spondylodiscitis | ALARM SIGNALS ("red flags")! |
| Sacroiliitis | Inflammatory low back pain |
| Metastases | Localized pain |
| Referred pain | Nocturnal pain |
| Interspinous ligamentitis | Fever, weight loss,… |
| Neurological compromise | History of neoplasm |
| Osteoporotic fracture | Associated visceral manifestations |
| | Risk or evidence of osteoporosis |
| | Onset before age 30 or after 50 |
| | Neurological manifestations |
| | Limitation of movement in all directions |

Table 11.1.
Common causes of low back pain and suggestive manifestations and alarm signals.

## THE ENQUIRY

### How and when did it start?

Pain that appears for the first time before the age of 30 or after 50 requires attention, as it is much more likely to be due to a specific condition. The same goes for an acute change in the characteristics of chronic back pain.

The onset of muscle spasm, sciatica and osteoporotic fractures is usually sudden and related to flexion or forced rotation. The onset of inflammatory, infectious or even metastatic lesions is progressive, reaching its peak in a few weeks or months.

Conversely, patients with common, chronic back pain usually go to the doctor after months or years of suffering with recurrent, intense episodes superimposed.

### Where is the pain? Does it radiate?

The location of the pain can tell us a lot.

> The more precise the location of the pain, the more likely a specific diagnosis.

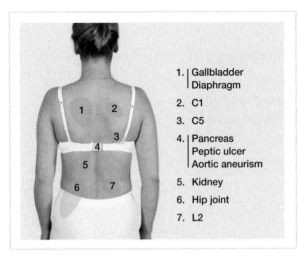

| | |
|---|---|
| 1. | Gallbladder<br>Diaphragm |
| 2. | C1 |
| 3. | C5 |
| 4. | Pancreas<br>Peptic ulcer<br>Aortic aneurism |
| 5. | Kidney |
| 6. | Hip joint |
| 7. | L2 |

**Figure 11.5.** Areas of pain referred to the lumbar and gluteal areas.

Chronic backache and the pain caused by fibromyalgia tend to be diffuse and imprecisely located. On the other hand, in discitis, metastasis or osteoporotic fracture, the patient usually identifies a focal painful area. Pain due to sacroiliitis is felt mainly in the sacrolumbar region, radiating to the buttocks.

The location of the pain can also suggest the origin of referred pain (Figure 11.5.).

> The patient should always be asked about radiation of the pain, paresthesia and its distribution, disturbances of the sphincters or localized weakness.

Pain radiating along a dermatome suggests radicular compression. The most common of these conditions is so-called *sciatica*, which is caused by irritation of the L5 and/or S1 roots. Paresthetic pain radiates down the outer aspect of the thigh, down the leg and may reach the foot. Compression of roots higher up is rare.

A description of weakness in the legs is very common in back-pain patients and should not be ignored if the neurological examination confirms it.

### What is the rhythm of the pain?

In most cases the pain will be typically mechanical, i.e. it is worse with movement (flexion and extension, walking or standing upright) and is alleviated at rest, especially lying down. Obesity and increased lumbar lordosis are often present.

> Any inflammatory pain requires special attention. It is an alarm signal. Low back pain that persists or predominates at night, with or without morning stiffness, means, until proven otherwise, an inflammatory condition (spondylitis, spondylodiscitis,...), metastasis (breast, prostate, kidney,...) or osteoporotic fracture.

### What exacerbates or relieves the pain?

We have already mentioned exercise, but there are other aspects that also deserve our attention. Pain that is alleviated by movement is probably related to an inflammatory process.

Exacerbation of the pain by Valsava's maneuvers (deliberate or when coughing, sneezing or defecating, for example) suggests nerve root irritation, especially if there is typical radiation.

Patients with radiculopathy often also say that the pain is more intense when they are standing still than when they are walking.

Lumbar stenosis, which is more common in the elderly, is associated with a suggestive, but not always clear, clinical pattern. The pain is deep, diffuse and ill defined (like "tiredness"), involving the lumbar region and the proximal part of the limbs. It worsens when walking and may be dysesthetic. As a rule, it appears after walking for some time and forces the patient to rest for a few minutes. The pain is usually more intense when the patient walks downhill than uphill. Strange, isn't it? Why should that be?[1]

Impairment of the sphincters is rare and appears late in lumbar stenosis, but the patient often complains of weakness in the lower limbs.

## The systematic enquiry

> An alarm signal in a back-pain patient makes the systematic enquiry particularly important.

Signs of peptic, pancreatic, intestinal, gynecological or urological disease can be the key to diagnosis. A description of psoriasis may reinforce the possibility of psoriatic spondylitis, etc.

We must ask about important constitutional symptoms like fever or weight loss if we have not already done so.

## Psychological and social evaluation

These aspects are particularly important in a context of chronic, mechanical low back pain. Indeed, it has been shown that the patient's psychological profile is one of the most decisive factors in determining whether an acute episode evolves into a chronic condition. The patient's convictions as to the nature and prognosis of the disease and the ways of dealing with the problem (coping strategies) are decisive elements that we must consider. Labor or legal disputes (e.g. suing for compensation after an occupational accident) can make back pain particularly resistant to treatment, and an integrated approach to these aspects should be adopted.

These factors have been called "yellow flags" (Table 11.2.).

| Questions | Indicators of a bad prognosis |
|---|---|
| Previous sick leave for low back pain? | Yes |
| What do you think is causing the pain? | Focus on a structural cause |
| | Pessimistic or catastrophic attitude |
| What do you think can help you? | Nothing |
| | Others, doctors, but not the patient |
| | They are hostile |
| How do others react to your pain? | Over-protective |
| What do you do to make the pain bearable? | Passive attitudes: rest, escape, avoiding activities, etc. |
| Do you think you'll work again? When? | No, or don't know |

**Table 11.2.** "Yellow flags" in low back pain, psychosocial criteria for a bad prognosis.

---

[1]When we walk down a slope we assume a position of lumbar hyperlordosis to keep our balance. When we go up, we tend to flex our spine. Hyperlordosis reduces the diameter of the lumbar canal, exacerbating the symptoms…

## THE REGIONAL CLINICAL EXAMINATION

The general rheumatologic examination described in Chapter 6 gives us an immediate indication of the existence of pain or limited mobility in the lumbar spine. Pain that appears particularly during flexion suggests pathology of the disks or vertebral bodies. Pain that appears particularly during extension points to disease of the facet joints or spondylolisthesis.

Pain on all types of movement is an alarm signal.

If the patient complains of low back pain or the examination shows anomalies, we need to look into it further.

### Inspection

Look at the curves of the spine when the patient is standing (Figure 11.6.). The lumbar spine normally shows mild physiological lordosis.

Common, non-specific low back pain is often associated with an exaggeration of this curvature – hyperlordosis. This condition is more common in women and may be aggravated by wearing high

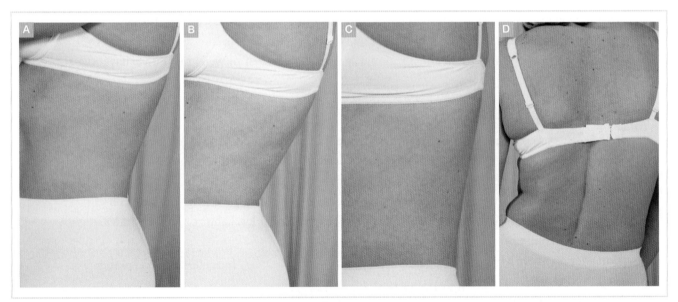

**Figure 11.6.** Normal and abnormal curves of the lumbar spine. **A.** Normal. **B.** Hyperlordosis. **C.** Lost lumbar lordosis. **D.** Scoliosis.

heeled shoes and lack of muscle strength in the abdominal wall. Whatever the cause, hyperlordosis means that the spine's support structures are overloaded and, presumably, there are conflicts of space on the extension surface that lead to exacerbation and maintenance of the pain. One of the aims of treatment is to correct this.

Reduced lordosis or straightening of the lumbar spine is most commonly seen in advanced cases of ankylosing spondylitis.

Scoliosis is also a cause of pain. It may be merely postural or be caused by rotation of the vertebrae (congenital or acquired). If severe, structural scoliosis should be referred to a specialist. Postural scoliosis can normally be corrected by physiotherapy or by compensating for leg-length discrepancy. To distinguish between the two, we ask the standing patient to flex his spine completely and touch the floor with his fingers, keeping knees extended. Postural scoliosis is corrected in this position: the spine is aligned and the shoulders are at the same height. In fixed, structural scoliosis the deviation remains and the shoulders or thoracic wall are asymmetrical (Figure 11.7.).

One of the most common causes of scoliosis and low back pain is leg-length discrepancy. This condition should be found during the clinical examination. While observing the patient from the back, with his knees extended, put your index fingers on the iliac crest on each side and evaluate their relative position (Figure 11.8.). Scoliosis caused by leg-length discrepancy disappears when the patient is sitting. If we suspect significant discrepancy, a precise measurement of the lower limbs can be obtained with x-rays. Correction of significant differences (>1 cm) using insoles or built-up heels can relieve scoliosis, thus treating and preventing back pain.

### Palpation

The joints in the spine are not accessible to direct palpation, as they are too deep.

With the patient lying face down, press the spinous processes from L1 to S2 with the tips of your fingers. Some authors suggest percussion of the spine with a closed fist. Also palpate the paravertebral muscles on either side. Note the location of the pain. The more localized it is, the more relevant it is to the diagnosis.

If the pain is localized, try to distinguish between pain in the longitudinal ligaments (ligamentitis) and vertebral body pain. In the former case, the pain is more intense when you palpate between the spinous processes. This evaluation may be more reliable with the patient sitting with the lumbar spine flexed, using the edge of the chest piece of the stethoscope to palpate the ligaments between the processes (Figure 11.9.).

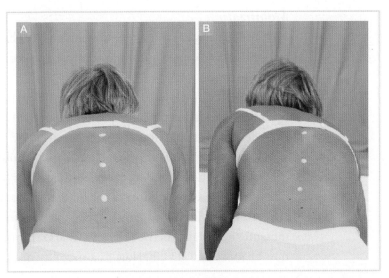

**Figure 11.7.** Postural scoliosis (**A.**) is corrected by flexing the lumbar spine: the spinous processes are aligned and the shoulders level. In structural, fixed scoliosis (**B.**), the abnormal curve persists in flexion and the shoulders and chest wall are assymetrical.

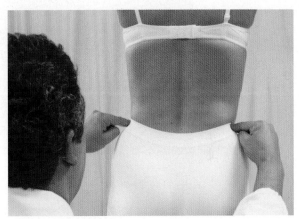

**Figure 11.8.** Clear identification of the iliac crests helps detection of lower limb length discrepancy, a common cause of scolliosis and low back pain.

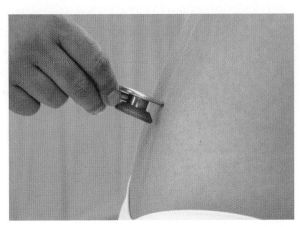

**Figure 11.9.** Exerting pressure between the spinous process with the stethoscope head will cause pain in interspinous ligamentitis.

### Mobilization

When the general rheumatologic examination shows limited mobility of the lumbar spine, it can be useful to quantify it more accurately, especially to assess the results of treatment at subsequent visits.

Lateral flexion of the lumbar spine can be quantified by measuring the distance between the tips of the fingers and the floor when the patient leans to one side and the other with his legs extended and his palm touching his leg.

The best way to quantify flexion is to use **Schober's test** (Figure 11.10.).

With the patient standing at ease, use a marker to indicate the spot where the line joining the iliac crests crosses the middle of the lumbar spine (L4–L5). Using a tape measure, make another mark 10 cm above this point. Ask the patient to flex his spine forward as far as possible and measure the distance between the two marks. In young, healthy individuals, the distance should now be more than 15 cm. Note that mobility of the spine diminishes naturally with age.

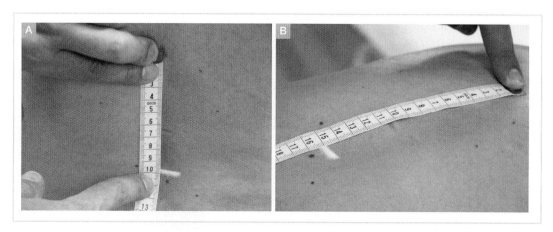

**Figure 11.10.** Schober's test: quantification of lumbar spine flexion. The lower reference is at the level of the iliac crests.

### Examination of the sacroiliac joints

If the back pain is inflammatory, also palpate the sacroiliac joints with the patient lying face down (Figure 11.11A.). Then exert posteroanterior pressure on the median line of the sacrum to see if it causes sacroiliac pain (Figure 11.11B.). After this, ask the patient to lie on his back. Cross your arms and lean your hands on the anterior superior iliac spines (i.e. if you are facing the patient, your left hand on the patient's left anterior superior iliac spine and vice-versa. Push posterolaterally, springing the sacrum on and spread the patient's pelvis (Figure 11.11C.). The manoeuver is positive if it causes pain in the sacral region, suggesting compromise of the sacroiliac joints (the pain under your hands is not significant… but it can be particularly intense in patients with fibromyalgia).

When you have finished examining the abdomen and lower limbs, ask the patient to get up, raising his body without using the arms. The difficulty he experiences gives you an idea of the state of his abdominal muscles, which are the lumbar spine's best friends!

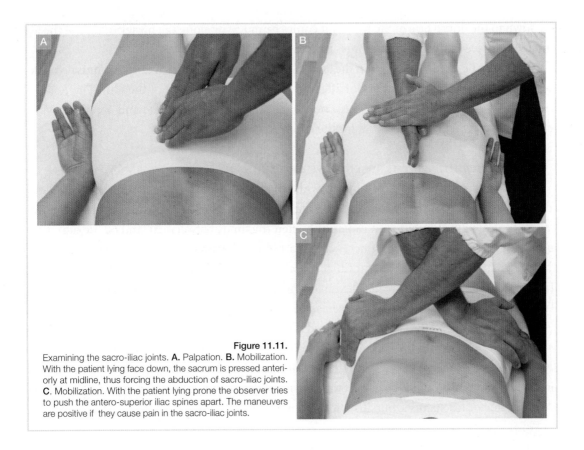

**Figure 11.11.**
Examining the sacro-iliac joints. **A.** Palpation. **B.** Mobilization. With the patient lying face down, the sacrum is pressed anteriorly at midline, thus forcing the abduction of sacro-iliac joints. **C.** Mobilization. With the patient lying prone the observer tries to push the antero-superior iliac spines apart. The maneuvers are positive if they cause pain in the sacro-iliac joints.

## Neurological examination

Any suggestion of neurogenic compromise should lead to a neurological examination of the lower limbs.

The distribution of the sensitive dermatomes of the lumbar roots is shown in Figure 11.12. Table 11.3. shows the muscle strength corresponding to each root.

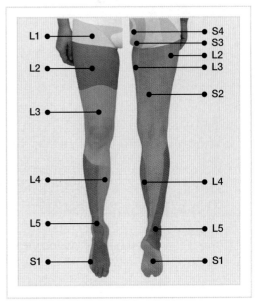

**Figure 11.12.** Skin dermatomes of lumbar nerve roots.

|      | Anterior face          | Posterior face          |
|------|------------------------|-------------------------|
| Hip  | L2, L3 (flexion)       | L4, L5 (extension)      |
| Knee | L3, L4 (extension)     | L5, S1 (flexion)        |
| Foot | L4, L5 (dorsiflexion)  | S1, S2 (extension)      |

**Table 11.3.** Radicular dependence of the strength in the lower limbs.

The patellar reflex depends on L3–L4 and the Achilles reflex on S1.

Sciatic pain is caused by irritation of the roots of L5 and/or S1. It is characterized by its lumbar location with radiation along the posterolateral aspect of the thigh to below the knee. If the pain does not go below the knee, it is called cruralgia, not sciatica. The radiated pain often continues along the antero-lateral face of the leg down to the dorsal face of the foot (if it comes from L5) or along the posterior face of the leg and plantar face of the foot (if it comes from S1).

There may be a sensory deficit in the area of the corresponding dermatome or muscle weakness: reduction of the strength of dorsiflexion (L5) or extension (S1) of the foot. The Achilles reflex may be reduced or absent. These neurological deficits appear late and are highly variable, however, and are not essential for the diagnosis.

***The sciatica stretch tests*** are effective earlier.

The patient is relaxed lying on his back, while you raise his extended leg by the heel and watch for signs of pain (straight leg rising test – Figure 11.13A.). The test is positive if the maneuver causes typical pain (lumbar with radiation) when the hip is between 30 and 60 flexion. Pain appearing above this angle is not necessarily pathological. Pain only in the posterior aspect of the knee may be due to short ischiotibial muscles (common in men) and should be ignored. Then flex the knee to allow greater flexion of the hip and induce passive extension of the knee. Typical pain with radiation constitutes Las gue's sign (Figure 11.13B.).

The diagnosis of sciatica can be reinforced if Bragard's test elicits typical pain. The lower limb is passively elevated, with the knee extended, to the *maximum tolerated without pain*. The foot is then forced into dorsiflexion (Figure 11.13C.). If these signs are inconsistent, we should suspect anxiety or manipulation on the part of the patient or also pseudo-sciatica (due to piriform muscle syndrome or trochanteric bursitis, for example).[2]

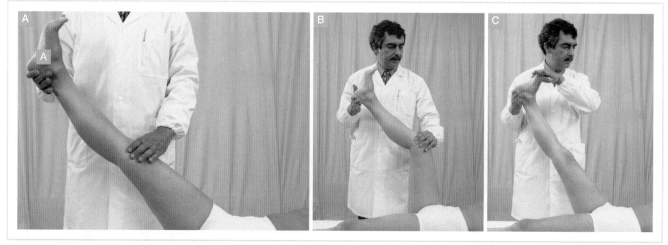

**Figure 11.13.** Sciatic nerve stretch tests. **A.** Passive elevation of the lower limb, with knee extended. **B.** Lasègue's test. **C.** Bragard's test. (Vd. text for explanations.)

[2]One way of distinguishing manipulation by the patient is to cause flexion of the leg with extension of the knee, while the patient is sitting. The manoeuver reproduces Lasègue's test, but is not so well known…

After the enquiry and the clinical examination, the common causes of low back pain can be divided into five main clinical groups.

- Mechanical back pain
- Inflammatory back pain
- Neurogenic back pain
- Back pain of systemic origin
- Psychogenic back pain

## Mechanical back pain

The pain is related to movement and exercise and is relieved by rest. Prolonged standing or sitting can exacerbate the pain. It does not get worse with Valsava's maneuvers. The pain may radiate to the knee but not below it, and is not of a dysesthetic nature. There is no neurological deficit.

Spinal osteoarthritis, postural impairment and small muscle or ligament distensions are the most common underlying causes.

It represents about 90% of cases of back pain in ambulatory clinical practice today and is therefore extremely common.

## Inflammatory back pain

The pain is worse at night and in the morning, and is accompanied by prolonged morning stiffness. Exercise relieves the pain.

Seronegative spondyloarthropathies are the most common cause but do not account for more than 1% of all back pain seen in general practice.

## Neurogenic back pain

The pain is mechanical, but radiates to below the knee following a dermatome (usually L5 or S1). There is often paresthesia and the pain is exacerbated by Valsava's maneuvers. A neurological examination may find impaired strength, sensitivity and myotatic reflexes. Sciatic stretch tests are usually positive. Very occasionally, neurogenic back pain can begin in higher roots, with corresponding radiation and neurological examination results.

Herniated disks are the most common cause, but it may also be due to osteophytosis, fractures, neoplasm, etc.

## Back pain of systemic orgin

The pain may have a varied rhythm but is not usually relieved by lying down. Clinical examination often reveals a clearly defined area of tenderness.

The pain may be referred from intra-abdominal viscera or reflect serious local bony or disc pathologies such as metastases or infection. Systemic manifestations like fever, weight loss or abdominal pain and onset before the age of 30 or after 50 should arouse suspicion.

**Psychogenic back pain**

Purely psychogenic low back pain is rare. Nevertheless, the patient may consciously or unconsciously exaggerate the manifestations of pain in situations such as depression, labor disputes, secondary gain or a manipulative personality.

A psychogenic component may naturally accompany clinical causes of pain and should be given due attention.

Our suspicions should be aroused when the description is particularly dramatic and colorful and the functional limitations described conflict too much with the physical examination of the patient. Multiple, spurious complaints, such as migratory paresthesia, a cold sensation in the back or intense pain on a superficial touch, are common and suggestive. The neurological examination is usually inconsistent.

Consider the possibility of fibromyalgia.

## TYPICAL CASES
## 11.A. CHRONIC BACK PAIN (I)

It was the third time that Manuel, a 68-year old pensioner, had come to emergency and always for the same reason: intense pain in the upper lumbar region that kept him awake at night. The pain was rather erratic: it never went away completely and was particularly intense early in the day, in the late morning and in the evening. He denied any local stiffness and insisted that the pain was not related to movement. There seemed to be some radiation to the abdomen.

In fact, the patient had been suffering from intermittent backache for many years but this was different. It used to be typically mechanical, related to exercise and went away completely on lying down. On his previous visits to emergency he had been given anti-inflammatories, which, according to the patient, seemed to exacerbate the pain. He denied any relevant systemic manifestations, other than slight weakness. He had a past medical history of "gastritis" and indigestion with no other relevant symptoms.

Examination of the spine showed slight limitation of flexion, without pain on local palpation or mobilization. Palpation of the abdomen elicited tenderness in the epigastric region, without guarding.

### Consider the differential diagnosis...

Let us make a list of the dominant characteristics in this clinical condition:

• Chronic, mechanical low back pain that has changed recently

• An uncharacteristic rhythm but perhaps... peptic?

• A perfectly normal local examination

• Exacerbated by anti-inflammatories

• A history of gastritis

### And... there is the possible diagnosis!

We decided to test the possibility before conducting an upper digestive endoscopy. We gave our patient 15 cc of antacid and… the pain soon got better.

An endoscopy the next day confirmed a perforated duodenal ulcer in the posterior wall, most likely causing irritation of the celiac plexus and lumbar pain.

## REFERRED BACK PAIN
### MAIN POINTS

This may appear at any age.

The pain is unrelated to movement.

The rhythm varies with the underlying disease.

An examination of the lumbar spine finds insufficient abnormalities to account for the pain.

The systematic enquiry and physical examination looking for visceral lesions that may lead to lumbar radiation are the key to the diagnosis.

## TYPICAL CASES
## 11.B. ACUTE LOW BACK PAIN (I)

I went to see a friend at his home. I found him surrounded by cushions in his dressing gown on the couch, to which he had moved with difficulty after 3 days in bed with acute low back pain that had appeared when he was trying to lift a heavy object from his car. The pain radiated strongly down the posterolateral aspect of his left thigh and leg down to the plantar aspect of his foot, like an electric shock. It was exacerbated by any attempt at movement, leaving a persistent burning sensation along his lower limb. I asked him if the pain was worse when he coughed or sneezed. "Excruciating," he said. He had never felt such pain in all his 38 years.

He had already taken diclofenac (a fast-acting non-steroidal) and intramuscular injections of high doses of Vitamin B12. The relief he felt with the tablets lasted 3–4 hours. He was scheduled to have an MRI of his lumbar spine the following week.

On clinical examination I noted clear, painful limitation of flexion of the spine. There was a scoliotic deviation to the left with increased tension of the paravertebral muscles on the same side. Las gue's sign was positive on the left at about 50 flexion of the hip joint. His left ankle reflex was clearly reduced in comparison to the right. Muscle strength on extension of the left foot was diminished but there were no apparent changes in sensitivity to pain.

*Summarize the patient's condition.*[3]

*What is your diagnosis?*

*Would you ask for any diagnostic tests? Would an MRI be of any use?*

*What would you advise the patient to do?*

There could be no doubt that Alberto was suffering from sciatica. At his age, and in the absence of any previous pathology, he most likely had a herniated disk, with compression of the S1 root.

I suggested that he began to take a full dose of anti-inflammatory to cover all 24 hours. I recommended additional medication with a muscle relaxant and a further analgesic, as needed. I said that he might find relief lying down, with his spine, hips and knees flexed. Hot baths might also be useful.

[3]Acute low back pain with sciatic radiation and neurological deficit in a young man.

I recommended escalating gentle exercises for his lumbar spine spasm and suggested that he went back to his normal life as soon as possible. I saw no point in continuing the vitamins or having the MRI before seeing how his condition progressed. I did not arrange any diagnostic tests.

My friend went back to work after 3 days and discontinued all treatment after about a week. I strongly urged him to do regular exercises with particular attention to his lumbar and abdominal muscles. I advised him to lose some weight and gave him some advice about posture to protect the lumbar region.

## SCIATICA
## *MAIN POINTS*

Diagnosing sciatica involves:

- Lumbar pain radiating to below the knee with or without paresthesia
- Positive sciatica stretch tests
- Neurological deficit (inconstant)

It appears mainly in young people in association with a herniated disk or spondylolisthesis and, more rarely, in the elderly (compression due to osteophytes or expansive lesion – neoplasm?)

When it is typical, no diagnostic tests are necessary.

Initial treatment consists of short-term rest, analgesics and muscle relaxants.[4]

The patient should be encouraged to resume normal physical activity as soon as possible and to take regular exercise for the spine.

If the pain and neurological deficit persist after four to eight weeks of conservative treatment, it is worth considering physical therapy or even surgery.

## *TYPICAL CASES*
## 11.C. CHRONIC BACK PAIN (II)

Aurora, a 68-year old patient, had been suffering from low back pain for over four years. At first, the pain was recurrent with pain-free periods in between episodes but it got progressively more intense and continuous, forcing her to go to her doctor again. Recently, the pain was located diffusely in the lumbar region. When asked about radiated pain, she said that her buttocks and thighs sometimes hurt too. She had not noticed any paresthesia, but she felt some "weakness" in her legs. The pain was exacerbated by walking and the little exercise that she was still able to take. It was relieved by lying flat on her back.

She also described mechanical pain in both knees, especially when going up and down stairs.

She had had non-insulin-dependent diabetes for about 10 years and was taking medication for hypertension and cardiac insufficiency. She denied any recent weight loss (the opposite…) and had not noticed any changes in her digestive or intestinal habits, or in the appearance of her stools or urine.

Our clinical examination showed an obese woman (weighing 84.2 kg and 1.51 m tall) with difficulty walking. Examination of her chest, abdomen and breasts was normal. The lumbar curvature of her spine was highly accentuated, but without scoliosis. The iliac crests were symmetrical. Active mobilization of the cervical and lumbar spine was painfully limited, especially in extension. There was patellofemoral crepitus, but no other anomalies in the examination of her legs.

Palpation of the lumbar spine and the paravertebral muscles was diffusely painful. A summary neurological examination showed no loss of muscle strength. There were absent ankle reflexes bilaterally. There was a symmetrical loss of sensitivity to pain in her lower legs and feet. The patient was unable to get up from the examining table without supporting herself on her arms, even when starting from 45 flexion.

---

[4]Around the compressed root, there is always some inflammatory reaction that exacerbates and perpetuates the pain. The fullest possible analgesia is important to prevent the vicious circle of pain and muscle spasm that plays an important role in these situations. Early, gentle exercise is important in facilitating the withdrawal of the herniated core. Regular, long-term exercise and care with posture are essential in preventing recurrences.

*What is the most probable diagnosis?*

*What tests and treatment would you suggest?*

We decided that this was a case of chronic, non-specific mechanical back pain. The patient's age and pain on extension made it likely that she was suffering from Spinal osteoarthritis. This would not affect the treatment, however, so we did not request any imaging. The reduced ankle reflexes and the apparent loss of distal sensitivity were probably related to her diabetes mellitus.

Her obesity, hyperlordosis and weakness of the abdominal muscles were exacerbating factors, justifying specific intervention.

We explained the situation to our patient, stressing the effect of her obesity both on the pain and on the diabetes. She was strongly advised to go on a low calorie diet. We reassured the patient as to the likely prognosis of backache, emphasizing the need to stay active and do regular exercises at home to strengthen the spinal and abdominal muscles. We gave her a leaflet of low back exercises and advice as to the best way to protect her back: the right footwear, a firm mattress, how to pick up heavy items, etc.

We prescribed a simple analgesic to be taken as required and arranged to see her again in about two months, hoping to find her thinner and more energetic…

*We have indicated some extra-articular characteristics for this patient. Could any of them have an impact on the way we examined and treated her?*[5]

## COMMON CHRONIC BACK PAIN
### MAIN POINTS

This is a very common condition in clinical practice, especially in the elderly.

It is defined as lumbar pain lasting more than six months with no specific diagnosis.

This diagnosis requires the exclusion of any suggestions of specific pathology ("red flags").

The pain is mechanical, with periods of exacerbation and relief. It often radiates to the buttocks.

A local examination may show reduced mobility, especially in flexion and extension. Palpation is diffusely painful. The neurological examination is normal.

It is often associated with depression, postural deficiency and occupational factors.

No additional diagnostic tests are necessary.

Treatment focuses on mobility and not the pain: analgesia, appropriate regular physical exercise, advice on posture, reaching ideal weight and continuing normal physical activity.

---

[5]Yes. Hypertension and heart failure can be aggravated by non-steroidal anti-inflammatories which can also result in edema and nitrogen retention. The diabetes would contraindicate the use of corticosteroids, if any other situation made them necessary. Type II diabetes and obesity reduce the risk of osteoporosis, which we should always consider in a patient aged 68.

### TYPICAL CASES
### 11.D. ACUTE BACK PAIN (II)

Jorge Esteves, a generally healthy office worker aged 36, went to the emergency department because of acute-onset back pain after heavy lifting when moving house. The pain radiated to the buttocks and the posterior aspect of the thigh, but not lower. It was exacerbated by any attempt at movement and by coughing and sneezing. Clinical examination showed scoliosis concave to the left, with obvious contracture of the left paravertebral muscles. Movements of the spine were painful in all directions. The summary neurological examination was normal. Sciatica stretching tests exacerbated the lumbar pain, with no typical radiation.

### What would you do in this situation?

We assured the patient and his wife that there was nothing seriously wrong with him and that the pain would go away in one or two weeks. We recommended rest for only a day or two and suggested that he gradually went back to his daily routine as soon as possible, even if he still had some pain. We prescribed paracetamol (1 g, four times a day) and a muscle relaxant (for 1 week) and suggested hot baths for relaxation. We gave him advice on posture and a regular exercise plan, which he should start after the acute episode had resolved.

### ACUTE, MECHANICAL BACK PAIN
### MAIN POINTS

It occurs frequently in young individuals, generally associated with lifting.

Muscle contracture, frequently obvious on palpation, plays a decisive role in the initiation and continuation of the process.

In the absence of any unusual clinical elements, no diagnostic tests are necessary.

Treatment is designed to relieve the pain and enable the patient to resume normal physical activity as soon as possible.

Prolonged rest is counterproductive as it facilitates progression to chronicity.

Manipulation of the lumbar spine by an experienced practitioner may be useful in the first four weeks of pain.

Most cases resolve in four to eight weeks. If pain persists for longer the patient should be reassessed or sent to a specialist.

It is important to reassure the patient, and initiate a long-term plan for protecting the joints.

*TYPICAL CASES*
## 11.E. CHRONIC BACK PAIN (III)

Francisco Garção, a 58-year old farmer, was referred urgently to our department because of low back pain with some unusual characteristics. The pain was unrelated to movement and was more intense at night. It had originally been related to farm work but was not relieved by rest or anti-inflammatories. His doctor requested some tests, which showed some surprising alterations. Although the spinal x-ray suggested osteoarthritis in L4–5, his ESR was elevated (45 mm in the first hour).

*Does this seem like ordinary low back pain? Why?*

*What additional information would you try to get?*

When we examined this patient, we were able to confirm the information obtained from his referral letter. Systematic enquiry revealed that he had had a feeling of fever for a few months. He had also noted some weight loss (about 5 kg in the last 3 months). His work involved frequent contact with goats and he regularly drank goat's milk.

The pain was clearly located over L4–L5. Our summary neurological examination was normal.

*What possible diagnoses are there?*

*What diagnostic tests might be useful?*

The x-ray was clearly compatible with discitis (Figure 11.14.). A CT-guided biopsy produced material from which *mycobacterium* tuberculosis was identified.

The patient underwent prolonged treatment which resulted in clinical improvement and normalization of the lab results. However, he still has persistent mechanical low back pain.

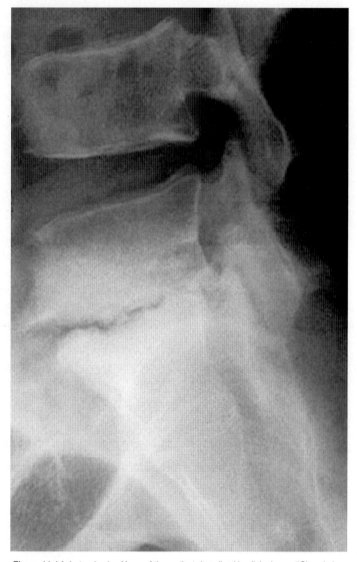

**Figure 11.14.** Lateral spine X-ray of the patient described in clinical case "Chronic low back pain (III)." There is loss of disk height, irregularity and sclerosis of vertebral end-plates. An anterior osteophyte in L5 demonstrates associated osteoarthritis.

## SPONDYLODISCITIS
### *MAIN POINTS*

Discitis (vertebral disk infection) is relatively rare but constitutes a rheumatologic emergency.

It requires rapid diagnosis and treatment to avoid the risk of irreversible neurological sequelae. On suspicion of this disease, the patient should be referred to a specialist immediately without waiting for any radiological alterations, which appear late.

Note the inflammatory rhythm of the pain, its precise location and any association with systemic symptoms of infection.

The acute-phase reactants are high and aid diagnosis and follow-up of treatment.

*Staphylococcus aureus*, streptococci, *Mycobacterium tuberculosis* and *Brucella mellitensis*, are the agents most commonly involved.

In later stages, a plain film of the spine shows loss of intervertebral space and lack of definition of the vertebral endplates sometimes with erosions. The picture may, however, be indistinguishable from ordinary spondyloarthropathy.

It is essential to conduct a biopsy for culture and antibiotic sensivities.

### *TYPICAL CASES*
### 11.F. CHRONIC BACK PAIN (IV)

Carlos, a 21-year old student and a keen amateur cyclist, came to us because of low back pain that had been developing for about two years. At the beginning, the pain was occasional and related to long periods studying at his desk or with more intensive sport. More recently, however, he noticed that the pain was becoming more persistent and was particularly severe in the morning, associated with stiffness. The pain would sometimes wake him up at night. It also got worse after sitting for a long time, but was relieved by exercising the spine.

The pain affected the lower lumbar region and radiated to both buttocks, but no lower. He denied any clinical manifestations of the skin, mucosa or digestive tract.

*Are there any alarm signals in this enquiry?*

*What are the potentially most important aspects of the physical examination?*

Mobility of the spine was painless but slightly reduced (Schober 10–13.8 cm). Assessment of the sacroiliac joints was positive, causing pain in the lumbosacral region. No abnormalities were founding in the skin.

*Summarize this clinical condition.[6]*

*Consider the most probable diagnoses and the diagnostic tests required.*

The clinical information provided pointed strongly to the possibility of ankylosing spondylitis (Chapter 24). This diagnosis was confirmed by an x-ray of the pelvis which showed typical changes in both sacroiliac joints (Figure 11.15.). The hemoglobin and ESR were normal.

*What treatment would you prescribe?*

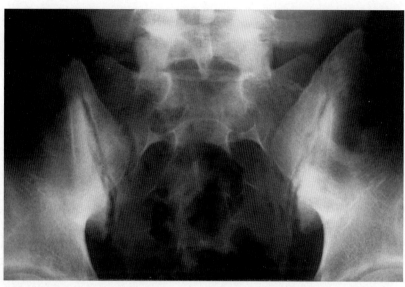

**Figure 11.15.** Anterior view of the lumbar spine. Clinical case "Chronic low back pain (IV)." Note the bone sclerosis surrounding the sacro-iliac joints associated with blurring and erosions of the joint margins: bilateral sacroiliitis.

We began therapy with non-steroidal anti-inflammatories. We explained the nature of the condition and its foreseeable development to the patient, taking an optimistic attitude about his prognosis. We particularly stressed his own role in the treatment: care with posture, regular flexibility exercises for the lumbar spine, breathing exercises, giving up smoking, watching for side effects of the medications, and regular medical checkups. We suggested that he might want to join the Association of Patients with Ankylosing Spondylitis.

## SERONEGATIVE SPONDYLOARTHROPATHIES
### MAIN POINTS

The inflammatory rhythm is an important alarm signal in low back pain – it always warrants careful attention.

Ankylosing spondylitis is the most common of the seronegative spondyloarthropathies (types of arthritis classified together because of their tendency to involve the axial skeleton – Chapter 24).

Males are more commonly affected and the manifestations normally begin in their late teens or twenties.

A careful examination of the sacroiliac joints with specific maneuvers is crucial in identifying sacroiliitis.

The systematic enquiry is important in identifying features associated with the different diseases: psoriasis, urethritis, conjunctivitis, diarrhea, etc...

Radiological alterations appear relatively late, but confirm the diagnosis.

[6]Inflammatory lumbosacral pain in a young man with no systemic manifestations. Probable sacroiliitis.

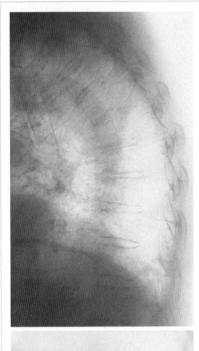

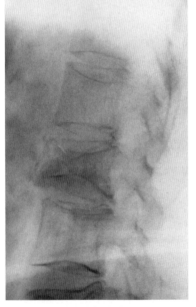

**Figure 11.16.** Clinical case "Acute low back pain (III)." **A.** Compression deformity of L2 and radiological osteopenia of the dorsal and lumbar spine. **B.** Osteoporotic fractures.

### *TYPICAL CASES*
### 11.G. ACUTE BACK PAIN (III)

Celeste Craveiro, a 67-year old housewife, came to the emergency department with severe thoracic and lumbar pain that had appeared the day before following a minor fall at home, with no other consequences. The pain was continuous, only slightly relieved by rest and exacerbated by all movements, including taking deep breaths.

She described occasional chronic low back pain for more than seven years, which responded to analgesics, though it had never been as intense as now. She had been monitored by her family doctor in a remote village for about 10 years for inflammatory joint pain in her hands, wrists, shoulders and feet. She was taking nonsteroidals regularly and was given injections during flare-ups. Although she did not know the name of the injections, she said their effect was "miraculous" for 2–3 months. She described considerable difficulty in walking and was practically housebound. She had had a spontaneous menopause at the age of 48 and had been diabetic for three years. She denied any other symptoms in the systematic enquiry.

*She's your patient! Is this common low back pain? Why?*

*What possible diagnoses can you think of? How would you investigate them?*

Our examination showed a frail patient, with hand deformities typical of rheumatoid arthritis: ulnar deviation of the fingers and swan-neck deformations. The skin of her hands was atrophic with some hemorrhagic suffusion. She had slight Cushingoid facies and a buffalo neck.

An examination of her spine showed accentuated thoracic kyphosis. Mobilization of the thoraco-lumbar spine was extremely painful in all directions. Palpation caused pain at the thoracolumbar junction.

A lateral x-ray of her thoracic and lumbar spines showed accentuated thoracic kyphosis with generalized radiological osteopenia and wedge-shaped deformation of the T12 and L1 vertebral bodies (Figure 11.16.). A radioisotope bone scan showed that these fractures were recent. Her ESR was elevated, but the protein electrophoretic strip was normal.

*What is your final diagnosis?*

*How would you treat it?*

The patient was hospitalized for treatment of the acute episode and the introduction of appropriate therapy for her rheumatoid arthritis and osteoporosis.

*Now think a little:*

- What risk factors for osteoporosis could we identify in this patient?

- What signs of iatrogenic hypercortisolism did this patient have?

- How important is the protein strip is this context?[7]

## OSTEOPOROTIC FRACTURE
### *MAIN POINTS*

This is a common situation in the elderly, especially women.

Although most osteoporotic vertebral fractures are progressive and clinically silent, they can cause acute, intense, incapacitating pain.

Osteoporotic vertebral fractures may occur spontaneously or as the result of a minor trauma.

Symptomatic osteoporotic vertebral fracture requires urgent treatment and often hospitalization.

An osteoporotic fracture indicates a very high risk of further fractures and requires aggressive treatment of the osteoporosis.

Always assess the patient's risk factors for osteoporosis or signs suggesting its existence thus ensuring appropriate treatment.

Prolonged treatment with corticosteroids must always be associated with osteoporosis prophylaxis.

## *TYPICAL CASE*
## 11.H. ACUTE BACK PAIN (IV)

Irene was clearly an obese, highly anxious patient who repeatedly described her pain in dramatic terms ("horrible, ghastly..."), making it difficult to focus our enquiry. Her history seemed to be dominated by pain located in the buttocks and radiating down the outer face of the left thigh and lower leg as far as her foot. The pain had started insidiously three months before. It was exacerbated by a variety of movements, but persisted at night, especially when lying on her left side. Valsava's maneuvers did not exacerbate the pain. She denied any paraesthesia, but felt that she "had no strength at all" in her left leg. The pain had been not been relieved by anti-inflammatory or other analgesic medication, or a course of physiotherapy with application of heat and mobilization of the lumbar spine.

Although our systematic enquiry abounded with all kinds of complaints it was inconsistent.

*Are there any alarm signals?*

*Into what type of low back pain does this condition fit?*

*What aspects of the clinical examination would you focus on most?*

---

[7]Signs: dorsal kyphosis, Cushingoid facies, cutaneous atrophy, diabetes, hypertension. Protein strip: in a patient of this age, with bone pain associated with severe osteoporosis, the possibility of multiple myeloma requires appropriate studies.

Walking was difficult, with manifestations of pain at each step. Flexion of the spine triggered pain in the left hip, thigh and lower leg but was not limited. Palpation of the lumbar spine was diffusely painful. The sciatica stretch tests were contradictory and difficult to interpret: elevation of the limb caused pain at about 80 flexion of the hip. Laségue and Bragard triggered pain in the calves but not the spine. Her ankle reflexes were normal. Sensitivity to pain seemed intact. The strength of extension of the feet seemed reduced on the left side but the patient was able to walk on tiptoe.

Examination of the hip and knees showed no abnormalities, but deep palpation of the left greater trochanter was extremely painful and, according to the patient, reproduced the characteristics of the spontaneous pain.

*What is your diagnosis?*

*What would you suggest to the patient?*

We administered an injection of local anesthetic and corticosteroid into the painful points around the trochanter. Two minutes later the pain was less intense and the patient was able to make previously "impossible" movements.

Our diagnosis was trochanteric bursitis. We suggested bed rest for 24 hours and prescribed a topical anti-inflammatory to be massaged in lightly after the application of heat. We saw the patient again 2 weeks later and she was practically asymptomatic. We stressed the need to lose weight and take regular exercise.

## PSEUDO-SCIATICA
### *MAIN POINTS*

There are a number of situations that can simulate sciatica:

- Trochanteric bursitis;
- Piriform muscle syndrome;
- Iliotibial fascia syndrome.

The clinical examination suggests sciatica but the pain is not normally exacerbated by Valsava's maneuvers.

The neurological examination is negative or inconsistent.

Specific maneuvers for alternative causes in the physical examination are the key to the diagnosis (Chapter 12).

## SPECIAL SITUATIONS

### *Spinal osteoarthritis*

This is osteoarthritis of the joints in the spinal column, involving the intervertebral joints, the facet joints or both.

It is one of the most common findings on plain spine radiographs of patients with (and without!!) low back pain and is almost universal after the age of 55–60, although to varying degrees.

The radiograph may show osteophytes, which are sometimes large, with a reduction in the articular space and subchondral sclerosis (Figure 11.17.). The osteophytes of the facet joints may narrow the intervertebral foraminae leading to nerve root compression. The same is true for intervertebral osteophytes in a posterolateral location. The most obvious osteophytes in a standard film, however (marginal anterior and lateral), cannot cause nerve compression and are important mainly as indicators of general alterations in the morphology and function of the spine and not as individual sources of symptoms.

The radiological appearance of spinal osteoarthritis may easily lead us to attribute the symptoms to it. We should, however, bear two basic aspects in mind:

1. The correlation between the radiological appearance and clinical signs and symptoms is very poor. We are just as likely to examine patients with few or no symptoms and a "disastrous" plain film or to come up against just the opposite. The severity of the situation depends on the symptoms, not on the x-ray.

2. Spinal osteoarthritis only justifies specific treatment in exceptional cases (if there is a neurological deficit). Even in these cases, we have to give this careful thought as it requires surgery, which is not always successful. In most patients with low back pain and spinal

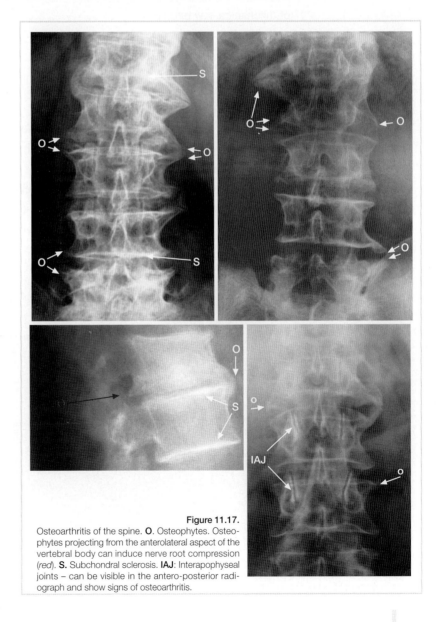

**Figure 11.17.**
Osteoarthritis of the spine. **O**. Osteophytes. Osteophytes projecting from the anterolateral aspect of the vertebral body can induce nerve root compression (*red*). **S**. Subchondral sclerosis. **IAJ**: Interapophyseal joints – can be visible in the antero-posterior radiograph and show signs of osteoarthritis.

osteoarthritis the treatment is the same as for other chronic mechanical low back pain without radiological alterations: focusing on mobility and not on the pain, on the patient's quality of life and not on his or her x-ray, and essentially aiming at relieving the symptoms and protecting the joints (exercise and keeping up normal physical activity).

---

### NOTE THAT

**Spinal osteoarthritis:**

- The correlation between the clinical examination and the x-ray is very poor.

- Specific treatment is only justified if there is neurological deficit or untreatable pain.

- For practical purposes it should not be considered a specific diagnosis. The clinical examination is decisive. Assessment and treatment follow the same principles for any kind of mechanical low back pain.

---

### Diffuse idiopathic skeletal hyperostosis

Diffuse idiopathic skeletal hyperostosis (DISH), also called Forrestier's disease, is a common condition and may be mistaken for spinal osteoarthritis or ankylosing spondylitis in clinical or radiological examinations.

This disease involves calcification of the intervertebral ligaments, forming bony bridges between adjacent vertebrae and limiting their mobility. The calcifications form excrescences between adjacent vertebral bodies, usually predominating on the right side of the thoracic spine. A profile x-ray often shows calcification of the anterior vertebral ligament, in front of the anterior face of the vertebral body and intervertebral disks. To satisfy the radiological criteria of the disease at least four adjacent vertebral bodies must be involved.

Unlike spinal osteoarthritis, the height of the disk spaces is unchanged and there is no subchondral sclerosis (Figure 11.18.).

It is most common in middle-aged and elderly men and the statistics associate the risk with alcoholism and diabetes mellitus. The symptoms are few, usually limited to mechani-

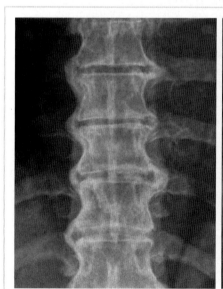
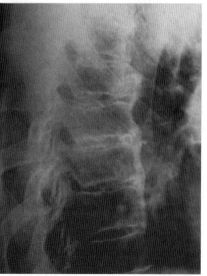

**Figure 11.18.** Diffuse Idiopathic Skeletal Hyperostosis (DISH). "Bone bridges" between adjacent vertebral bodies may suggest osteophytes but the disk space is preserved. Abnormalities frequently predominate on the right side of the body.

cal axial discomfort and reduced mobility.

Peripheral joints may be involved in this hyperostotic tendency, leading to early osteoarthritis with exuberant osteophytosis and often calcification of periarticular ligaments and entheses.

Treatment is essentially symptomatic.

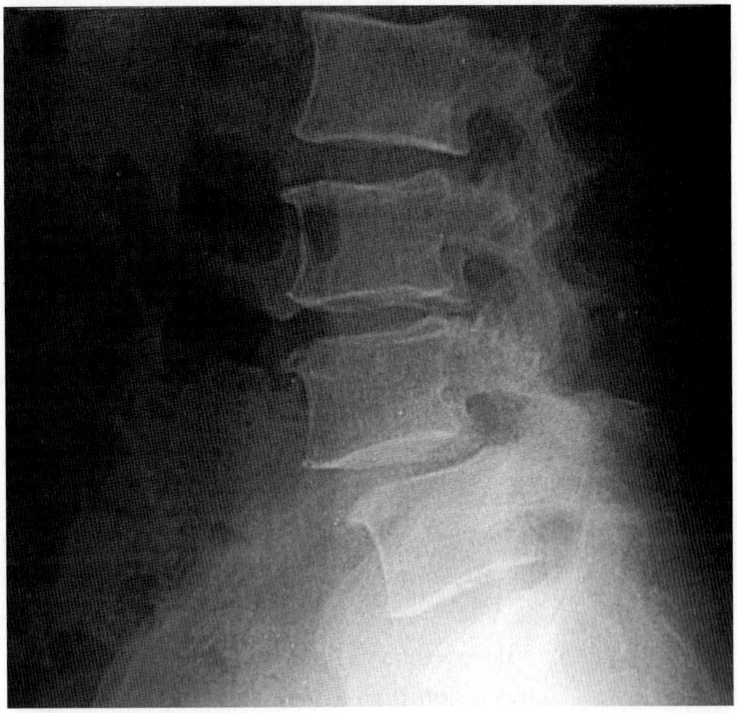

### Spondylolisthesis

This is caused by a defect in the vertebral isthmuses allowing the vertebral body to lose the fixation represented by the facet joints and slide over the underlying vertebra (Figure 11.19.). It is often congenital, but may be caused by trauma.

**Figure 11.19.** Spondylolisthesis. Anterior dislocation of one vertebral body over the underlying one.

The relationship with clinical manifestations is highly variable. The patient may mention lumbar pain that is generally worse in extension. The greater the degree of dislocation, the greater the probability of its causing symptoms. On rare occasions it may cause nerve compression.

Treatment is essentially conservative (exercise, posture, reassurance), resorting to surgical stabilization in cases of severe symptoms.

### Spina bifida

This is caused by a congenital defect in the development of the lumbar spine, which consists of the duplication of the spinous processes, leaving the posterior wall of the spinal canal without complete coverage by bone.

It is very common and is a frequently reported radiological finding. In most cases, it is benign and asymptomatic, and should not normally be considered the cause of painful or neurogenic symptoms.

### Fibromyalgia

Although the typical symptom of fibromyalgia is generalized pain (Chapter 15), many patients with this condition locate the pain predominantly in the lumbar region. If the patient is not questioned carefully, we may focus our attention on this region and the underlying diagnosis is missed and thus the appropriate treatment not offered.

# DIAGNOSTIC TESTS

A common mistake in clinical practice is to request too many tests in cases of low back pain.

Most cases of low back pain are mechanical, with no alarm signals, and do not require any tests, as the clinical examination provides enough information to diagnose and treat it. If we request spine radiographs for all these patients, we will find some kind of structural abnormality in many of them, especially varying degrees of spinal osteoarthritis. These findings should not, however, change our choice of treatment, as we do not have specific measures for each condition and the relationship between radiology and clinical examination is very weak. An investigation that does not change treatment is unnecessary!

In addition, unnecessary x-rays are far from harmless. The dose of radiation in repeated x-rays is by no means negligible, but the most important thing is the impact that these investigations and their findings have on the patients' approach to their condition. When faced with a structural diagnosis that they find hard to interpret, patients naturally focus on the disease and not on their mobility. This may reinforce their tendency to avoid exercise, which is the opposite of what is required, and also to justify their "role as a patient" or secondary gains.

If we want the patient to remain active in spite of the pain, it is better to play down irrelevant x-ray results than to lend them too much importance.

Diagnostic tests should depend on the clinical types of low back pain described above:

## *Mechanical low back pain*

In most cases no diagnostic tests are justified. If they are necessary to reassure an overanxious patient, we should limit them to the essential and avoid repeating them. The focus should remain on mobility and not on the pain or its cause.

## *Inflammatory low back pain*

As ankylosing spondylitis is the most common cause of this condition, it is worth requesting a anteroposterior x-ray of the pelvis to study the sacroiliac joints and two x-ray projections of the lumbar spine to look at vertebral morphology and detect any syndesmophytes (see Chapter 24). These plain films are also appropriate for other types of seronegative spondyloarthropathy. The abnormal findings are, however, relatively late and their absence should not rule out a clinically grounded diagnosis.

## *Neurogenic low back pain*

Clinical history and the physical examination are the basis of diagnosis. Electrophysiological studies may be warranted when we are in doubt as to neurological function. An ordinary x-ray of the spine in no way confirms or rules out radicular compression or its location. It may be useful only to ascertain the general state of the spine and the advisability of surgery.

CT or MRI scans are only justified if surgery is being considered. Otherwise, they can bring more problems than solutions. For example, MRI scans identify small disk anomalies in a large percentage of totally asymptomatic people. They can only be interpreted in the light of a clearly defined neurological deficit.

## Low back pain of systemic origin

Tests will depend on the nature of our clinical suspicion (metastases, local infection or osteoporotic fracture), and can include a wide range of diagnostic studies: full blood count, acute phase reactants, plain films, bacteriological tests, biopsy, gastro-intestinal endoscopy, bone scintigraphy (metastases), densitometry, etc.

## Psychogenic low back pain

This is the situation in which unnecessary tests pose the greatest iatrogenic risk. Once we are sure of our diagnosis, we should be firm in establishing the limits to further investigations and in defending a clear, consistent plan of action.

# TREATMENT

The treatment of low back pain with a specific diagnosis has already been addressed or will be dealt with in the appropriate chapters.

The comments below focus on the treatment of the most common condition, mechanical low back pain.

### 1. Educating the patient and preventing recurrences and chronicity

This is a fundamental aspect in treating low back pain.

We must first be aware of the patients' psychological relationship with their illness, encouraging them and their families to take a positive, proactive attitude in which the patients try to lead as full and normal a life as possible in spite of the pain. Overprotective attitudes, despondency and dependence on others should be fought. Optimism and self-sufficiency above all else!

The quality of the doctor-patient relationship has been scientifically identified as one of the most important factors in the progression of low back pain.

## 2. Rest and exercise

Contrary to traditional belief, it has been shown that prolonged rest actually extends the duration of acute low back pain episodes and promotes progression to chronicity. In acute, incapacitating low back pain the patient should be advised to rest for a short time (no more than 48–72 hours) and encouraged to return to normal life as soon as possible. Physiotherapy may be necessary in some cases.

We should make sufferers from chronic low back pain aware of the crucial importance of regular exercise and care with posture, if possible giving them leaflets like that shown in Figure 11.20. These exercises are also the best way of preventing the recurrence of acute episodes.

We should also explain the importance of body weight and the best way of protecting the spine during daily activities as this helps the patient to adhere to the treatment. Patients must be made to feel that they play the most important role in their own treatment.

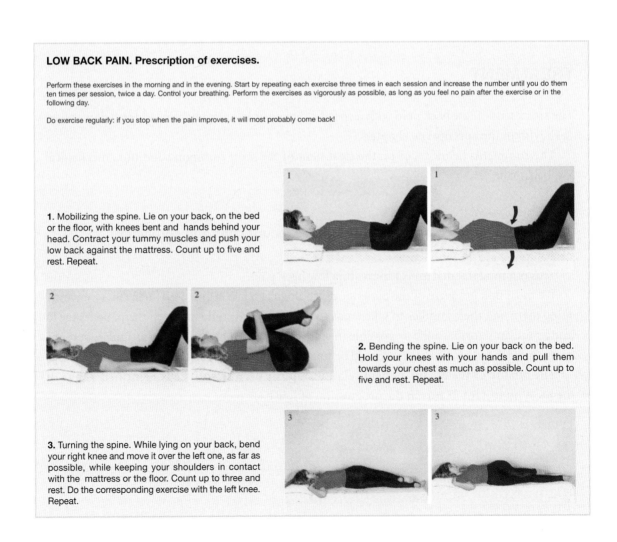

**LOW BACK PAIN. Prescription of exercises.**

Perform these exercises in the morning and in the evening. Start by repeating each exercise three times in each session and increase the number until you do them ten times per session, twice a day. Control your breathing. Perform the exercises as vigorously as possible, as long as you feel no pain after the exercise or in the following day.

Do exercise regularly: if you stop when the pain improves, it will most probably come back!

**1.** Mobilizing the spine. Lie on your back, on the bed or the floor, with knees bent and hands behind your head. Contract your tummy muscles and push your low back against the mattress. Count up to five and rest. Repeat.

**2.** Bending the spine. Lie on your back on the bed. Hold your knees with your hands and pull them towards your chest as much as possible. Count up to five and rest. Repeat.

**3.** Turning the spine. While lying on your back, bend your right knee and move it over the left one, as far as possible, while keeping your shoulders in contact with the mattress or the floor. Count up to three and rest. Do the corresponding exercise with the left knee. Repeat.

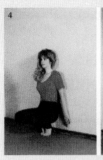
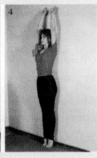

**4.** Stretching. Try to stretch your body as much as possible. Force your heels, buttocks, shoulders and back of the head against the wall. Bend your knees and stand again, reaching as high as possible, while keeping in touch with the wall.

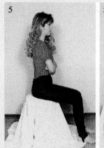
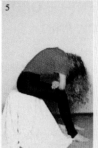

**5.** Sit down with your arms around the waist. Bend forward until your elbows touch the knees. Count up to five and rest. Repeat.

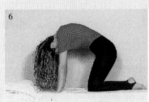
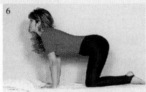

**6.** Place yourself as in picture 6. Bend your low back upwards and hold. Now bend it down and hold. Repeat.

**7.** Strengthening your abdominal muscles (a). Lie on your back with your arms alongside you. Keep your knees straight and rise your heels about 20cm above the floor. Count up to five. Rest, relax and repeat.

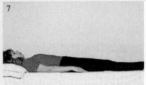
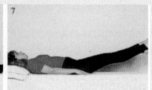

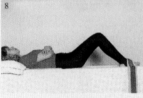
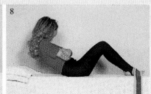

**8.** Strengthening your abdominal muscles (b). Lie on your back and strap your feet. Keep your knees bent to about 40 to 50°. Cross your arms in front of you and rise slowly from the bed as far as possible. Count up to five and slowly return to the initial position. Repeat.

**9.** Bend over a table, with a pillow under your tummy. Hold to the table and rise your legs from the floor. Count up to three and rest. Rise your body from the table. Rest. Repeat.

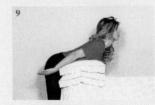
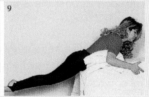

### Other means of protecting your back

**1. Body weight.** Excess body weight demands too much effort from your back, wearing out your bones and tiring your muscles. It is essential that you keep an appropriate body weight. (As an approximate rule, your weight in Kg should not exceed the number of cm of your height, above 1 m. Example: height 156cm. Ideal maximum weight ~56Kg)

**2. Mattress and pillow.** Be aware of soft mattresses! They may seem comfortable but they will not keep your back in a healthy position. Avoid sleeping on your stomach. Your will appreciate it.

**3. Seating.** Try to seat up straight, hold your back against the seat and get it close to the table. Use a lumbar support if needed. Always try to seat facing your working area, especially for prolonged tasks.

**4. Bending down.** Whenever possible, try to bend your knees and keep your back straight.

**5. Standing.** When required to stand up for long periods, use a a support to keep one of your feet about 15cm above the floor level. This will help your back to rest.

**6. Footware.** Give preference to shoes with about 2 cm of heel height.

**7. Carrying weights.** To shift and carry weights, use rule nº 4. Carry the weight close to your body. Whenever possible distribute the weight equally between your arms.

**8. Rest.** Try to distribute your workload during the day and plan periods of rest. Lie on your back and stretch out. A pillow under your knees may help your back to relax.

*Perform these exercises regularly.*
*Help yourself!*

**Figure 11.20.** Exercises for low back pain patients. Example of a patient leaflet. We suggest that the proposal is presented as a formal "prescription" (Produced in cooperation with Prof. J. Pascoa Pinheiro).

## TREATMENT OF ORDINARY MECHANICAL LOW BACK PAIN
### *General Guidelines*
Royal College of General Practitioners, UK[8]

**Assessment**

- Carry out diagnostic triage.
- X-rays are not routinely indicated in simple backache.
- Consider the psychological factors.

**Medication**

- Prescribe analgesics at regular intervals and not p.r.n.
- Start with paracetamol. If inadequate, replace with NSAIDs. Finally consider adding a short course of muscle relaxant.
- Avoid strong opioids if possible.
- Bed rest.
- Do not recommend or use bed rest as a treatment in simple low back pain.
- Some patients may be confined to bed for a few days as a consequence of their pain, but this should not be considered a treatment.

**Advice on staying active**

- Advise patients to stay as active as possible and to continue normal daily activities.
- Advise patients to increase their physical activities progressively over a few days or weeks.
- If a patient is working, then advice to stay at work or return to work as soon as possible is probably beneficial.

**Manipulation**

- Consider manipulative treatment in the first six weeks of an acute episode for patients who need additional help with pain relief or who are failing to return to normal activities.

**Physical therapy**

- Referral for physiotherapy/rehabilitation should be considered for patients who have not returned to ordinary activities and work by 6 weeks.

**Psychological aspects**

- Psychological, social and economic factors play an important role in chronic low back pain and physical disability. They influence the patient's response to treatment and rehabilitation.
- Psychological factors are important much earlier than we first thought.

## 3. Analgesics, anti-inflammatories and muscle relaxants

In low back pain, a vicious circle of pain and muscle spasm often sets in: intense, repeated nociceptive stimuli caused by the disease result in exaggerated reflex muscle contraction, which accentuates and perpetuates the pain. This phenomenon is particularly important in cases of acute low back pain in which the muscle spasm may be clinically apparent. In these circumstances, it is important to relieve the pain as much as possible, not only for the patient's comfort but also for the physiopathological resolution of the clinical condition. We should opt for ordinary analgesics and save anti-inflammatories for more resistant cases. Muscle relaxants are particularly useful for exaggerated reflex muscle contraction.

In persistent, chronic cases, small doses of antidepressants (e.g. amitriptyline) may be very helpful in pain control.

## 4. Physical therapy

The local application of wet heat has a very useful relaxing effect, especially in acute low back pain. In the same way, a gentle local massage can help to relieve muscle contracture. Patients and their families can do this themselves at home with very little instruction (in a hot bath for example). Physical therapy may be necessary in cases that are particularly severe or resistant to simple measures. Manipulation of the spine by an experienced therapist may be very useful in the initial stages (<4 weeks) of an acute episode.

[8]For more information or to access the latest version: http://rcgp.org.uk

Physiotherapy sessions can be useful in dealing with chronic low back pain with incapacitating flare-ups, but the patient must also be committed to exercises regularly. Visits to physical therapy centers should always be used to educate the patient and not only for passive treatment sessions.

### WHEN SHOULD THE PATIENT BE REFERRED TO A SPECIALIST?

(Most patients with low back pain can and should be treated by their GP.)

All inflammatory back pain of unexplained causes.

Whenever there is reason to suspect an underlying systemic cause.

When there is neurological deficit that persists after conservative treatment.

In acute mechanical back pain if intense pain persists after 4–6 weeks of conservative treatment.

In chronic mechanical low back pain, if incapacitating pain persists in spite of an integrated plan of general care.

## REGIONAL SYNDROMES. LOW BACK PAIN
### ADDITIONAL PRACTICE

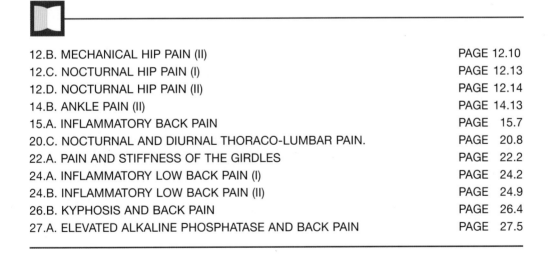

# REGIONAL SYNDROMES
## THE HIP

**12.**

J.A.P. da Silva, A.D. Woolf, *Rheumatology in Practice*, DOI 10.1007/978-1-84882-581-9_12,
© Springer-Verlag London Limited 2010

# 12. REGIONAL SYNDROMES THE HIP

The hip joint and the adjacent muscles and ligaments are often the site of disease. Given the importance of these structures in walking, their involvement can be an important cause of disability and suffering. Regional conditions can also seriously impair sexual activity. Given its deep location, physical examination of the hip is more about examining the joint movements than palpation but history and examination remain the pillar of most common diagnoses involving the hip.

## FUNCTIONAL ANATOMY

The hip joint consists of the femoral head and the acetabulum of the iliac bone (or hip bone). The depth of the acetabulum is increased by the acetabular labrum, a ring-shaped fibrocartilaginous structure that forms a tight collar around the femoral head. The labrum has a space in its lower part through which the transverse ligament passes, taking blood vessels to the inside of the joint.

The joint is covered by a resistant capsule that inserts around the acetabulum and the lateral end of the femoral neck, which is thus located inside the joint. The capsule is reinforced anteriorly, inferiorly and posteriorly by strong ligaments. Stability is increased by the muscles and ligamentum teres, an intra-articular ligament which arises from the acetabular rim and inserts into the vertex of the femoral head.

The joint is deep-set and surrounded by powerful muscles that join the iliac bone and the proximal femur. Figure 12.1. shows the local muscle insertions. Several muscles insert into the

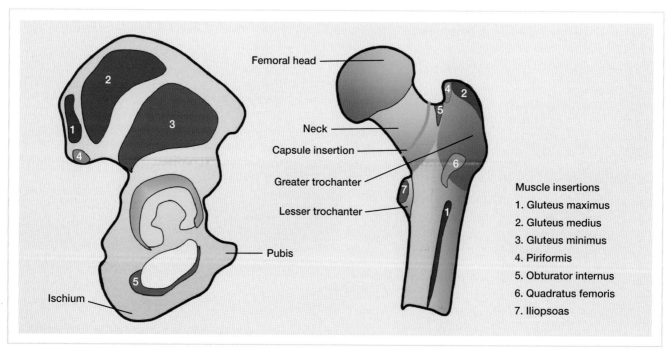

**Figure 12.1.** Muscle insertions on the iliac bone and proximal femur. Simplified scheme posterior aspect, right side).

superior, posterior and internal face of the trochanter. These muscles are responsible for abduction and external rotation of the thigh (piriform, internal obturator, superior and inferior gemelli, and quadriceps femoris). The external aspect of the greater trochanter is covered by the trochanteric bursa with extensions between the insertion fibers of the external rotators at the posterior and superior edge of the trochanter (Figure 12.2.). This area is often the site of painful inflammation. Given that it is not easy to distinguish bursitis from tendonitis on clinical grounds, we will use the expression "burso-tendonitis."

The sciatic nerve, which originates in the roots of L4 to S3, leaves the pelvis through the great sciatic foramen formed between the iliac bone and the sacrum, passing under the piriform muscle, which can produce pseudo-sciatic pain when inflamed.

The ischiotibial muscles (semimembranous, semitendinous and femoral biceps) insert into the ischium. The first two join the iliac to the anterointernal face of the tibia. The biceps inserts into the lateral condyle of the tibia and head of the fibula. The ischium is covered by a bursa that can become inflamed causing local pain when sitting.

The iliotibial fascia, which is the direct continuation of the tensor fascia lata, extends along the lateral face of the thigh from the iliac crest to the external tubercle of the tibia. Powerful muscles insert into it and can cause excessive tension and pain.

The joint is capable of flexion (120°, diminishing with age), extension (about 30°), external rotation (60°), internal rotation (30°–40°), abduction (about 45°) and adduction (about 30°).

Flexion depends mainly on the iliopsoas muscle, which is innervated by L2/3. Extension is mainly the task of the gluteus maximus and the ischiotibials, which depend on L4/5 and S1/2, respectively. External rotation is induced by the gluteus maximus, piriform and quadriceps femoris (L4/5 and S1). Internal rotation is mainly the responsibility of the gluteus minimus (L4/5 and S1). Figure 11.12. shows the dermatomes of the hip.

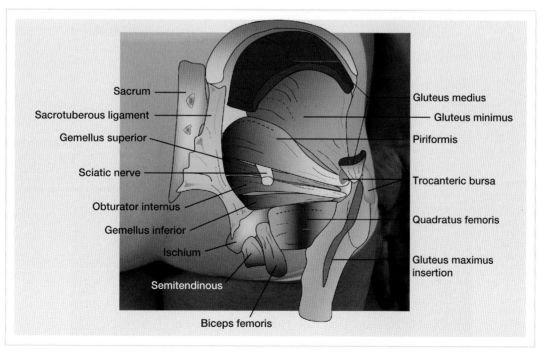

**Figure 12.2.** Muscles inserted posteriorly to the great trochanter and trochanteric bursa.

## Radiological anatomy

From an anteroposterior view (Figure 12.3A.) we can see the hip joints: size and regularity of the articular space and surfaces, morphology of the femoral head, and coverage of the head by the acetabulum. This is also the best routine angle for evaluating the sacroiliac joints. Look at their lower third and assess the size of the space and the definition, density and regularity of the articular surfaces. Look for focal alterations in the bone density of the iliacs and proximal femur (lytic or sclerotic lesions).

The lateral radiograph (Figure 12.3B.) shows changes in the joint space and the morphology of the head or even fractures that may not be evident when viewed anteroposteriorly.

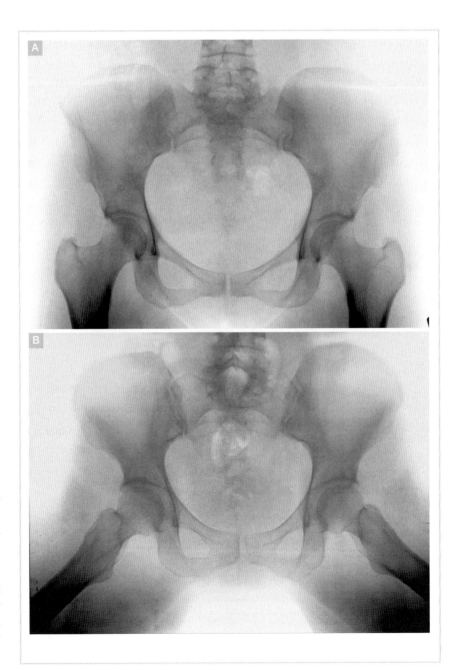

**Figure 12.3.**
Radiological anatomy of the pelvis. **A.** Antero-posterior view – the hip and sacro-iliac joints. Search for lytic or sclerotic focal lesions, as well as fractures, in the iliac bones and proximal part of the femurs. **B.** Frog-leg view. Additional evaluation of the hip joints and of the femoral head. Some fractures of the proximal femur will only be detected with this view.

# COMMON CAUSES OF PAIN IN THE HIP AREA

Referred pain, burso-tendonitis and osteoarthritis are the most common causes of isolated hip area pain (Table 12.1.). The joint is often involved in polyarticular disease, in which case the clinical context suggests the diagnosis and suitable investigation. A thorough local examination is always essential, not only to clarify the nature of the local involvement, but also to assess the indication for local therapy adjuvant to the systemic treatment.

| Etiology | Clinical clues |
|---|---|
| Referred pain | Pain radiating from the lumbar spine, sacroiliac joints, appendix and urinary tract |
| | Poorly defined |
| | Associated manifestations |
| | Normal local examination |
| Trochanteric burso-tendonitis | Pain in the lateral aspect of the hip |
| | Worse at night (lying on ipsilateral side) |
| | Frequent pseudo-sciatic radiation |
| | Typical pain on local pressure |
| Osteoarthritis | Mechanical pain |
| | Progressive onset |
| | Limited active and passive mobility |
| | Predominates in the elderly |
| Arthritis | Rarely monoarthritis |
| | Inflammatory pain |
| | Suggestive general context |
| | Limited active and passive mobility |
| Tendonitis of the adductors | Pain in the inguinal region |
| | Exacerbated by forced abduction |
| | Often accompanies hip disease |
| | Typical pain on local pressure |
| | Specific provocation maneuvers |

**Table 12.1.** Common causes of hip pain.

## THE ENQUIRY

### *The exact location of the pain*

The location of the pain is an important clue for diagnosis. Hip joint pain is usually located deep in the groin along the inguinal ligament, although in some patients it is felt deep in the buttocks.

Pain referred from the spine and sacroiliac joints, which is probably the most common in clinical practice, affects the buttocks diffusely. Occasionally pain of this origin is accompanied by dysesthesia.

Trochanteric burso-tendonitis may be extremely misleading. Usually, the patient (typically an obese, middle-aged woman), locates the pain in the lateral aspect of the hip. In some cases, however, the pain radiates to the buttocks and even down to the knee, along the external aspect of the thigh. In tendonitis of the adductors, the pain is confined to the medial aspect of the inguinal region.

### *The rhythm of the pain*

Pain due to osteoarthritis and synovitis has the expected mechanical and inflammatory rhythms, respectively. The rhythm of referred pain depends on the cause. In most cases it is mechanical, and is often associated with chronic mechanical backache. The pain from sacroiliitis, however, often involves the buttocks, with a typically inflammatory rhythm.

Pain caused by lesions of the soft tissues is more variable in rhythm and is mostly associated with walking and postures that cause tension or compression of the inflamed structures.

### *Exacerbating factors*

Exacerbation of pain when the patient is lying on their side in bed is strongly suggestive of ipsilateral trochanteric burso-tendonitis. The pain from tendonitis of the adductors worsens with abduction, when getting into a car for example. Both may be exacerbated by walking, but not by flexion of the spine.

On the contrary, this last symptom suggests pain radiating from the lumbar spine. Exacerbation of the pain by Valsava's maneuvers also suggests a lumbar cause. Note, however, that more anxious patients may describe this feature in other situations.

### *Form of onset and clinical context*

The onset of osteoarthritis is usually very slow and progressive. As a rule, the patient goes to the doctor only after several years of recurrent episodes of pain of growing intensity. Most patients with hip osteoarthritis have the same disease in other load-bearing joints, particularly the knees. It usually affects the elderly.

Monoarthritis of the hip is very rare. In most cases, hip synovitis appears in the context of an oligo- or polyarticular inflammatory disease and can be found in practically all types of arthritis. Monoarthritis of the hip should be considered septic until proven otherwise. In either case, the onset is relatively quick (days or weeks).

Radiating pain is usually accompanied by chronic or recurrent acute low back pain, which should be taken into account, even if the patient focuses his or her description on the hip area. Occasionally, a patient with hip region pain and fever may have appendicitis or a urinary infection.

Trochanteric burso-tendonitis is extremely common in clinical practice and often appears with no associated pathology. It may simulate sciatica. Remember to exclude this possibility whenever you are thinking of sciatic pain!

Conversely, tendonitis of the adductors most often accompanies a recent exacerbation of hip joint disease. Even in these situations, it often dominates the patient's clinical condition, making its identification and treatment very rewarding, even if the joint disease persists.

Hip region pain is also common in patients with fibromyalgia. Four of the typically sensitive points of fibromyalgia are located around this area (Chapter 15). Pay attention to the context of generalized pain.

## THE REGIONAL EXAMINATION

### Inspection

Inspection is not very productive in diseases of the hip, as it is a deep joint protected by muscle. Periarticular lesions are not usually accompanied by visible swelling or redness. Clinical assessment of the hip joint is based essentially on mobilization.

Leg length discrepancy, described in the previous chapter, may also cause hip pain and should be considered.

### Mobilization

Mobilization of the hip as described in the general rheumatologic examination is sufficient for exploring this joint. Mobilization is passive while the patient is lying on their back relaxed.

> 1. We first induce passive elevation of the leg, thus testing the sciatic nerve, then assess flexion, extension, internal and external rotation, abduction and adduction, as described in Chapter 6.

Note that angles given as normal for these movements vary from one person to another, and tend to diminish with age. Always make a comparison with the other side.

Hip osteoarthritis starts with painful limitation of internal rotation and abduction, and affects the other movements later. Do not forget that extension is assessed while forcing flexion of the contralateral hip (Thomas's test).

In hip joint synovitis, all movements are painful.

In referred pain, mobilization of the hip, especially forced flexion, may cause pain in the lumbar region, possibly radiating to the buttocks.

Patients with trochanteric bursitis-tendonitis often complain of pain on forced internal rotation, though it is not always present.

In tendonitis of the adductors, the pain is more intense during forced abduction. Where appropriate, this condition should be explored with more specific maneuvers:

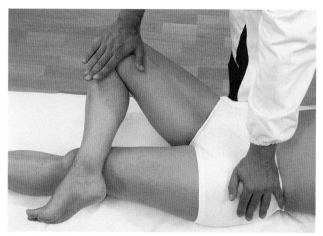

**Figure 12.4.** Forced abduction with external rotation. Pain in the insertion of the adductor muscles close the pubic symphysis suggest adductor tendonitis.

2. The patient crosses his legs, placing his foot on the outside of the contralateral knee. The observer then forces abduction (Figure 12.4.). This maneuver causes pain on the inside of the inguinal region, in the presence of tendonitis of the adductors.

3. With his knee flexed to about 90° and his foot on the examining table, the patient is asked to adduct his knee, against the observer's resistance (Figure 12.5.). Pain in the inguinal region suggests the diagnosis, especially if it is exacerbated by direct palpation.

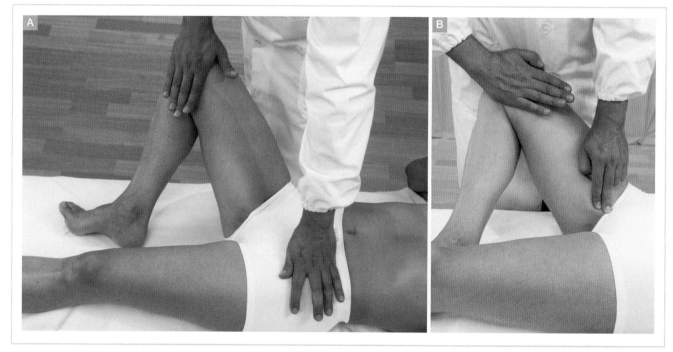

**Figure 12.5. A.** Resisted adduction of the thigh. Pain the inguinal area suggests adductor tendonitis. **B.** Tenderness at the tendon insertion also supports the diagnosis.

### Palpation

The hip joint is not directly palpable, and so we cannot directly assess the existence of swelling, effusion, heat or even crepitus.

Palpation is used mainly to examine the points of common periarticular involvement:

4. Bursa and trochanter muscle insertions. Slide your fingers over the external aspect of the hip from the iliac crest, palpating deeply. Note the bony promontory formed by the greater trochanter. Exert firm pressure on the external face of this promontory. This is where the trochanteric bursa is located. Also palpate along the superior and posterior edges of the trochanter. This is the most common location of pain, suggesting inflammation of the muscle insertions of the abductors (Figure 12.6.). Quite often this area of tenderness extends distally well into the fascia lata.

If in doubt as to the intensity of the pain and palpation, examine the other side.

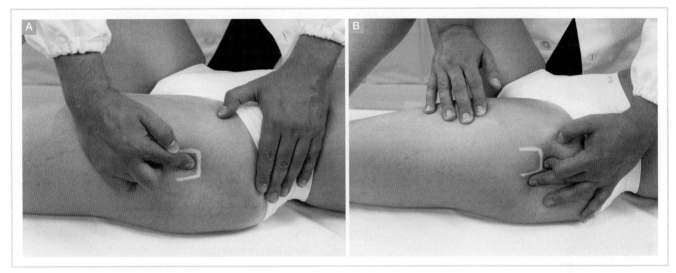

**Figure 12.6.** Palpating the trochanteric bursa (**A.**) and muscle insertions in the vicinity (**B.**).

Note that there may be pain on palpation in the absence of local inflammation. It is a frequent finding in fibromyalgia.

Clinical assessment of the hip is not complete without an examination of the lumbar spine and the knee. A careful abdominal and pelvic examination is also indicated on occasions.

### TYPICAL CASES
### 12.A. MECHANICAL HIP PAIN (I)

Alfredo Porfírio, an 82-year old farmer, had been monitored by his doctor for years with polyarticular osteoarthritis involving the spine, hips and knees, which was being treated with analgesics and anti-inflammatories. The pain was typical: exacerbated by exercise and walking and relieved by rest, with no significant morning stiffness. He had been offered replacement surgery for his right hip, but he had declined because of the many associated diseases that he had as well as the advice of his cardiologist. He came to us because the pain in his right hip had recently worsened, further limiting his walking and also making it difficult to drive. He also said that the pain persisted at night in the right inguinal region.

He walked with small steps and rotation of the pelvis. An examination of his hips showed extreme limitation of mobility in abduction, adduction, internal and external rotation and extension. He could manage about 90 flexion. There were no doubts about the diagnosis from the pelvic x-ray that he had with him (Figure 12.7.).

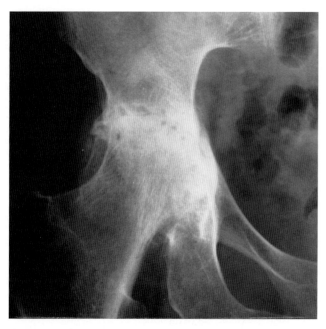

**Figure 12.7.** Radiograph of the right hip – Clinical case "Mechanical hip pain (I)". Note the complete loss of joint space associated with subchondral sclerosis, focal radiolucent areas (geodes or subchondral cysts). These are typical features of osteoarthritis.

*Was the situation completely clear?*

*What could have caused the recent deterioration?*

Abduction triggered intense pain in the anterior aspect of the right hip and particularly in the internal part of the inguinal region. Resisted adduction was very painful. Palpation identified intense pain at the superior insertion of the adductors of the right thigh. Most of his pain could be caused by tendonitis of the adductors, a common complication of hip osteoarthritis.

*What treatment would you suggest?*

We carefully administered a local injection of methylprednisolone and xylocaine around the tendon. He noticed the difference almost immediately with a significant reduction in pain on passive mobilization and when walking. This relief, which enabled him to go back to his normal daily activities, lasted for about a year, after which we repeated the procedure. For economic and personal reasons, Mr. Porfírio had not taken the physical therapy that we had recommended.

## OSTEOARTHRITIS OF THE HIP
### MAIN POINTS

This condition is common in men and women over 50, though it can appear earlier.

Predisposing factors include childhood hip disease (Legg-Perthes disease, slipped femoral epiphysis, and congenital hip dysplasia), acetabular dysplasia and hard physical labor (farmers, miners).

It causes mechanical pain in the inguinal region, which can radiate to the knee or buttocks. Brief stiffness after rest is common. It is often accompanied by osteoarthritis of other weight-bearing joints.

Clinical examination reveals pain and limited mobility, especially of internal rotation. Secondary shortening of the affected leg may occur.

Progression varies: most patients will worsen slowly with growing limitations to mobility.

X-rays show typical signs of osteoarthritis: polar loss of articular space, subchondral sclerosis (sometimes with subchondral geodes and cysts), and osteophytes.

Treatment is conservative in the initial stages:

- Analgesics or anti-inflammatories
- Well cushioned footwear to absorb the shock of walking
- A walking stick or crutch on the opposite arm
- Encouraging physical exercise and self-sufficiency
- Physical therapy in more advanced cases

Although there are no solid criteria as to the best time for a total hip replacement, we consider that it is indicated if the patient cannot sleep, walk or work because of the osteoarthritis despite suitable analgesia. The results are usually highly satisfactory.

## TENDONITIS OF THE HIP ADDUCTORS
### MAIN POINTS

It appears most commonly in patients with hip osteoarthritis, but can occur on its own in athletes, for example.

It causes pain in the internal part of the inguinal region, aggravated by abduction of the hip.

The diagnosis can be made if there is pain over the tendon on palpation, forced abduction and resisted adduction.

Inguinal pain may be caused by a hernia.

Treatment is conservative, aiming at strengthening the muscles and local rest. It is important to relieve the local and hip pain to facilitate muscle relaxation.

In more intense or stubborn cases, a careful local injection can be administered.[1]

[1]See Chapter 30 for guidance on the technique.

*TYPICAL CASES*
## 12.B. MECHANICAL HIP PAIN (II)

Leonor Rodrigues, a retired teacher aged 58, came to us with pain in her right hip, that had been getting progressively worse over the last three years. It hurt when she walked, getting progressively worse with continued use and preventing her from taking the evening walks she enjoyed so much. The pain was relieved by rest. It was diffuse and imprecisely located in the groin and the buttocks, sometimes radiating to the posterior aspect of the thigh. She also complained of an old, fluctuating mechanical backache, which "she was used to." Occasionally, she had pain in her knees when walking upstairs but it was bearable. She took anti-inflammatories when the pain was more intense, with moderate relief.

The systematic enquiry revealed no relevant findings.

The general examination showed an obese, good-humored woman (weight 72 Kg, height 1.50 m), with slow, difficult movements of the lower limbs. Forced flexion of the lumbar spine caused pain. Extension was also painful, radiating vaguely to the buttocks. Her arms were normal. Mobility of the hip joints was notably preserved. Forced flexion caused lumbar pain and reproduced the spontaneous complaints. An examination of her knees revealed crepitus in the patellofemoral compartment. Palpation around the hip did not reveal any painful areas. The summary neurological examination was normal.

*How would you explain this patient's hip pain?*

*Were any diagnostic tests necessary?*

This information led us to consider that it was probably radiated pain from the chronic mechanical back pain, most likely associated with spondyloarthrosis and osteoarthritis of the facet joints. We gave the patient appropriate advice, stressing the need for regular exercise and care with her posture because of her spine. We carefully explained the need to lose weight, emphasizing the relationship between obesity and osteoarthritis of the spine and knee. We suggested she take simple analgesics as required to relieve the pain and enable her to exercise. We recommended that she join an exercise or stretching class.

### REFERRED HIP PAIN
*MAIN POINTS*

Hip pain can radiate from the lumbar spine, sacroiliac joints and abdominal organs (pelvis, urether, bladder, appendicitis or diverticulitis in contact with the iliopsoas muscle[2]).

Its location is diffuse and ill defined, predominating in the buttocks when it comes from the spine and in abdomen and groin if caused by intra-abdominal pathology.

Degenerative pathologies of the spine and hip often coexist, but they can occur separately, requiring different treatment.

When dealing with hip pain, always explore the lumbar spine and sacroiliac joints, along with the abdomen and pelvis.

A detailed local physical examination fails to explain the pain.

A general rheumatologic and abdominal examination is the key to the diagnosis.

Treatment is aimed at the underlying condition.

[2]Note that in these last cases the patient may mention painful limitation of mobility of the hip and the pain may worsen with active and passive mobilization of the hip due to inflammation of the iliopsoas…

*TYPICAL CASES*
## 12.C. NOCTURNAL HIP PAIN (I)

According to the patient, a 52-year old personal assistant, the worst thing about her pain was that it stopped her from sleeping. She was able to rest on her back, but could not bear the pain if she lay on her side. As this was her natural position, she would wake up several times during the night. The pain was bearable during the day. She had trouble getting up after sitting for a long time, but the pain soon went. She also had to be careful when sitting on the toilet, to avoid the pain, but the strain of defecation did not make it worse. She located the pain on the lateral face of both hip areas and denied any radiation.

She was generally healthy and was not taking any medication. Her doctor suspected that the cause was lumbar. However, a spinal x-ray did not show any significant anomalies, apart from a discreet degree of osteoarthritis.

Our examination of her spine revealed no alterations, although forced flexion caused slight pain in the posterior aspect of the thighs and knees.

Passive mobilization of the hips required great efforts to relax the patient, who was afraid that it would hurt. Having managed this, however, there was only slight pain in the posterolateral face of both hip areas during forced internal rotation. There was no limited mobility in any direction. Sciatic nerve stretch tests were negative.

## TROCHANTERIC BURSO-TENDONITIS
*MAIN POINTS*

This is an inflammatory process that affects the trochanteric bursa and/or the muscle insertions in the greater trochanter of the femur.

It is one of the most common causes of hip pain, predominating in middle-aged and elderly women.

The pain is felt in the external face of the hip and may radiate to the buttock and external face of the thigh.

It is exacerbated by lying on the ipsilateral side and walking.

It does not affect passive mobility of the hip, though it can cause some pain in extreme rotation. Firm local palpation reproduces the symptoms.

Obesity, leg length discrepancy, hip joint disease and demanding exercise like running predispose to this pathology.

No diagnostic tests are necessary (ultrasound scans often give false positives and negatives).

Treatment is conservative: local rest, relaxation, topical anti-inflammatories and heat. SEE ABOVE

Physical therapy or local injection may be necessary in cases with more intense symptoms or that are resistant to basic treatment.[3]

*What could be happening?*

*Would you look for any additional information from the physical examination?*

Palpation of the trochanteric region triggered intense pain, limited to the external face of the trochanter on the left side but much more extensive on the right (superior and posterior border of the trochanter and an adjacent area of the fascia lata).

The general examination and the examination of the other joints were normal.

*What is your diagnosis?*

*How would you proceed?*

We decided that it was bilateral trochanteric burso-tendonitis, more extensive on the right side. We explained the condition to the patient and reassured her. We prescribed a topical anti-inflammatory for her to apply three times a day after local heat. We referred her to a physiotherapy centre for muscle relaxation exercises. After the third week, the patient was much better and said that the pain on the left side had cleared up though there was still some discomfort on the right. An examination of this area revealed pain on pressure, now limited to the superior edge of the

[3]See Chapter 30 for guidance on the technique.

trochanter. We administered a local injection of anaesthetic and corticosteroid, which relieved the symptoms..

## TYPICAL CASES
## 12.D. NOCTURNAL HIP PAIN (II)

Pain in his left hip finally forced António, a 42-year old, self-employed carpenter, to take time off to go to the doctor.

The pain had begun about three months before and had deteriorated rapidly. It was located all around his hip region, predominating in the lateral and anterior face. It was particularly severe when he got up after rest and improved slowly with movement. It persisted at night, though it was less intense. It was accompanied by morning stiffness for about 40 minutes. Anti-inflammatories, which he had been taking for several years "for his back," did not help very much.

*Could the backache be related to the hip pain? How could we investigate this?*

Our enquiry into the back pain was interesting. It also had an inflammatory rhythm, similar to the hip pain. It had started three years before and responded well to the anti-inflammatory that he took at night.

He denied any complaints in other joints. Our systematic enquiry was negative, including questions about any skin, mucosal or intestinal changes. The rest of his personal history was not relevant. His father had suffered from psoriasis, however.

We found no anomalies on general examination, including signs of psoriasis. Mobility of the lumbar spine was frankly reduced, with a Schober of 10–13.2 cm. Palpation and mobilization of the sacroiliac joints triggered pain on the right.

The left hip joint was painful on active and passive mobilization in all directions. Passive mobility was limited by pain.

*What possibilities does this clinical condition suggest?*

*What additional studies would you request?*

The pain was typically inflammatory and accompanied by painful limitation of mobility, strongly suggesting arthritis. The back pain, which might seem quite normal in a physical worker, was also inflammatory – an alarm signal. The patient had no systemic manifestations, but his father's history of psoriasis was important. The possibility of psoriatic arthritis, with predominant axial involvement and affecting the hip had to be explored.

We requested plain films of the lumbar and thoracic spine (2 views), an anteroposterior view of the pelvis and lateral views of both hips. We also asked for routine blood tests, including acute phase reactants, full blood count and liver tests in preparation for disease-modifying treatment. We also ordered a technetium bone scan because of the difficulty involved in the physical examination of these deep joints.

His sedimentation rate was elevated at 47 mm in the first hour. The full blood count, liver enzymes and routine tests were normal. The spinal x-ray showed no alterations. His hips were also radiologically normal (which did not exclude synovitis, in view of the short time since onset). Figure 12.8. shows the x-ray of the pelvis. The bone scan performed three months later showed increased uptake in the right sacroiliac joint.

In view of these results, we decided that our tentative diagnosis had been confirmed. Given that the involvement was predominantly axial and, therefore would not be very responsive to disease-modifying drugs, we decided to continue treatment with anti-inflammatories and administer a local injection in the hip guided by ultrasound. We stressed the need for the patient to do regular exercises of the spine and to be aware of potential side effects of the medication.

The result was excellent, but we continued to monitor the patient, as the involvement of new joints might justify a different treatment.

## ARTHRITIS OF THE HIP
## *MAIN POINTS*

Synovitis of the hip is suggested by:

- Local inflammatory pain;

- Painful limitation of active and passive mobility;

- Elevated acute phase reactants;

- Circumferential loss of radiological articular space, with no subchondral sclerosis (appears later);

- Increased uptake of radiolabel on bone scintigraphy.

It normally appears in the context of more disseminated arthritis. When isolated, it should be considered septic until proven otherwise: a rheumatologic emergency.

It requires differential diagnosis with osteoarthritis, periarticular lesions, sacroiliitis, avascular necrosis of the femoral head, …

Treatment depends on the underlying disease. Septic arthritis requires bacteriological diagnosis and urgent, sometimes surgical, treatment.

Persistent arthritis of the hip may justify an imaging-guided corticosteroid injection as a rapid way of reducing the inflammation and preventing irreversible sequelae.

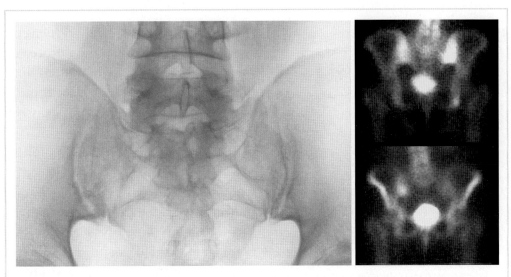

**Figure 12.8.** X-Ray of the pelvis – Clinical case "Nocturnal hip pain (II)." Note the blurring of the right sacroiliac joint margin, with subchondral sclerosis and erosions. This demonstrates the presence of asymmetrical sacro-iliitis, quite compatible with psoriatic arthritis. Bone scintigraphy reveals increased uptake of the radiotracer around the right sacro-iliac joint. **AV** – Anterior view. **PV** – posterior view.

## SPECIAL SITUATIONS

### Avascular (previously called aseptic) necrosis of the femoral head

This is a relatively uncommon condition in clinical practice but requires timely diagnosis. It involves the loss of viability of a part of the femoral head bone and overlying cartilage due to ischemia. The ischemia alone causes pain that is sometimes incapacitating. The dead tissue collapses, causing irregularity on the articular surface, with or without the release of free intra-articular bodies, which will lead to the relentless development of osteoarthritis (Figure 12.9.).

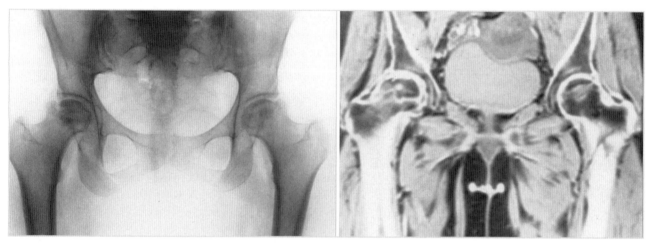

**Figure 12.9.** Bilateral aseptic necrosis of the femoral head. Note the deformity and sclerotic aspect of the femoral head. This patient, with systemic lupus, required bilateral hip replacement a few years later.

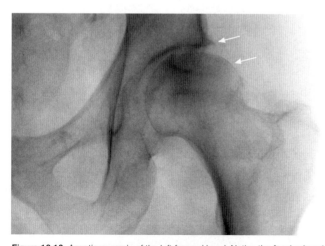

**Figure 12.10.** Aseptic necrosis of the left femoral head. Notice the focal sclerosis of the superior part of the femoral head with slight deformation and loss of continuity of the cortical layer. There are already features of secondary osteoarthritis: loss of joint space, subchondral sclerosis and early osteophytes (*arrows*).

It appears most frequently in young people with predisposing factors: chronic glucocorticoid treatment, systemic lupus erythematosus, antiphospholipid syndrome, alcoholism, diabetes mellitus, AIDS and local trauma. Sometimes no predisposing factors are identified.

Early diagnosis requires, above all, a high degree of suspicion. This condition is heralded by articular pain in the hip, with a variable rhythm, but often inflammatory. Mobility of the hip joint may be limited, even in the early stages of the disease. Radiographs should be from an anteroposterior projection and lateral, trying to identify subtle loss of the spherical shape of the femoral head (Figure 12.10.). This deformation becomes more marked over time. Ideally, however, the diagnosis should be made before any radiological changes, using magnetic resonance imaging (the earliest and most specific technique) (Figure 12.11.) or technetium bone scan.

If the diagnosis is confirmed a careful search for likely causes should be initiated. Treatment is based on analgesics. Ultimately, hip replacement may be required.

### Meralgia paresthetica

This is caused by compression of the lateral femoral cutaneous nerve in the vicinity of the anterosuperior iliac spine or where it exits the deep fascia in the anterior face of the thigh. It causes pain and paresthesia in the anterolateral aspect of the thigh (Figure 12.12.), often aggravated by certain positions, such as crossed legs. Accentuated obesity or tight clothes can precipitate the symptoms. The neurological examination may reveal hypo- or hyperesthesia in the affected area. Palpation or percussion of the nerve's exit point just below the anterosuperior iliac spine or at a point 10 cm below it can trigger pain. An electromyogram may confirm the diagnosis.

Treatment is aimed at removing the causes, if they have been identified. In their absence or if the symptoms persist, local injections or even surgical decompression may be necessary.

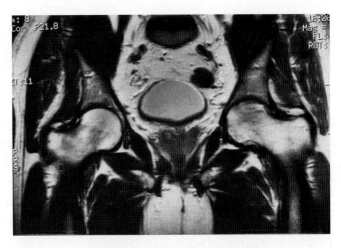

**Figure 12.11.** Aseptic necrosis of the femoral head – early phase. Magnetic resonance imaging shows a change of signal in the left femoral head – "crescent sign." The shape of the femoral head is still preserved and there are no signs of osteoarthritis.

### Iliopectineal bursitis

The iliopectineal bursa is deep within the median part of the inguinal region between the anterior face of the articular capsule and the iliopsoas tendon. It communicates with the synovium of the hip joint in about 15% of people and can be involved in its inflammatory processes.

It causes pain in the anterior face of the thigh and inguinal region, which is aggravated by flexion of the thigh. Local palpation is painful. Plain films are normal. The diagnosis requires ultrasound or MRI scans.

Treatment is directed towards the associated hip disease, if any. Ultrasound-guided local injections may be very useful.

### Fractures of the proximal femur and pelvis

Many fractures of the proximal femur or pelvis are obvious, not only because of violent trauma required to sustain them but also because of the immediate functional disability that they cause. The radiographs usually leave no doubt. Nevertheless, fractures of the proximal femur are one of the most common types of osteoporotic fracture. In these cases, the trauma may be minimal or even non-existent. Many osteoporotic fractures occurring under the patient's weight get "stuck," i.e.

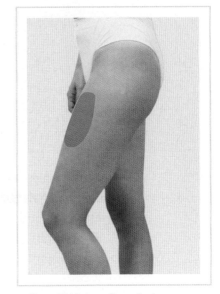

**Figure 12.12.** Area of hyposthesia or paraesthesia in meralgia paresthetica.

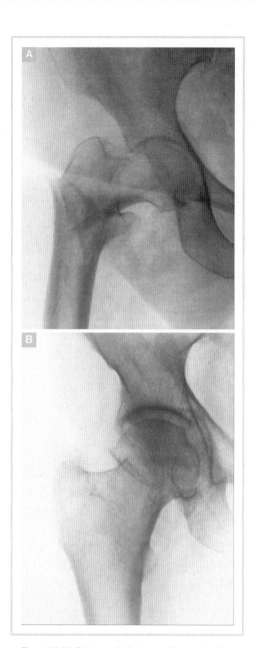

**Figure 12.13.** Osteoporotic fractures of the proximal femur. **A.** In most cases, the fracture is obvious on the x-ray. **B.** Bone endings may, however, be impacted making the diagnosis more difficult. Fractures may be obscurred by coexisting haematoma. (Courtesy: Prof. Fernando Fonseca).

the bone ends are compacted into each other. The disability is less marked and the fracture may not be detectable in a physical examination. We should consider this possibility whenever an elderly patient presents with acute pain in the inguinal region, especially if there are other risk factors for osteoporosis. Note that in an early x-ray, the fracture line may be concealed by a local hematoma (Figure 12.13.), especially in compacted fractures.

Severe osteoporosis is also associated with factures of the iliac bone (namely in the iliopubic branch) and sacrum, which may occur spontaneously or after minimal trauma. These fractures cause deep, sometimes continuous disabling pain with no apparent cause. A careful x-ray examination in at least two planes and bone scanning may provide the key to the diagnosis.

Metastases and Paget's bone disease are other causes of pelvic pain to be considered in the elderly.

## DIAGNOSTIC TESTS

As always, clinical assessment takes first place and, in most cases, it is all we need to make a diagnosis and prescribe treatment.

Referred hip pain, trochanteric burso-tendonitis and tendonitis of the adductors all fall into this category. The x-rays will be normal in these conditions. Peritrochanteric calcification or irregular bone at the insertion of the adductors is occasionally visible. This reinforces the diagnosis, but does not change the treatment.

### *Imaging*

An anteroposterior x-ray of the pelvis is usually sufficient for studying the hip and sacroiliac joints. Suspected aseptic necrosis, Legg-Perthes disease or slipped femoral epiphysis (see Chapter 28) may justify lateral films so that we can evaluate the sphericity or dislocation of the epiphysis.

Radiographs in osteoarthritis show the same typical characteristics of this condition in any location (Figure 12.14A.): focal loss of joint space, subchondral sclerosis and osteophytes. In some cases, such as aseptic necrosis, the femoral head may appear atrophic, reduced in size, with no osteophytes.

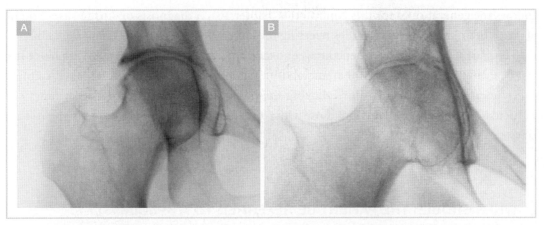

**Figure 12.14. A.** Hip osteoarthritis. Note the loss of joint space, predominating in the upper pole, subchondral sclerosis and osteophytes. **B.** Inflammatory arthritis of the hip: joint space loss is uniform and there is no subchondral sclerosis or osteophyte formation.

In osteoarthritis, the loss of articular space predominates in the superior pole of the femoral head and the adjacent area of the acetabulum. Conversely, in inflammatory arthritides, the loss of articular space is diffuse, without subchondral sclerosis or osteophytes, unless there is secondary osteoarthritis (Figure 12.14B.). In advanced cases, synovitis may be accompanied by erosions of the periphery of the femoral head. Septic arthritis causes rapidly progressive destruction, with loss of bone definition.

MRI scans are only justified to investigate possible aseptic necrosis or even rarer conditions, in the sphere of specialized care.

Situations involving persistent, incapacitating pain that are still undefined after a basic clinical examination and tests may benefit from bone scanning, which can help clarify situations of arthritis, aseptic necrosis or rarer conditions like osteoid osteoma and algodystrophy (circumscribed osteoporosis of the hip – see Chapter 14).

Ultrasound scans are most indicated in the study of soft tissue lesions. However, clinical examination of the hip is quite specific while ultrasound is relatively unreliable in this area.

### Other tests

Laboratory tests, such as the sedimentation rate, C reactive protein, rheumatoid factor, antiphospholipid antibodies, synovial biopsy and analysis of the synovial fluid may be indicated in cases of arthritis of unknown origin or aseptic necrosis, usually in a specialized context.

## TREATMENT

The initial treatment of most causes of hip pain is within the reach of General Practitioners and has already been described.

The use of simple analgesics and, possibly, anti-inflammatories is often justified and worthwhile. Treatment of referred pain is determined by the cause. Treatment of hip osteoarthritis follows the general rules for this condition (Chapter 16). A diagnosis or strong suspicion of arthritis of unknown origin justifies referring the patient to a specialist as soon as possible.

The patient should always be encouraged to take physical exercise compatible with his or her physical ability. Reinforcing lumbar and abdominal muscles and the quadriceps with simple exercises at home is excellent for relieving the pain and maintaining long-term function. Particularly debilitated patients and those with resistant tendonitis or bursitis may benefit from physical therapy.

---

### WHEN SHOULD THE PATIENT BE REFERRED TO A SPECIALIST?

Whenever arthritis of unknown cause is suspected.

Reasonable suspicion of aseptic necrosis of the femoral head.

Whenever the pain is still incapacitating in spite of appropriate basic treatment.

Physical therapy can be very useful for patients with persistent periarticular lesions or moderate or severe osteoarthritis, when surgery is contraindicated.

In cases of osteoarthritis or avascular necrosis, total hip replacement should be considered, when the pain and loss of mobility cause substantial functional limitation, after excluding periarticular causes of aggravation.

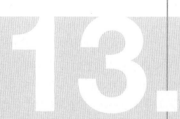

# REGIONAL SYNDROMES
## THE KNEE

J.A.P. da Silva, A.D. Woolf, *Rheumatology in Practice*, DOI 10.1007/978-1-84882-581-9_13,
© Springer-Verlag London Limited 2010

# 13. REGIONAL SYNDROMES THE KNEE

The knee is the largest and one of the most complex joints in the human body. With a large synovium and subject to extreme mechanical demands, it is highly prone to both mechanical and inflammatory lesions.Diseases of the knees, such as osteoarthritis, and lesions of the meniscus and ligaments, are some of the most common causes of disability.

## FUNCTIONAL ANATOMY

The knee joint brings together three bones: the distal end of the femur via the femoral condyles, the proximal end of the tibia, through the tibial plates (or condyles) and the patella, the largest sesamoid bone in the body. The menisci, which consist of crescent-shaped, triangular in section hyaline cartilages, partially separate the articular surfaces of the femur and tibia. They adhere to the interior face of the capsule and help the joint to glide and remain stable while absorbing a substantial part of the joint's mechanical load (Figure 13.1.). The menisci are subject to multiple trauma due to friction and "trapping," and are a common cause of symptoms.

We can think of the knee joint as having three compartments: medial tibiofemoral, lateral tibiofemoral and patellofemoral.

The articular capsule completely surrounds these joints, inserting in the borders of the patella and along the borders of the articular surfaces of the femur and tibia. On the anterior aspect of the distal femur, above the patella, it forms a large pouch, where articular fluid may accumulate. It is therefore an important area to include in the physical examination when looking for articular effusion or swelling (Figure 13.2.). The posterior face of the joint corresponds to the popliteal fossa. Here, the joint may communicate with the semimembranous bursa, forming a popliteal pouch. When this bursa is full of fluid, it forms a palpable, oval mass known as a Baker's cyst (Figure 13.2.).

The articular capsule is reinforced by resistant fibrous ligaments that join the femur to the tibia, forming the internal and external collateral knee ligaments. The cruciate ligaments are inside the joint. The anterior cruciate inserts above and behind on the internal face of the lateral femoral condyle and below and in front, on the anterior intercondyle area of the tibia. It therefore prevents the tibia from glid-

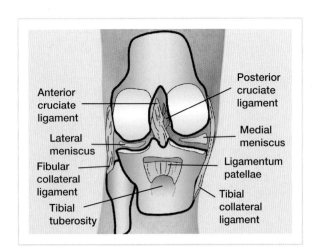

**Figure 13.1.** Bones and ligaments of the knee (*anterior view* – right knee).

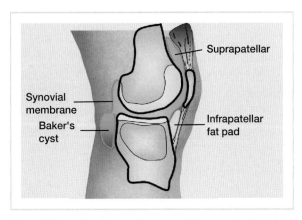

**Figure 13.2.** Synovial membrane of the knee and Baker's cyst (*medial view*).

ing anteriorly over the femur. The posterior cruciate is positioned the other way round and prevents the opposite movement (Figure 13.1.). The muscles that operate the joint play an important role in its stability and, when strong, can partially compensate for weakness of the ligaments.

The patella is suspended within the femoral quadriceps or patella tendon. The tendon inserts into its superior border and joins its inferior end to the tibial tuberosity. Two fibrous bands, the patellar retinacula, insert on each side of the patella and the corresponding faces of the femoral condyles, thus limiting the lateral mobility of the patella.

Load-bearing flexion and extension of the knee understandably cause firm compression of

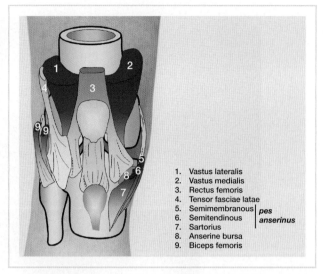

| | |
|---|---|
| 1. | Vastus lateralis |
| 2. | Vastus medialis |
| 3. | Rectus femoris |
| 4. | Tensor fasciae latae |
| 5. | Semimembranous *pes* |
| 6. | Semitendinous *anserinus* |
| 7. | Sartorius |
| 8. | Anserine bursa |
| 9. | Biceps femoris |

**Figure 13.3.** Muscle insertion around the knee (*anterior view* – right knee)

the patella against the femur. This may account for why patellofemoral osteoarthritis is more common in the obese and causes pain particularly when going up and down stairs. In cases of deviations of the patella (most often lateral) the pressure is exerted mainly on the condyle on that side, leading to rapid wearing of the cartilage and early osteoarthritis. Behind the patellar tendon is an fat pad known as Hoffa's fat pad, which may become inflamed.

The anterior face of the patella is covered by the prepatellar bursa, an occasional site of inflammation associated with repeated trauma ("clergyman's or housemaid's knee").

The knee is capable of flexion (about 135°), depending basically on the femoral biceps muscles, semitendinosus and semimembranosus, which are innervated by L5/S1. Extension (0°) is the responsibility of the femoral quadriceps, which are innervated by L3/L4. There are also discreet rotation and anteroposterior gliding movements. Figure 13.3. shows the muscle insertions around the knee. The sensory innervation in this area is shown in Figure 11.12.

A complex tendinous structure consisting of the tendons of the semitendinous and semimembranous muscles (coming from the iliac ischium) and the sartorius muscle (inserting superiorly in the anterosuperior iliac spine) inserts in the anteromedial face of the superior end of the tibia. This structure is called the *pes anserinus*. Arranged deeply between these tendons is the anserine bursa. These structures are often the site of painful, incapacitating inflammation (Figure 13.4.).

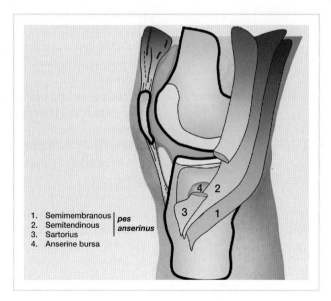

| | |
|---|---|
| 1. | Semimembranous *pes* |
| 2. | Semitendinous *anserinus* |
| 3. | Sartorius |
| 4. | Anserine bursa |

**Figure 13.4.** *Pes anserinus* and anserine bursa (*medial view* – right knee).

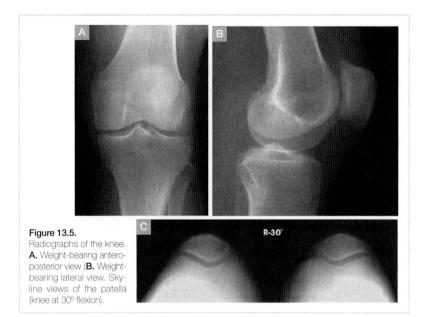

**Figure 13.5.**
Radiographs of the knee.
**A.** Weight-bearing anteroposterior view (**B.** Weight-
bearing lateral view. Skyline views of the patella
(knee at 30° flexion).

### Radiological anatomy

In a weight-bearing anteroposteri-or radiograph (Figure 13.5.), assess the size and regularity of the artic-ular space and bone edges, inside and around the joint. Note the den-sity of the subchondral bone. In profile, assess the same aspects and also the patellofemoral joint and tib-ial tuberosity.

Tangential projections of the patella at 30° of flexion (so-called "sky-line" views) compliment the study of the patellofemoral joint. Look for any external deviation of the patella, with sclerosis or a reduc-tion in articular space.

## COMMON CAUSES OF KNEE PAIN

Osteoarthritis is the most common cause of knee pain. Periarticular lesions often occur in isolation or in association with joint disease (Table 13.1.). Lesions of the ligaments and menisci are the main causes of knee pain in young people.

Chronic instability of the knee contributes to pain and aggravation of the articular process.

| Etiology | Clinical clues |
|---|---|
| Osteoarthritis. | Pain with mechanical rhythm<br>Associated with obesity |
| Baker's cyst. | Deep, moderate pain in the popliteal fossa<br>Palpable cyst |
| Anserine bursitis/tendonitis. | Pain in the medial face of the knee<br>Worse at night and with exercise<br>Painful local palpation<br>More frequent in obese women<br>Often associated with knee joint disease |
| Lesions of the menisci. | Recurring episodes of acute knee pain<br>The knee locks or g ives way<br>Predominant in young people and athletes |
| Instability of the knee. | Unsteadiness and pain while walking<br>Associated with trauma or chronic joint disease |
| Arthritis. | Inflammatory knee pain<br>Swelling, effusion or local heat |
| Referred pain. | Diffuse pain<br>Local examination inconclusive<br>Pathology of the lumbar spine or hip |
| Anterior knee pain syndrome. | Pain in the anterior face of the knee<br>Variable rhythm, generally exacerbated by walking<br>Examination generally inconclusive<br>Predominant in young women |

**Table 13.1.** The most common causes of knee pain.

## THE ENQUIRY

### Age

The age of onset of a complaint gives us important clues as to the most probable diagnosis, as shown in Table 13.2.

### Rhythm of the pain

In most cases the pain has a mechanical rhythm, associated with movement and relieved by rest. Exceptions are inflammatory synovitis and anserine bursitis/tendonitis, in which it usually predominates at night or in the morning.

### Onset and progression

While the onset of pain related to osteoarthritis or Baker's cyst is usually insidious and progressive over months or years, pain caused by synovitis or bursitis/tendonitis appears in days or weeks. Ligamental lesions are very often acute and related to trauma.

Meniscal lesions in most patients are reflected by recurrent episodes of self-limit-ing pain often related to rotation on a load-bearing foot. Patients may say that their knee "gives way" (sudden weakness), or locks, i.e. the knee "gets stuck" in semi-flexion and then resumes movement after a while. These occurrences may be associated with transient swelling (a few days).

| Age group | Predominant causes |
|---|---|
| <15 | Juvenile idiopathic arthritis |
|  | Anterior knee pain syndrome |
|  | Osgood-Schlatter's disease |
|  | Hypermobility syndrome |
|  | Hip diseases |
| 10–30 | Lesions of the meniscus |
|  | Lesions of the ligaments |
|  | Hypermobility syndrome |
|  | Anterior knee pain syndrome |
| 30–50 | Lesions of the meniscus |
|  | Lesions of the ligaments |
|  | Anserine bursitis/tendonitis |
|  | Patellofemoral osteoarthritis |
|  | Baker's cyst |
|  | Arthritis |
| >50 | Osteoarthritis |
|  | Baker's cyst |
|  | Anserine bursitis/tendonitis |

**Table 13.2.** Most common causes of knee pain, by age groups.

### Signs of inflammation

Descriptions by the patient of signs of inflammation of the knee (swelling, heat or redness) are highly suggestive of local inflammation. Note, however, that advanced osteoarthritis is often accompanied by indolent joint effusion. Meniscal lesions and chronic instability of the knee may also cause joint effusion.

### Involvement of other joints

Many diseases of the knee are associated with similar developments in other joints, and their nature and location may help make the diagnosis. Knee osteoarthritis may be the first sign, but many patients also have mechanical back pain and degenerative change of the spine and, less commonly, the hip. Isolated acute or subacute synovitis of the knee should be considered septic until proven otherwise and referred urgently for the appropriate tests and treatment.

Remember that pain originating in the hip or the spine can radiate or even present as pain in the knee. It is important to examine these joints, especially if the examination of the knee is inconclusive.

## REGIONAL EXAMINATION

### *Inspection*

Watch the way the patient walks when coming into the room or climbing onto the examination couch and check the alignment of the knees while the patient is standing. In normal conditions, the axis of the thigh with the lower leg forms an angle of about 5°. With an accentuation of this angle the patient is said to be knock-kneed (*genu valgus*). A deviation in the opposite direction is called *genu varus,* i.e. the patient is bowlegged, a very common deformity in patients with osteoarthritis.

Note the spontaneous position of the knees when the patient is lying down. Normally, the popliteal fossa is in contact with the couch. Any inability to do this indicates limited extension due either to pain or a fixed flexion deformity (Figure 13.6.).

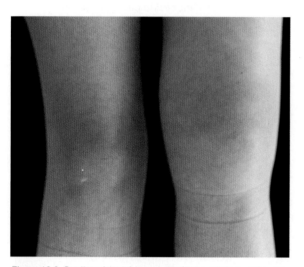

**Figure 13.6.** Swelling of the *left knee*: loss of bone contours  and suprapatellar swelling. Patients usually keep the knee in flexion.

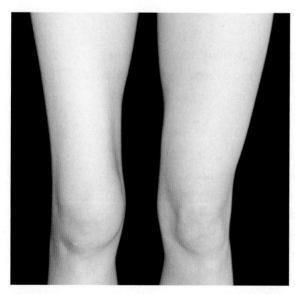

**Figure 13.7.** Muscle atrophy of the *right thigh* in association with ipsilateral knee arthritis.

Swelling or effusion of the knee is suggested by the disappearance of the bony contours (compare with the other knee – Figure 13.6.). A rounded swelling may be seen superior to the patella. These signs must be confirmed by palpation, however. Articular redness is rarely visible, even in cases of active arthritis. Skin redness overlying the joint is more commonly associated with septic, microcrystalline or reactive arthritis.

Look for signs of muscle wasting, which is common in chronic diseases of the knee and in neurological lesions (Figure 13.7.). The skin covering the anterior aspect of the knees is often the site of psoriasis.

### *Palpation*

Feel the local temperature with the back of your hand and compare it to that of the thigh, lower leg and contralateral knee.

Palpate the joint space on either side of the patella (the articular space is at the level of the lower edge of the patella, when the patient is lying down). Synovial inflammation is suggested by the presence of elastic tissue covering the contour of the bone. Osteophytes, typical of osteoarthritis, feel like irregular bony spurs.

In synovitis, palpation usually causes pain along the whole articular space. In osteoarthritis, it is more typical to find various diffuse points of pain.

Also palpate the superior and inferior insertion points of the internal and external collateral ligaments to identify pain suggesting ligamentitis.

Palpate the *pes anserinus*, following it along the anterome-dial face of the tibia and posteromedial edge of the knee. In cases of anserine bursitis/tendonitis, the patient will complain of intense pain (Figure 13.8.).

### Looking for knee joint effusion

**1.** Firmly mold your palm to the upper part of the patient's knee, with the fold between your thumb and index finger slightly above the upper edge of the patella. Squeeze the medial and lateral aspects of the knee with your fingers. This pushes the synovial fluid to the posterior face of the patella. With the thumb of your other hand, push the patella against the femur (Figure 13.9.). Normally, the patella should now be in contact with the femur and will not move. If there is effusion, there will be anteroposterior movement of the patella until it hits the femur (the "piano key sign").

Identifying joint effusion is a crucial aspect of the clinical assessment of the knee.

Note that the thumb must be in the centre of the patella, pushing it posteriorly. If it is not in the centre, the patella will swing and this can simulate effusion. A systematic check for this sign in all patients can do a lot to increase your sensitivity in detecting small volume effusions.

The following technique may be more effective for discrete effusions.

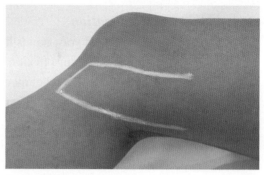

**Figure 13.8.** Área of tenderness associated with pes anserinus tendonitis (*Right knee*, medial aspect.)

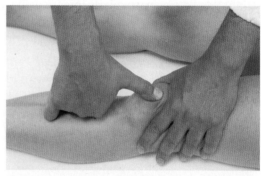

**Figure 13.9.** Looking for knee effusion (**1**). The *left hand* has been drawn down over the suprapatellar bursa forcing any fluid to accumulate under the patella. The *right thumb* is checking for fluctuation of the patella.

### Looking for knee joint effusion

**2.** Run the back of your hand firmly along the medial face of the knee so that any fluid accumulated there is pushed outward. Now run your hand along the outer face while watching the medial face of the knee carefully. Any effusion that is not under pressure will cause a small swelling to appear on the internal face of the knee, inside and above the patella (Figure 13.10A. and B.).

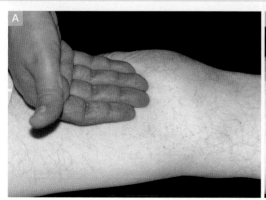
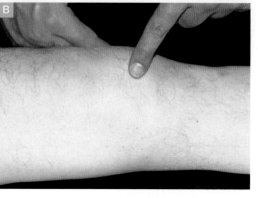

**Figure 13.10.**
Looking for knee effusion (**2**). **A.** Palpate firmly the medial aspect of the knee to move any effusion. **B.** Now sweep the hand over the lateral aspect while examining the medial aspect: the relocation of a rounded swelling reveals the presence of moderate volume effusion.

### *Mobilization*

Place one of your hands lightly on the knee. Hold the patient's leg with your other hand and induce maximum flexion and extension of the knee. Repeat these movements. The hand on the knee will detect any crepitus or snapping in the knee compartments. Osteoarthritis is accompanied by coarse crepitus. Light crepitus may also be perceptible in some other cases of arthritis.

Note the range of movements. Both osteoarthritis and other arthritides may involve painful and/or structural limitation of mobility. Extension is normally 0°. In many normal young people, especially women, there may be hyperextension of up to −10°. Further than this, the movement is clearly excessive and may be part of the benign hypermobility syndrome.

Lesions of the posterior face of the patella (osteoarthritis, patellar chondromalacia) cause particularly intense pain when the patella is forced against the femur.

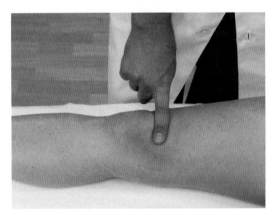

**Figure 13.11.** Patello-femoral maneuver. The index finger forces the patella against the femur while the patients contracts the quadriceps, pulling the patella upwards.

### Examination of the patellofemoral joint

With the patient lying on their back and the knee relaxed and in extension, firmly press your index finger along the upper edge of the patella. Ask the patient to contract his quadriceps (or press his heel against the examining table) (Figure 13.11.). Intense pain when the patella is moved upward suggests a patellofemoral lesion.

### Assessing joint stability.

### 1. Collateral ligaments

Firmly hold the knee by its internal face with one hand and the lower leg with the other, keeping the knee at about 30° flexion. Try to induce external deviation of the knee (genu varus).

Repeat the maneuver in the opposite direction (Figure 13.12.).

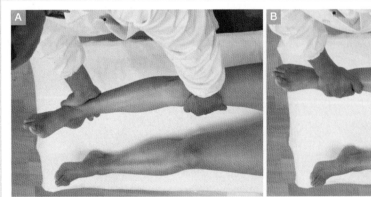

**Figure 13.12.** Checking knee stability. **A.** Fibular collateral ligament. **B.** Tibial collateral ligament. (Vd. Explanations in text.)

In the first maneuver, we test the competence of the external collateral ligament, while the second assesses the medial ligament. These maneuvers require training to avoid mistaking flexion of the knee for instability. Make sure that the movement is on the patient's coronal plane.

Instability of the lateral ligaments is very common in patients with advanced osteoarthritis, contributing decisively to the pain and progression of the degenerative process. This anomaly requires its own specific treatment. It may also be the result of trauma.

### 2. Cruciate ligaments

Ask the patient to flex his knee to 90°, with his foot resting on the examination couch. Sit gently on the foot to immobilize it.

Firmly grasp the proximal end of the tibia with both hands. Try to induce anterior and then posterior movement (Figure 13.13.).

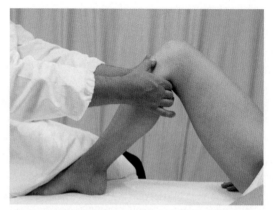

**Figure 13.13.** Assessing cruciate ligament integrity. With the knee flexed at 90° and the foot immobilized, the observer tests the antero-posterior mobility of the tibia on the femur.

In these maneuvers we assess the dislocation of the tibia in relation to the femur. Excessive movement indicates impairment of one of the cruciate ligaments. Rupture or laxity of a cruciate ligament is usually secondary to trauma, but can also be found in patients with chronic arthritis of the knee.

**Examining the menisci.**

### 1. McMurray's test

Start with the knee flexed at 90°. One of your hands holds the patient's foot in internal rotation. The other holds the knee by its internal face pushing it outwards. While maintaining this pressure, induce repeated extension and flexion of the knee (Figure 13.14A.).

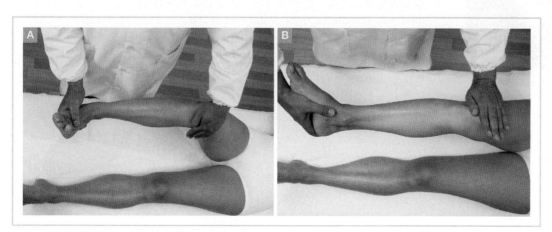

**Figure 13.14.**
Assessing meniscus integrity. McMurray's test. **A.** Medial meniscus. **B.** Lateral meniscus. (Vd. explanations in text.)

Pain in this maneuver indicates a lesion of the internal meniscus, which, with this method, is compressed between the femur and tibia. There is sometimes a snap or click in the joints, which reinforces the diagnosis.

> Repeat the above maneuver, now rotating the foot outwards and pushing the knee inwards (Figure 13.14B.). This tests the external meniscus.

## TYPICAL CASES
## 13.A. KNEE PAIN (I)

Carlos Rodrigues was a cheerful 67-year old man who liked parties and outings. Unfortunately, he was no longer able to enjoy these pleasures in the same way because of growing pain in her knees seriously limiting her ability to walk. The pain was typically mechanical, appearing with exercise, especially walking and climbing stairs, and disappearing completely while lying down. It was particularly intense when he got up and walked after sitting for some time. This caused him to say initially that it was worse with rest! He described intense morning and post-rest stiffness lasting 5–10 minutes, known as "gelling."

The pain had begun 5 or 6 years before and worsened progressively. Anti-inflammatories and local heat were increasingly ineffective. He complained of chronic, mechanical backache, which was reasonably controlled. He was being treated for hypertension and non-insulin dependent diabetes. He had a history of gastritis and anemia.

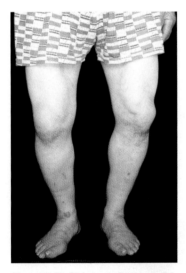

**Figure 13.15.** Clinical case "Knee pain (I)." Note the distance between the knees while the patient stands – *Genu varum*.

*What possible causes are you thinking of?*

*Program the clinical examination in your mind.*

> On clinical examination we found the patient limped and was clearly bow-legged (Figure 13.15.). He was plainly obese (weight 72 kg, height 1,47 m).
>
> Examination of the lumbar spine showed a painful reduction in mobility on flexion and extension. The hip joints were normal. The knees presented about 10° genu varus. Inspection suggested deformation of the joint. Palpation showed no increase in local temperature. We noted pain and osteophytes on palpation of the medial joint space bilaterally and discreet joint effusion on the right. Palpation of the pes anserinus was painless. The external collateral ligament was impaired bilaterally. Mobilization revealed a painful reduction in flexion to about 90° on the right and 80° on the left with accentuated crepitus of the patella and internal compartment.

*Briefly summarize the main problems.*[1]

*What is your diagnosis?*

*Were diagnostic tests necessary? What would you expect from them?*

*What treatment would you recommend?*

We concluded that the patient had advanced osteoarthritis, with probable involvement of the knees and lumbar spine. An x-ray of the knees confirmed this diagnosis (Figure 13.16.). We also requested a full blood count and kidney function tests to monitor the treatment.

We explained the situation to the patient, stressing its etiological relationship with his obesity and recommending a "radical" change in his eating habits. We suggested and explained some exercises for strengthening the quadriceps and ischiotibial muscles, to be done twice a day.

Unfortunately, the analgesic that we would have preferred to prevent the side effects of the anti-inflammatories,[2] had already proved ineffective. We therefore prescribed an anti-inflammatory drug combined with a proton-pump inhibitor and advised a regular monitoring of his blood pressure. We suggested local heat and massages with a topical anti-inflammatory during flare-ups. Mr. Rodrigues refused to use a stick. We may have to consider a joint prosthesis depending on his progress.

## OSTEOARTHRITIS OF THE KNEE
### MAIN POINTS

It is very common in patients over 60 years of age although it may appear before.

More common in women.

Its starts insidiously and may get progressively worse.

It causes typically mechanical pain, though there may be periods of inflammatory exacerbation, with effusion and nocturnal pain.

Clinical examination may reveal crepitus, painful limitation of mobility and osteophyte excrescences. Joint effusion may be present.

There is often instability of the knee ligaments, which exacerbates the situation.

It most commonly affects the medial tibiofemoral compartment and the patellofemoral joints.

It is closely related to being overweight. Local trauma or inflammation and hard physical labor are other risk factors.

X-ray changes are typical of osteoarthritis.

The treatment of osteoarthritis is described in Chapter 16.

[1] Progressive-onset knee pain and mechanical backache in an obese middle-aged man. Objective alterations of a degenerative nature. *Genu varus.*

[2] What risk factors for anti-inflammatories can you identify in this patient? Aged over 65, history of gastritis, anemia and hypertension.

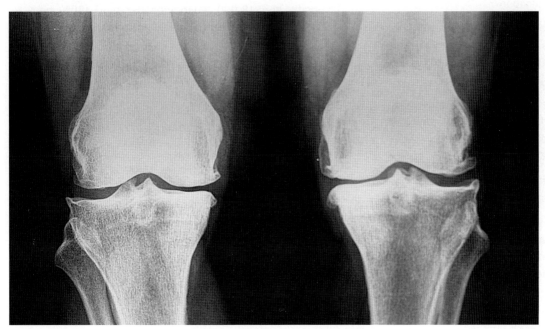

**Figure 13.16.** Knee X-rays. Clinical case "Knee pain (I)."

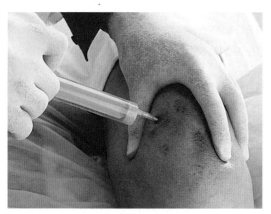

**Figure 13.17.** Clinical case "Knee pain (II)." Arthrocentesis revealed a clowdy synovial fluid.

## ACUTE SYNOVITIS OF THE KNEE
### MAIN POINTS

The following indicate an acute synovitis[4] of the knee:

- Inflammatory pain
- Synovial swelling and/or joint effusion
- Local heat
- The diagnosis is clinical: it only requires laboratory tests for etiological investigation

It often appears in a context of poly- or oligoarthritis. It is the joint most often affected by idiopathic juvenile arthritis.

Monoarthritis of the knee should be considered infectious until proven otherwise. Reactive arthritis and microcrystalline arthritis are other possibilities. It is essential to aspirate and examine synovial fluid.

In cases of unexplained monoarthritis consider the possibility of algodystrophy (see Chapter 14).

Treatment depends on the clinical and etiological context and should always be guided by specialists.

### TYPICAL CASES
### 13.B. KNEE PAIN (II)

Joana Castelão, a 21-year old student, came to the emergency department because of intense pain in her left knee that had begun 2 days before and rapidly become incapacitating. Her knee was hot, swollen and slightly red. Palpation was painful all around the joint and there was a large, tense effusion (Figure 13.6.). Her axillary temperature was 38.2°C.

Three weeks earlier she had gone on a school trip, and she and other members of the group had developed febrile gastroenteritis, for which they had been treated successfully with antibiotics.

*Give a brief description of the problem.*[3]

*What is the most probable diagnosis?*

*How would you proceed in terms of additional investigation?*

There could be no doubt as to the diagnosis of acute arthritis. Her history of infection strongly suggested post-dysenteric reactive arthritis or, less likely, septic arthritis.

A stool culture conducted in hospital was negative. Serological studies revealed high levels of anti-Salmonella typhi antibodies. Her sedimentation rate was 56 mm in the first hour. We aspirated the joint (Figure 13.17.) and the fluid had the expected inflammatory characteristics: cloudy, low viscosity, and 18,000 leukocytes per mm³ (80% neutrophils). A bacteriological examination and crystal test were negative.

These findings were consistent with a diagnosis of **reactive arthritis**.

### What treatment would you suggest?

We administered an intra-articular injection of 40 mg triamcinolone hexacetonide, which rapidly alleviated the symptoms. There were no recurrences in the following three months.

We explained the nature of the disease, emphasizing that it generally cleared up completely. There was, however, still a risk of recurrence due to reinfection, as the previous episode had demonstrated a genetic predisposition to this type of reaction.

---

[3] Acute, post-infectious monoarthritis in a young woman.
[4] By "synovitis" we understand "inflammatory arthritis" as opposed to osteoarthritis.

*TYPICAL CASES*

**13.C. KNEE PAIN (III)**

Maria Rosa had already been treated at our clinic for moderate osteoarthritis of the knees for several years. She called and asked for an emergency appointment because the pain had become worse 2 weeks previously. She also had pain at night now, especially in her right knee, which kept her awake. The pain was more intense lying on her side. Normally morning stiffness was negligible but now it lasted about 30 minutes. Her usual simple analgesics were no longer effective and her knee was more swollen.

Examination of her right knee showed a discreet increase in skin temperature, accompanied by pain along the joint space and large effusion. Palpation of the pes anserinus caused extreme pain as far as the postero-superior edge of the medial femoral condyle.

*How would you explain this condition?*

*What treatment would you recommend?*

We concluded that our patient was suffering an **inflammatory flare of her knee osteoarthritis**, which was now associated with **anserine tendonitis**.

We recommended partial rest and temporarily replaced the simple analgesics by a full dose of anti-inflammatories. We added a topical anti-inflammatory to be applied to the medial knee three times a day. Three weeks later she was much better. The stiffness and the articular effusion had gone. Although it was not too bad, she still had some pain on lying down and with some movements. A local examination confirmed the persistence of the anserine tendonitis, though the painful area was much smaller. We administered a local injection of a mixture of local anesthetic and glucocorticoid, which relieved the pain. The patient went back to her normal analgesic and was reminded to do the muscle-strengthening exercises we had advised.

**ANSERINE BURSITIS/TENDONITIS**

*MAIN POINTS*

It is a very common cause of pain, especially in obese middle-aged women.

It appears most often as an aggravation of a known joint disease, but may occur in isolation.

The pain predominates on the medial aspect of the knee and is aggravated by sudden movements of the lower limbs and lying on the side.

Pain on palpation is the key to the diagnosis.

Treatment is based on rest and the application of local anti-inflammatories.

In stubborn cases, provided that the painful area is not too large, a local injection may be effective.[5]

Physiotherapy can be used in difficult cases.

In exceptional cases, surgery may be necessary.

[5]See Chapter 30 for technical guidance.

### TYPICAL CASES
### 13.D. KNEE PAIN (IV)

Madalena Rosado, a 21-year old student, came to the clinic because of pain in her left knee. It had first occurred about 8 years before when she was doing ballet, sometimes forcing her to wear an elastic bandage. The pain was intermittent, appearing suddenly and lasting 2 or 3 days, sometimes with joint swelling. After giving up her favorite physical activity, it occurred less frequently, when she was getting into or out of a car, for example. She felt discomfort in her knees after sitting for a long time. When asked, she described one or two episodes when her knee "gave way," but she denied that it locked.

A more detailed enquiry revealed that she also had transient pain in other joints, like her wrists and shoulders though it was rare. She had a history of several "sprains," which she attributed to ballet.

General examination showed she had great articular flexibility and agility (she placed her palms on the floor with ease, keeping straight legs). Examination of the knees found no deviations, swelling, pain, crepitus or limited mobility. We noticed knee hyperextension of about 20° and appreciable instability of the collateral ligaments. The cruciates were competent.

*What possible explanations were there for this situation?*

*Was there some pathology underlying the more dispersed pain?*

*How would you complete the physical examination?*

The maneuvers for assessing the left internal meniscus caused intense pain, while the others were normal.

We conducted a specific examination for hypermobility of other joints. The patient had no trouble in putting her palms on the floor, and there was about 15° hyperextension of the elbows. We could get her thumb to touch her forearm and the fifth metacarpophalangeal joint easily achieved 90° extension (Figure 13.18.). The skin was normal.

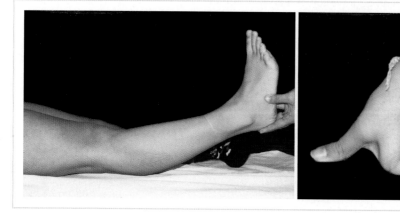

**Figure 13.18.** Clinical case "Knee pain (**IV**)." Two of the criteria for hypermobility syndrome: hyperextension of knee and metacarpo-phalangeal joints.

Our patient very probably had a **lesion of the internal meniscus** of the left knee in association with the benign **hypermobility syndrome**, which was confirmed by the above criteria. This condition probably played an important role in the lesion of the left internal meniscus and *explained the intermittent, migratory pain as well as the tendency to suffer sprains*.

We explained the situation to the patient, stressing that the hypermobility that had been so useful in ballet facilitated repeated articular subluxations with transient pain in several joints. It could also have contributed to the lesion of the meniscus. We reassured her about the prognosis and made it clear that it was not the polyarticular inflammatory disease that she feared. We suggested that the physical exercise, which she continued to do, should be devoted to strengthening her muscles, though she should avoid extreme range of joint movements. Elastic bandages on the most susceptible joints might also be useful as well as specific exercises to strengthen supporting muscles.

Where the meniscus was concerned, we agreed that it was not serious enough for surgery. We therefore did not request an MRI at this stage, which is the best way of formally diagnosing this condition.

## MENISCAL LESIONS
### MAIN POINTS

They occur mainly in young individuals, and especially in athletes. They can contribute considerably to pain and disability in chronic knee conditions.

They cause acute-onset, recurring pain, with spontaneous recovery. With time, the pain becomes more persistent.

It may be accompanied by joint effusion during flares.

Many patients describe their knee "giving way" (sudden weakness) or locking (the knee gets stuck in semi-flexion, recovering gradually and painfully to normal mobility).

There may be pain on deep palpation of the anterior part of the joint space, on either side of the patellar tendon. McMurray's test is essential in confirming a suspected diagnosis.

Sports, instability of the knee and hypermobility syndrome are important risk factors.

Tolerable cases do not require diagnostic tests and are treated with measures to strengthen the muscles and elastic supports.

Persistent or incapacitating pain warrants confirmation by MRI, in preparation for a meniscectomy.

Meniscectomy increases the risk of later development of osteoarthritis, and should not be undertaken lightly.

## HYPERMOBILITY SYNDROME
### MAIN POINTS

This condition consists of generalized laxity of the ligaments and skin in otherwise healthy people.

It may cause recurring episodes of transient pain in several joints, with no signs of inflammation or criteria for fibromyalgia.

The knees (patella), shoulders, and tibiotarsal, metacarpophalangeal and temporomandibular joints are often affected.

The repeated episodes favor the occurrence of secondary osteoarthritis.

The diagnosis is based on the patient's ability to carry out a number of "exaggerated" movements. Give one point to each sign:

- Passive extension of the fifth MCP > 90°
- Passive contact of the thumb with the forearm — Right and left
- Hyperextension of the elbow > 0° — 1 point
- Hyperextension of the knee > 0° — for each
- Touching the floor with the palms, with the knees in extension — side

Diagnosis: 4 or more points + joint pain for more than three months in four or more joints.

Other syndromes involving hypermobility must be excluded, like Ehlers-Danlos syndrome, Marfan's syndrome and osteogenesis imperfecta.

Treatment is conservative, without medication.

## TYPICAL CASES
## 13.E. KNEE PAIN (V)

A colleague from vascular surgery referred 56-year old Alberto Falcão to us. He had come to the emergency department because of suspected deep vein thrombosis in the right leg. The Echo-Doppler was negative, however. Was there a rheumatologic cause?

The patient believed he had knee osteoarthritis, for which his GP had prescribed anti-inflammatory analgesia. His symptoms were compatible with this diagnosis: typically mechanical, slowly progressive pain. Sometimes, the joint would swell, forming a painful "lump" at the back of the knee, which made walking difficult. The week before, he had taken a long walk during which he had intense pain in the right calf, which prevented him from continuing. The next day, the pain was even worse and accompanied by accentuated swelling of the whole leg below the knee.

## BAKER'S CYST
## MAIN POINTS

This is the collection of synovial fluid at the semimembranous bursa , which communicates with the knee joint forming a cul-de-sac.

It can appear in isolation, but usually accompanies diseases of the knee.

It can cause pain and discomfort in the popliteal fossa, where it is palpable (and sometimes visible) as an oval swelling in the superomedial part of the popliteal fossa.

An ultrasound scan is a sensitive method of confirming the diagnosis.

If the patient is symptomatic, it may require ultrasound-guided drainage with a large needle, followed by infiltration or even surgery.

A ruptured Baker's cyst causes symptoms similar to deep vein thrombosis and may, rarely, develop into compartmental syndrome with edema, ischemia and muscular necrosis.

In a rupture, the echo-doppler may show alterations compatible with vein thrombosis. Ultrasound and arthrography of the knee are the best examinations, though it may be necessary to conduct a venography to exclude the differential diagnosis.

*Give a brief description of this condition.*[6]

*What are the possible diagnoses at this stage?*

An examination of the knees confirmed the presence of coarse crepitus and palpable osteophytes, with slight bilateral limitation of extension. On the left, there was clearly a large Baker's cyst, but not on the right. There was no joint effusion. Palpation of the right calf was extremely painful and there was accentuated edema and pitting in the median and lower third of the leg. Hommans' sign was positive (passive dorsiflexion of the foot caused pain in the calf). Everything pointed to vein thrombosis except the Doppler...

*How would you explain the situation?*

*Would you request any diagnostic tests?*

We asked for an ultrasound scan of the knees and calf, which confirmed bilateral Baker's cysts. In the right calf, there was a layer of liquid outside the muscles suggesting a probable rupture of the Baker's cyst on that side. The echo-Doppler showed diffuse vascular compression caused by edema of the gastrocnemius, but no vein thrombosis. We avoided ordering an arthrography of the knee, as there is usually clear loss of the contrast agent into the lower leg muscles.

We admitted the patient for rest, articular injection of corticosteroids and physical therapy, for rapid relief of the symptoms and to prevent the (real) risk of deep vein thrombosis induced by muscular edema in reaction to the synovial fluid.

Symptoms suggesting deep vein thrombosis of the calf in a patient with a disease of the knee should always raise the possibility of rupture of a Baker's cyst. They may be clinically indistinguishable!

[6]Condition suggesting deep vein thrombosis in a patient with knee osteoarthritis.

## SPECIAL SITUATIONS

### Anterior knee pain syndrome

This is an ill-defined condition affecting mainly young women. It is characterized by pain in the anterior aspect of the knee, growing progressively worse and having a variable relation to movement, rest and cold weather. The clinical examination is perfectly normal. Diagnostic tests, including arthroscopy, are also normal.

In some cases, the pain seems to be caused by a ***synovial plica*** that can insinuate itself between the patella and the femur, where it is compressed and occasionally causes intra-articular hemorrhage. The diagnosis is not evident even on MRI, and is only possible after an arthroscopy, though even then there are limitations.

In other situations there is pain when applying pressure on the medial or lateral border of the patella, suggesting inflammation of the alae of the patella, which it is impossible to confirm.

***Chondromalacia patella*** consists of a softening of the posterior cartilage of the patella. It causes mechanical pain, particularly exacerbated by going up or down stairs and generally beginning in adolescence. The usual maneuvers for this joint cause pain. Only arthroscopy can confirm the diagnosis. It has no specific treatment, but tends to resolve spontaneously after the age of 20–25.

A relatively common condition is ***lateral deviation of the patella***. It is caused by an increase in the Q angle (> 20º – Figure 13.19.), which results in accentuated compression of the patella against the lateral condyle of the femur, with patellar pain and accelerated wear, leading ultimately to osteoarthritis. Clinical suspicion of this condition should lead to a skyline film of the patella with the knee flexed at 30º. An outward deviation of the patella in relation to the intercondylar axis, sometimes already associated with a reduction in joint space or subchondral sclerosis, strengthens the diagnosis. Treatment involves physiotherapy exercises to strengthen the *vastus medialis*. It is, however, sometimes associated with a retraction of the internal ala of the patella. Surgical correction of this anomaly is simple and often relieves the symptoms. It is important to note, however, that it is not known whether this procedure reduces or increases the risk of patellofemoral osteoarthritis in the long term.

In spite of the above, a high percentage of cases of anterior knee pain persist in the medium term with no precise diagnosis and therefore without specific treatment. Analgesics or anti-inflammatories are used as needed. Muscle-strengthening exercises for the quadriceps and distension of the ischiotibials are often useful. The use of an elastic knee band has contradictory results from one case to another. Patients should avoid high heels as they increase the pressure of the patella against the femur. These conditions tend to resolve spontaneously by the age of 25–30.

### Osteochondritis dissecans

This is a relatively rare cause of knee pain and is found in young men. A fragment of cartilage and subchondral bone detaches itself from the rest of the bone and becomes an intra-articular foreign body causing pain and recurrent locking of the knee joint.

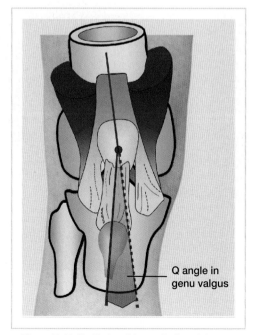

Q angle in genu valgus

**Figure 13.19.** Positioning of the patella: Q angle in genu valgus.

Plain films show a radiolucent area where the fragment has separated. MRI is required to demonstrate intra-articular loose body. Treatment is surgical.

### Algodystrophy

This is a localized vasomotor disturbance causing local pain, swelling, redness and heat, simulating monoarthritis. It often follows trauma but this is not always apparent in the history. See Chapter 14 for a more detailed description.

### Osgood-Schlatter's disease and referred pain

Particularly in children, pain in the knee may be caused by diseases of the hip. Osgood-Schlatter's disease typically presents in adolescence and consists of osteitis and enthesitis of the inferior insertion of the patellar tendon into the tibial tuberosity. It causes pain, which is aggravated by walking. Both Osgood-Schlatter's and referred knee pain are explained in more detail in Chapter 28.

## DIAGNOSTIC TESTS

As the knee joint is superficial, it lends itself to a detailed, highly informative clinical examination. This limits the need for diagnostic tests to situations in which we wish to assess the degree of structural alteration in the joint or evaluate the aetiology of arthritis.

### Imaging

A plain film of the knees is indicated whenever clinical examination suggests an unexplained articular problem. It should be conducted with the patient standing, weight-bearing and is usually from two angles. Under these circumstances, the distance between the bones is a good indication of the thickness of the articular cartilage.

In osteoarthritis, a sharpening of the tibial spines is one of the earliest signs. Loss of articular space tends to be asymmetrical, more pronounced in the medial compartment. Whether this is due to pre-existing *genu varum* or whether this develops secondary to disease, is the subject of current studies. Subchondral sclerosis, the formation of cysts and osteophytosis become more pronounced over time (Figure 13.20.).

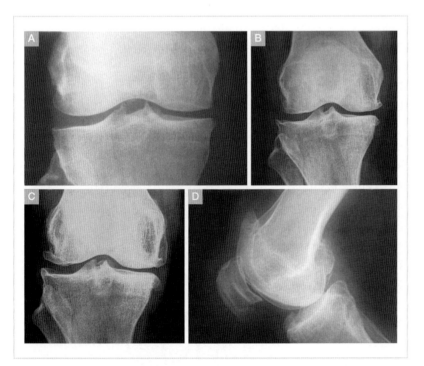

**Figure 13.20.** Radiological features of osteoarthritis. **A.** Sharpening of the tibial spines is one of the earlier signs. **B.** Joint space loss and osteophyte formation start at early stages of the disease. **C.** Joint space loss tends to be assymetrical. Subchondral sclerosis, geodes and osteophytes become more prominent with time. Please note that a marginal osteophytes can simulate an erosion immediately above or below. **D.** The patello-femoral joint is assessed with the lateral (and skyline) views.

The study of the patellofemoral joint requires a profile of the knee and a skyline view at 30º flexion.

In the inflammatory arthritides, radiological changes appear late. As in osteoarthritis, there is loss of joint space reflecting cartilage loss, which may be more diffuse. It is usually accompanied by periarticular osteopenia (unlike subchondral sclerosis). Erosions are rarely visible (Figure 13.21.).

Ultrasound scans are particularly useful in identifying small Baker's cysts (Figure 13.22.). Ultrasound scans are frequently normal in clinically manifest *anserine bursitis/tendonitis*. Ultrasound is not a good method for studying the menisci, MRI is much better.

An MRI is only justified when an unexplained, incapacitating situation justifies consideration of surgery.

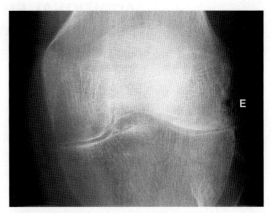

**Figure 13.21.** Knee X-rays in advanced inflammatory arthritis. Note that joint space loss is homogeneous and symmetrical. There is subchondral osteopenia (as opposed to sclerosis) and erosions can be present (**E**).

### Other tests

Any synovial fluid aspirated from the knee should be sent for testing, even if the etiological diagnosis has already been clearly established as secondary infection is always a possibility. This test is clearly mandatory and urgent in the case of monoarthritis of the knee. A total and differential cell count is always important, to distinguish between a mechanical and an inflammatory process. Testing for crystals and bacteriological culture are indicated whenever clinical assessment admits the possibility of microcrystalline or septic arthritis.

Diagnostic arthroscopy may be necessary in complex cases.

Blood and urine tests will be guided by the clinical context, in an appropriate differential diagnosis strategy.

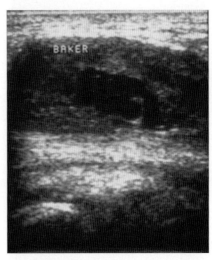

**Figure 13.22.** Baker's cyst revealed by ultrasonography of the popliteal area.

## WHEN SHOULD THE PATIENT BE REFERRED TO A SPECIALIST?

Whenever there is arthritis of unknown cause.

When the degree of pain or disability is not explained by the clinical examination and plain films.

When there is effusion, if the study of synovial fluid is deemed important for differential diagnosis (e.g. in the suspicion of gout).

In cases of meniscal lesions or bursitis/tendonitis that are resistant to standard treatment.

In severe functional disability, with significant limitation of mobility (physiotherapy).

In acute ruptures of the ligaments or chronic, accentuated joint instability (orthopedics).

In osteoarthritis, whenever doubts persist as to the diagnosis (rheumatology) or if surgery is indicated (orthopedics).

## ADDITIONAL PRACTICE
### REGIONAL SYNDROMES. THE KNEE.

# REGIONAL SYNDROMES
## THE FOOT AND ANKLE

**14.**

J.A.P. da Silva, A.D. Woolf, *Rheumatology in Practice*, DOI 10.1007/978-1-84882-581-9_14,
© Springer-Verlag London Limited 2010

# 14. REGIONAL SYNDROMES THE FOOT AND ANKLE

Pain in the foot and ankle is a very common reason for a visit to the doctor. It can cause considerable suffering and disability, as walking is one of the activities that most influences a person's functional capacity and quality of life. Anatomically speaking, the foot combines great strength with a remarkable adaptability. A diagnosis is usually quite clear after a well focused enquiry and careful clinical examination, opening the way to successful treatment.

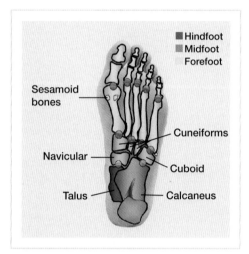

**Figure 14.1.** Bones and joints of the ankle and foot. Functional units.

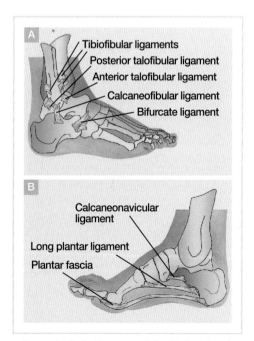

**Figure 14.2. A.** Ligaments of the hindfoot (lateral aspect). **B.** Antero-posterior arch and its ligaments.

## FUNCTIONAL ANATOMY

The ankle and foot constitute a highly complex structure which lends itself to remarkable versatility and strength. The main function of the foot and ankle is to support the body's weight and distribute it throughout the weight-bearing structure as well as generating a spring effect to facilitate locomotion. At the same time, the structure is able to adapt itself to irregular surfaces and constant variations in the mechanical requirements that are imposed upon it.

The ankle and foot are made up of three functional units (Figure 14.1.):

a) The **hindfoot**, consisting of the distal extremities of the tibia and fibula, the talus and calcaneus and their joints and ligaments

b) The midfoot or **tarsus**, consisting of five small bones

c) The **forefoot**, consisting of the metatarsals, proximal, medial and distal phalanges, and their joints

The joints of the hindfoot are stabilized by a complex set of ligaments (Figure 14.2.). These ligaments, especially those of the ankle joint, are frequently the site of traumatic lesions, with sprains or ruptures, which may result in chronic articular instability.

### The arches of the foot

Under normal conditions, the bony structure is kept arched, a shape essential for distributing loads and achieving the spring effect. The anteroposterior arch is more accentuated in the medial aspect of the foot. It is maintained both by the form of the bones and by the ligaments that provide both resistance and elasticity (Figure 14.2.). The most superficial of these ligaments is the plantar fascia, a strong, fibrous band that connects the lower edge of the calcaneus to the transverse ligament of the metatarsals (under their distal extremities). This fascia is understandably exposed to very powerful distending forces and to repeated trauma by compression, which may lead to inflammation at its posterior insertion – a common condition known as plantar fasciitis.

The loss of this anteroposterior arch results in so-called pes planus or flat foot. It may be accompanied by an outward deviation of the forefoot. It may be congenital, but is often found in patients with chronic arthritis as a result of laxity of the ligaments and collapse of the talonavicular joint.

There is also a transverse arch, which is more accentuated in the region of the tarsus and then continues more discreetly in the region of the metatarsophalangeal joints. Under normal conditions, the third and fourth metatarsophalangeal joints are not in contact with the ground. In patients with chronic arthritis such as rheumatoid arthritis, laxity of the ligaments may lead to collapse or even inversion of this arch, which results in painful calluses under the medial metatarsophalangeal joints.

## Movements

The hindfoot is capable of dorsiflexion and plantar flexion or extension, which are based at the tibiotarsal (ankle) joint. The subtalar joint between the talus and the superior aspect of the calcaneus plays an essential role in the inversion and eversion of the foot, in which it is helped by the tarsal joints.

The metatarsophalangeal and interphalangeal joints are capable of flexion and extension.

Dorsiflexion of the foot is performed by the anterior tibial muscle (root L4/L5, deep peroneal nerve) (Figure 14.3.). Extension of the foot depends essentially on the contraction of the gastrocnemius, which inserts into the posterosuperior edge of the calcaneus through the powerful Achilles tendon (root S1/S2, tibial nerve). On either side of this tendon are an anterior bursa and a posterior bursa. The tendon and bursae may be the site of painful inflammation.

Eversion is induced by contraction of the long and short peroneal muscles whose tendons pass behind the lateral malleolus, surrounded by a tendinous sheath, and insert through a common tendon at the base of the fifth metatarsal. Inversion is mainly the result of the action of the posterior tibial muscle, whose tendon passes behind the medial malleolus and inserts in the cuneiform bone.

Figure 11.12. shows the distribution of the cutaneous innervation of the foot.

The cutaneous and motor innervation of the toes is carried by nerves that are arranged

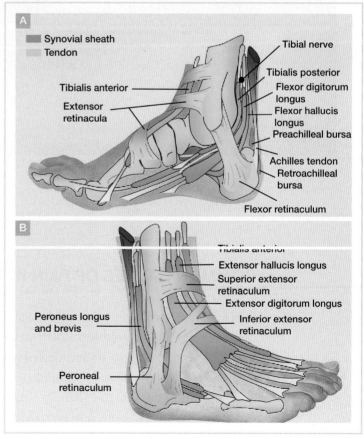

**Figure 14.3.** Tendons, synovial sheaths and bursae of the ankle and foot. **A.** Medial aspect. **B.** Lateral aspect.

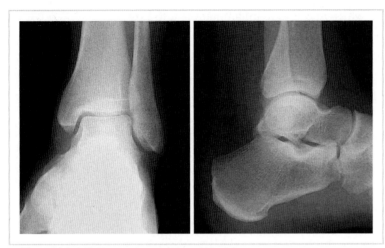

**Figure 14.4.** Ankle X-rays: antero-posterior and lateral view.

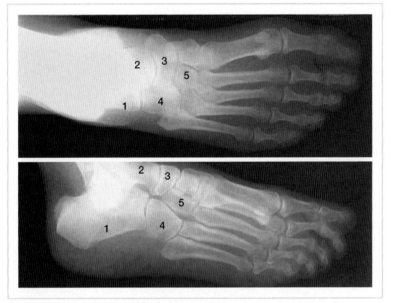

**Figure 14.5.** Foot X-rays: antero-posterior and oblique views. **1.** Calcaneus. **2.** Talus. **3.** Navicular. **4.** Cuboid. **5.** Cuneiforms.

between the metatarsals and metatarsophalangeals, where they may be subject to repeated traumatic lesions caused particularly by tight-fitting footwear. This causes Morton's metatarsalgia.

### Radiological anatomy

Anteroposterior and lateral radiographs of the ankle (Figure 14.4.) give a clear view of the articular space, cortical edges and subchondral bone. On the lateral, the insertion of the Achilles tendon is clearly visible and erosions and calcification may be evident. The subtalar and talonavicular joints may also be assessed from this plane.

An anteroposterior film of the foot gives a good view of the tarsometatarsal and metatarsophalangeal joints. Note the articular space and look for erosions or osteophytes. An oblique angle complements this study and gives a better view of the tarsal joints (Figure 14.5.). The interphalangeals are not easy to see in standard x-rays.

## COMMON CAUSES OF PAIN IN THE FOOT AND ANKLE

Pain in the ankle and foot is frequently related to problems of footwear. Plantar fasciitis is commonly seen in middle-aged and elderly patients. In young people, traumatic lesions predominate. The most likely primary location of gout is in the first metatarsophalangeal joint (podagra), and is relatively common in middle-aged men (Table 14.1.).

The joints in this area are often involved in different types of degenerative and inflammatory polyarthropathy. Note, however, that primary osteoarthritis only affects the tarsus and the first metatarsophalangeal joint with significant frequency. Its presence in other joints, including the tibiotarsal (ankle) joint, is rare and suggests osteoarthritis secondary, for example, to trauma, infection or other causes.

# THE ENQUIRY

The enquiry should focus on the aspects that are typical of each condition and on those that distinguish between them.

## *Where does it hurt?*

Table 14.1. shows the importance of this information. Generally speaking, pain in the ankle and foot is confined to one place and points to the injured structure.

Diffuse pain in the tarsus may be caused by local osteoarthritis or, more often, by changes in the structure of the foot or inappropriate footwear. Morton's metatarsalgia may be described like this but, as a rule, is located further forward.

## *How did it begin?*

Acute onset of pain is to be expected in gout and sprains.

Plantar fasciitis, Achilles tendonitis or bursitis, non-microcrystalline arthritis and dactylitis usually develop in days or weeks.

The pain in osteoarthritis, Morton's metatarsalgia, and foot or toe deformities usually develops over months or years before the patient seeks medical attention.

| Location | Nature of the lesion | Suggestive manifestations |
|---|---|---|
| Hindfoot | Plantar fasciitis | Pain in the plantar aspect of the hindfoot |
| | | Exacerbated or triggered by load bearing |
| | | Local tenderness |
| | Tendonitis of the Achilles tendon | Pain in the posterior aspect of the ankle |
| | | Exacerbated by walking |
| | | Local tenderness |
| | Sprain | Acute, post-traumatic onset |
| | | Pain and functional disability |
| | | Swelling and/or bruising |
| | | Local tenderness |
| | Synovitis | Inflammatory pain |
| | | Pain on palpation and motion |
| | | Local warmth and swelling |
| Tarsus | Osteoarthritis | Mechanical pain |
| | | Exacerbated by inversion and eversion |
| | Flat foot | Deep, ill-defined mechanical pain |
| | | Flattening of the anteroposterior arch of the foot |
| Forefoot | Cavovarus foot | Deep, ill-defined mechanical pain |
| | | Accentuation of the anteroposterior arch of the foot |
| | Morton's metatarsalgia | Mechanical, sometimes paresthetic pain |
| | | Aggravated by tight-fitting shoes |
| | | Pain on palpation between the metatarsals |
| | Hallux valgus | Mechanical pain over the big toe |
| | | Valgus deformity of the first metatarsophalangeal joint |
| | | Often associated with bursitis (bunions) |
| | Gout | Acute, recurring monoarthritis |
| | | Predilection for the first metatarsophalangeal joint |
| | Metatarsophalangeal arthritis | Inflammatory pain |
| | | Usual context of polyarthritis |
| | | Local tenderness |
| | Dactylitis | Swelling and rubor of the whole toe ("sausage toe") |
| | | Suggestive of psoriatic arthritis |
| | Toe deformities | Mechanical pain aggravated by footwear |
| | | Visible deformity |

**Table 14.1.** The most common causes of pain in the ankle and foot.

### What is the rhythm of the pain?

Almost all the pain in this area is mechanical, either because of the degenerative nature of its source or because it is triggered by compression or distension of an inflamed structure, as in Achilles tendonitis and plantar fasciitis.

> Note that the pain caused by structural abnormalities of the feet is often accentuated at the first steps in the morning, gets better after a while and worsens again by the end of the day.

When the pain persists at rest, especially during the night, arthritis should be suspected.

### Exacerbating factors

Understandably, standing and walking are common exacerbating factors for pain in this area. Pain associated with the use of specific types of footwear (high heels, tight-fitting shoes) points to changes in structure or metatarsalgia. Arthritis of the metatarsophalangeals is also exacerbated in these circumstances.

### Usual footwear

Footwear plays a fundamental role in protecting the feet and unsuitable shoes are an extremely important factor in triggering acute pain and promoting chronic structural alterations. High heels overload the forefoot by transferring a lot of the weight to this area. Stiletto heels cause accentuated instability in the hindfoot and overload the local ligaments, frequently leading to repeated, chronic sprains. Tight-fitting, pointed shoes can obviously cause hallux valgus, facilitate the development of Morton's metatarsalgia and exacerbate pain related to deformities of the toes and arthritis of the forefoot.

Thin, hard soles cause repeated trauma of the soft structures and bones of the feet causing pain that may be relieved by wearing soft yet supportive, springy soles.

Repeated trauma of the Achilles tendon leading to tendonitis or bursitis may also be due to poor shoes.

### Habits

Many occupations and leisure activities place intense, prolonged loads on the feet and demand superhuman resistance from them. This can be aggravated by irregular surfaces, tight, inflexible footwear and being overweight. Sometimes such simple facts need to be made clear to the patient.

### Associated manifestations

In general medicine, only rarely will ankle or foot swelling be related local inflammation. Venous insufficiency, heart, kidney or liver failure, and other causes of water retention are, by far, the commonest causes of lower limb edema. Typically, in these cases the edema tends to be bilateral and to predominate at the end of the day and after standing, and is improved in the morning or after resting with the legs raised. In arthritis of the ankle, the swelling is usually moderate and limited to the joint area. It is not relieved by rest. Gout causes accentuated local swelling with intense local heat and redness. In cases of concomitant pain and edema of the ankles or feet, it is essential to clarify the aspects.

The systematic enquiry will look mainly for articular manifestations in other places, especially when enthesopathy or arthritis is suspected as the cause of local pain (see manifestations of seronegative spondyloarthropathy). Associated diseases are also obviously important: heart failure in cases of edema, kidney stones in cases of gout, history of peptic ulcers, trauma, etc. Diabetes mellitus very often causes accentuated discomfort in the feet.

> **NOTE**
>
> In the presence of recurring enthesopathy of the feet in a young patient, seronegative spondyloarthropathy should always be considered.

## THE LOCAL AND REGIONAL EXAMINATION

We suggest that you first conduct the general rheumatologic examination described in Chapter 6. An examination of the foot must include an assessment of the whole lower limb. If the patient complains about his or her ankle and foot, examination of this area should be more detailed. While paying special attention to the painful area, it is important to examine the patient's whole foot and his or her footwear.

### Inspection

Localized redness is almost exclusive to gout, dactylitis and infection. A diffuse purplish color or paleness, is a rare observation that suggests algodystrophy (see below) or Raynaud's phenomenon. The skin of the feet is a preferential location for lesions of vasculitis, which may consist of palpable purpura, bloody vesicles or even ulceration and gangrene (Figure 14.6.). Vasculitis is, however, very rare overall.

Ankle joint synovitis causes discreet swelling, which obliterates the normal depressions anterior and inferior to the medial and lateral malleoli.

Dystrophy of the toenails may be due to mycosis or psoriasis.

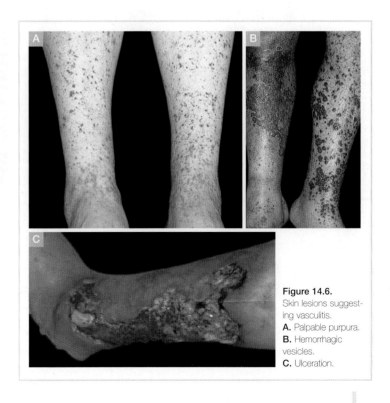

**Figure 14.6.**
Skin lesions suggesting vasculitis.
**A.** Palpable purpura.
**B.** Hemorrhagic vesicles.
**C.** Ulceration.

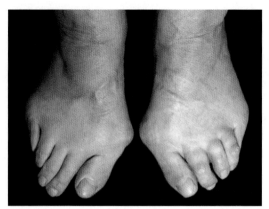

**Figure 14.7.** Hallux valgus in a patient with rheumatoid arthritis. Note also the loss of the transverse arch of the forefoot.

Note the alignment of the hallux: accentuated lateral deviation (hallux valgus) is a common cause of local pain (Figure 14.7.). It is often accompanied by an inflammatory reaction of the bursa that covers the medial face of the first metatarsophalangeal joint: the associated bursitis is commonly known as a bunion. Assess the other toes for deformities that may explain pain (Figure 14.8.). Examine the soles of the feet, looking for calluses. They are important especially if they are not in the usual places (under the calcaneus, the first or fifth metatarsophalangeal joints). Outside these locations, calluses suggest deformity of the foot or inadequate footwear. Flatness or inversion of the transverse arch of the forefoot may be evaluated with the patient lying on his back and is almost always associated with calluses under the third and/or fourth metatarsophalangeal joints (Figure 14.7.).

Alterations in the structure or dynamics of the foot are easier to assess when the patient is standing:

- Examine the position of the axis of the heel in relation to the lower leg. External deviation (calcaneus valgus) is very common, especially in patients with chronic arthritis (Figure 14.9.);
- Under normal conditions, the medial edge of the foot is arched so there is a space between it and the ground when the patient is standing. Absence or reduction of this distance means flat foot. An exaggerated longitudinal arch is typical of cavovarus foot.

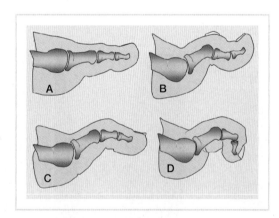

**Figure 14.8.** Deformities of the toes. **A.** Normal. **B.** Hammer toe. **C.** Mallet toe. **D.** Claw toe.

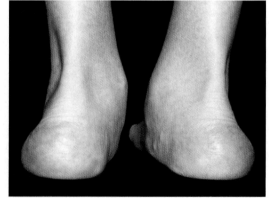

**Figure 14.9.** Calcaneo valgus in a patient with rheumatoid arthritis.

### Palpation

Explore the articular space on the anterior aspect of the tibiotarsal joint. The edges of the joint curve backwards, making them hard to palpate. In cases of synovitis this space is full with an elastic and tender tissue. Swelling and pain around the malleoluses are also common. Firm palpation of inflammatory swelling does not leave any "pitting," unlike vascular edema.

In the case of hindfoot pain, carefully palpate the inferior insertion of the Achilles tendon and adjoining structures. In tendonitis or bursitis, palpation is painful, and is sometimes accompanied by local edema. In plantar fasciitis there is pain on deep palpation at its posterior insertion in the calcaneus (Figure 14.10.).

If these areas are painless, palpate along the posterior face of the internal and external malleoli looking for tenosynovitis of the posterior tibial and peroneal muscles, respectively. The tibial nerve passes behind the medial malleolus. Rarely, its compression here can cause tarsal tunnel syndrome, with paresthetic pain in the sole of the foot. This is the place for Tinel's test.

Perform the metatarsal "squeeze" test, applying pressure across the metatarsophalangeal joints transversely. This maneuver is painful in local synovitis, metatarsalgia, hallux valgus and bunions. If there is pain, you should then focus the palpation on each individual MTP joint, putting your thumb on its dorsal face and your index finger on the plantar face (Figure 14.11A.). Look for swelling, deformity and pain.

In Morton's metatarsalgia, transverse compression of the foot causes pain between two adjacent metatarsals. Deep palpation along the spaces between the metatarsals is painful, and may be accompanied by paresthesia of the corresponding toes (Figure 14.11B.).

The first metatarsophalangeal is often the site of osteoarthritis, generally associated with hallux valgus. The bursa that covers it is often inflamed and painful. It is also a common site for gouty tophi.

The interphalangeal joints of the feet are difficult to examine, but may be painful in cases of arthritis or repeated trauma.

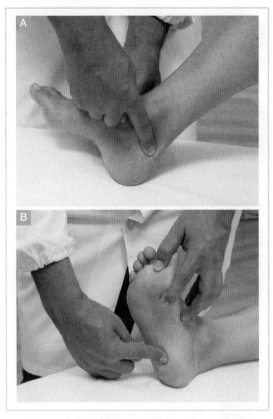

Figure 14.10. A. Palpation of the Achilles tendon and preachillean bursa. B. Palpation of the posterior insertion of plantar fascia.

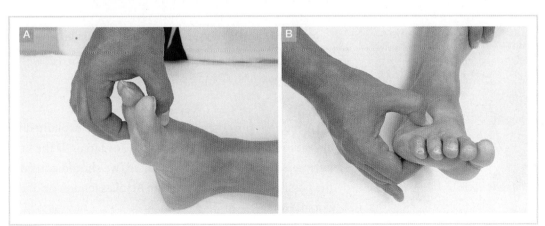

Figure 14.11.
A. Individual palpation of metatarsophalangeal joints.
B. Palpation of intermetatarsal spaces – painful in Morton's metatarsalgia.

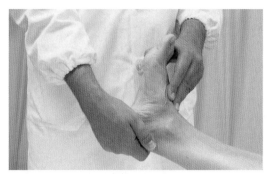

**Figure 14.12.** Mobilization of the ankle joint. The hand that grasps the heel moves the ankle joint, distinguishing it from that of the mid-foot.

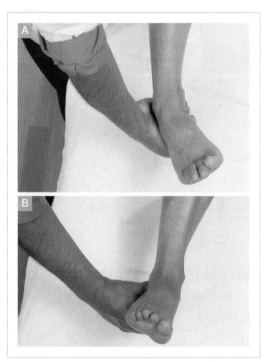

**Figure 14.13.** Mobilization of the subtalar joint. Hold firmly the heel and induce movements of inversion (**A.**) and eversion (**B.**).

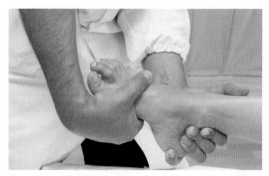

**Figure 14.14.** Mobilization of the midfoot. The heel is immobilized while the other hand rotates the midfoot into inversion and eversion.

## *Mobilization*

### 1. Mobility of the ankle joint

To assess the mobility of the tibiotarsal joint, hold the heel firmly with one hand and the tibia with the other, keeping the knee semi-flexed. Induce dorsal and plantar flexion and evaluate the movements of the heel (Figure 14.12.).[1] Compare with the other side.

Normal dorsiflexion goes up to 15–25° and extension from 40 to 50°: limited mobility indicates articular and not periarticular abnormality.

### 2. Mobility of the subtalar joint

Firmly holding the heel, induce inversion and eversion (Figure 14.13.). Compare with the other side.

A reduction in inversion (about 40°) and eversion (about 15°), or pain during these maneuvers, suggests local synovitis, which is common in rheumatoid and psoriatic arthritis.

### 3. Mobility of the tarsus/midfoot

Immobilize the heel with one hand. Hold the tarsus with the other and induce inversion and eversion (Figure 14.14.).

These movements depend on the tarsal joints and are limited or painful in the presence of local arthritis. It is essential to immobilize the heel to distinguish the mobility of the tarsus from that of the subtalar joint.

### 4. Global active motion of the foot and ankle

Now ask the patient to turn his feet up and then down as far possible. Compare the two sides.

A reduction in these movements can be explained by alterations already found in the ankle or tarsus. If the limitation is much more than expected, we should consider the possibility of retraction of the Achilles tendon or of the dorsiflexors.

[1]The tarsus also has flexion and extension movements. Immobilizing the heel enables us to isolate the movements of the tibiotarsal joint and evaluate them separately.

### *The neurological examination*

Pain in the foot may be caused by nerve root compression (sciatica). Lesions due to peripheral neuropathy, which are common in diabetes, for example, can also cause local pain, which is usually paraesthetic and diffuse. Both neuropathies and sciatica can be accompanied by reduced or absent Achilles reflexes. When the alteration is unilateral, its pathological significance is more certain, reflecting a root or peripheral nerve lesion. In peripheral neuropathies, the alteration is usually bilateral. We should, however, bear in mind that the Achilles reflexes of many elderly patients are almost or completely unreactive, even in the absence of disease.

If you suspect a neurogenic lesion, test the sensitivity to pain of the feet and lower legs: a symmetrical, sock-shaped distribution of loss is typical of peripheral neuropathy. Localized loss affecting a dermatome may be due to nerve root or peripheral nerve lesion, depending on the affected area (Figure 11.12.).

It is easier to assess muscle strength with the patient standing. Ask him to take a few steps on tiptoe (gastrocnemius, S1/S2) or on his heels (anterior tibial, L4/L5).

Please note: It can be useful to look at the patient's shoes, provided that they are not new. Asymmetrical wear of the heel indicates a dynamic imbalance. Deformation of a shoe can be a clear indication of a varus or valgus deviation of the hindfoot, hallux valgus, deformed toes or a collapsed transverse arch, for example.

---

### *TYPICAL CASES*
### 14.A. HEEL PAIN (I)

Rosário Domingos, a normally healthy 52-year old cook, went to her doctor because of pain in her left foot that was making it difficult to work. The progressive onset of the pain, which was mainly located in the heel, had begun two months before, increasing in intensity until she could not stand on it for any length of time. It was particularly intense when she took the first steps in the morning and went away soon after. It was exacerbated by prolonged standing. She had not noticed any relationship with footwear. She was much better wearing trainers.

She denied any other important manifestations and had had no treatment.

On clinical examination, we found her to be obese, with no other relevant alterations.

The foot, examined with the patient lying down and standing, had no apparent deformities and the arches were normal. There were accentuated calluses on the inferior face of both heels. Articular mobility was normal and painless.

## PLANTAR FASCIITIS
### MAIN POINTS

Consists of the inflammation of the posterior insertion of the plantar fascia in the calcaneal tuberosity, with or without associated bursitis.

It is common in middle-aged men and women.

Being overweight, having flat feet, prolonged standing and walking and irregular surfaces are risk factors.

It may occasionally be a manifestation of seronegative spondyloarthropathy.

It is reflected by plantar pain in the hindfoot, aggravated by weightbearing.

The local examination makes the diagnosis.

In the absence of other manifestations, there is no place for plain films. Ultrasound and MRI scans may help with a doubtful diagnosis.

Treatment consists of reducing compression and local trauma through rest, weight loss and special insoles (Figure 14.15.). Suggest soft yet firm, supportive, properly shaped footwear.

In persistent situations, a local injection may be necessary.

*Did we know enough for a diagnosis?*

*What else would you have done?*

Palpation of the inferior face of the heel was diffusely painful, but triggered intense pain at the lower anterior edge of the calcaneus. The inferior insertion of the Achilles tendon was normal on inspection and palpation.

*What is your diagnosis?*

*What advice would you give the patient?*

We concluded that the patient had **plantar fasciitis**.

We explained the situation to her and stressed the relationship between her complaint and being overweight and prolonged standing and walking. Such conditions can cause pain even in the absence of fasciitis! We prescribed a pair of doughnut-shaped insoles to take the load off the insertion of the fascia. We recommended partial rest and loss of weight.

We suggested that she wear well-cushioned shoes with thick, flexible rubber soles providing support for the longitudinal arch (good-quality trainers/sneakers would be a good choice). We arranged to see the patient again if her condition did not improve and prepared her for the possibility of a local corticosteroid injection.

### Heel spur

We mention this merely to devalue it. This is a bony growth that is often seen in radiographs at the point of plantar fascia insertion in the calcaneus (Figure 14.16.). Although many doctors tend to consider this anomaly to be a source of pain or plantar fasciitis, in practical terms it is unrelated to the symptoms. The patient has plantar fasciitis if we find the above symptoms, even if the x-ray is normal. The patient does not have plantar fasciitis if the clinical examination does not indicate it, even if s/he has a spur. We therefore suggest that you not attach any significance to this radiographic finding.

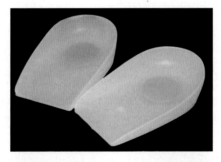

**Figure 14.15.**
Insoles used in the treatment of plantar fasciitis – the area corresponding to the posterior insertion of the fascia (*blue*) is softer, to avoid compressing the painful structure.

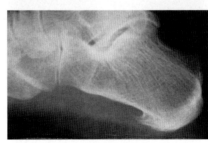

**Figure 14.16.**
Calcaneal spur. It is a common radiological image with no clinical relevance.

## TYPICAL CASES
## 14.B. HEEL PAIN (II)

David Paiva, a 21-year old student, came to us because of pain in the posterior face of his right heel, which had begun about three months before and had become progressively worse. The pain was more intense when he walked, and especially while playing football or going downstairs. He had nocturnal discomfort and it was much worse in the morning. He described swelling of the Achilles tendon/posterior aspect of heel.

Our systematic enquiry revealed that he had also been suffering back pain for two or three years, especially after long periods of immobility at his desk. He had occasional morning pain. He denied any other articular or extra-articular manifestations except for asthmatic bronchitis that he had had for a long time and was well controlled.

The clinical examination of his feet suggested slight swelling of the inferior insertion of the right Achilles tendon, with marked tenderness on local palpation. Mobilization caused pain on forced dorsiflexion of the right ankle joint, with painful limitation of the range of movement.

*Give a brief description of the relevant problems.*[2]

*What is your diagnosis?*

*What treatment would you suggest?*

We concluded that David had **tendonitis of the Achilles tendon with associated bursitis.**

We suggested that he wore shoes with a higher heel for some time to relax the tendon somewhat. We advised him to stop playing football and other strenuous exercise for a while and prescribed a topical anti-inflammatory.

We stressed the importance in the future of warming-up exercises and stretching the tendons before any more strenuous exercise.

We arranged to see him again 3 weeks later.

*Were we missing anything?*[3]

## ACHILLES TENDONITIS/BURSITIS
### MAIN POINTS

This is the inflammation of the inferior insertion of the Achilles tendon and/or of the pre- and retro-Achilles bursae.

It is most common in young males.

It causes local pain that is exacerbated by walking, especially going downstairs, as this involves greater distension of the tendon.

Strenuous sports, inappropriate footwear and seronegative spondyloarthropathy are important risk factors.

Pain on local palpation, exacerbated by forced dorsiflexion, confirms the diagnosis. There may be local swelling.

Repeated episodes weaken the tendon and may lead to partial or total rupture.

Ultrasound and MRI scans are useful in assessing the tendon's condition, especially in chronic inflammation or suspected rupture.

The initial treatment involves resting the tendon with raised heels, topical anti-inflammatories and partial physical rest.

Stubborn cases may benefit from oral NSAIDs or demand the use of physical agents, stretching exercises or a splint in physiotherapy.

Local steroid injections are associated with increased risk of tendon rupture and should only be avoided.

[2]Achilles tendonitis in a young man with a history of back pain.

[3]Very good! We have a young man with Achilles tendonitis with no apparent cause. But he has a suspicious backache. In fact, although we might think that his back pain was postural, from an incorrect position while sitting, it is inflammatory: after rest and sometimes in the morning. We had to consider the possibility of seronegative spondyloarthropathy, and especially ankylosing spondylitis, of which the tendonitis would another sign (enthesopathy). And this was, indeed, the case with our patient.

*TYPICAL CASES*
## 14.C. PAIN IN THE FOREFOOT (I)

It was the third time that it had happened: intense pain over the first metatarsophalangeal joint that appeared at night after going to bed quite well. The joint swelled and went red and the slightest touch caused excruciating pain. The first two episodes, which had occurred the year before, had been on the other foot and responded in about 4 days to NSAIDs prescribed at emergency. Manuel, a 45-year old farmer, wondered what the problem was and how it would develop.

He denied any similar episodes in other joints. He had a history of kidney stones (a single episode 3 years before) and well controlled hypertension. He confessed that he normally ate rather too much and often drank alcohol.

His late father had had severe articular problems similar to his, but they also affected other joints.

There were no other significant abnormalities in our clinical examination. The examination of the foot confirmed monoarthritis of the first right MTP, which was frankly swollen, hot and painful (Figure 14.17.). There did not seem to be any articular effusion, so we did not conduct an arthrocentesis.

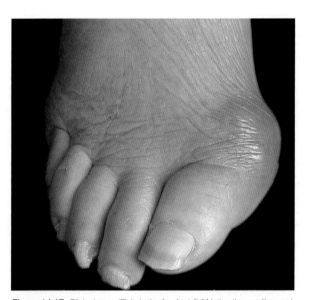

**Figure 14.17.** Clinical case "Pain in the forefoot (I)." Notice the swelling and redness of the first metarso-phalangeal joint.

*What do you think are the probable diagnoses?*

*On what basis?*

*Would you request any tests?*

*How would you treat this situation?*

We reached a diagnosis of **acute gouty arthritis**, and prescribed a full dose of anti-inflammatories to be taken regularly until the pain ceased.

We requested routine lab tests, including serum urate level, serum lipids, liver enzymes, creatinine and 24-hour uricosuria. The patient was instructed to have these tests a few weeks after the end of this crisis.

He came to clinic again 4 weeks later as agreed. The flare-up had responded to the medication with no recurrences. The lab tests showed elevated uricemia at 9.4 mg/dl, with hypertriglyceridemia and elevated $\gamma$-GT. The uricosuria was normal.

This confirmed our suspected diagnosis.[4] We discussed the highly probable relationship of the disease with his eating and drinking habits, stressing the need to moderate his protein intake and give up alcohol. Allopurinol would be started in the future if these measures proved insufficient. The patient promised to comply…

[4]A positive diagnosis had to wait for a sample of synovial fluid showing the presence of uric acid crystals.

## GOUTY ARTHRITIS
### MAIN POINTS

This is the inflammation of a joint in reaction to deposition of monosodium urate crystals.

It occurs most commonly in middle-aged men.

It is rare in post-menopausal women and exceptional in young women.

It usually starts with episodes of acute, recurring monoarthritis, with clear signs of inflammation, separated by asymptomatic intervals.

The first MTP is the site of the first episode in about 50% of cases (podagra). The tarsus is also often affected. With time it tends to involve more proximal joints and even the upper limb.

The diagnosis is essentially clinical and is reinforced by findings of hyperuricemia.

The final diagnosis is established by demonstration of monosodium urate crystals in the synovial fluid.

A more detailed clinical description of gout and its treatment is given in Chapter 18.


### TYPICAL CASES
### 14.D. PAIN IN THE FOREFOOT (II)

"My feet are killing me," answered the patient when I asked her why she had come to see us.

She described "excruciating" pain in both feet that had become worse over several years. It had recently become unbearable in her right foot, preventing her from working in her boutique. The longstanding pain was typically mechanical and was located in the first MTP. It was particularly bad in the morning when she put her shoes on and got worse again at the end of the day. It was distinctly less severe during the weekends, when she wore her favorite slippers.

Recently the pain in her right foot had changed significantly. It was more intense and affected the whole forefoot. Sometimes, she even had what felt like an electric shock and had to take off her shoes in the middle of the shop! The pain was less intense at night, though it sometimes woke her up.

She denied any other relevant symptoms.


*Think about the possible diagnoses at this stage.*

*Plan the clinical examination.*


In the clinical examination, I noted her elegant, high-heeled shoes with thin soles and pointed toes. The hallux deviated considerably in both feet, pushing against the second toe. The little toe was bent inwards. On the medial aspect of the right first MTP there was a slightly reddish swelling that fluctuated on palpation. Mobilization of the hallux was painful, with crepitus that was more accentuated on the left.

Examination of the left tarsus revealed no alterations. Deep palpation between the third and fourth right metatarsals, however, caused intense pain at a well defined point, reproducing the characteristics of the recent spontaneous pain.

## HALLUX VALGUS
### MAIN POINTS

This is a very common condition in middle-aged and elderly women.

It consists of the inward deviation of the first metatarsophalangeal joint.

It is associated with a congenital predisposition, but is further exacerbated by ill-fitting shoes.

Traumatic bursitis on the medial face of the joint ("bunions") is a common complication.

It causes local pain, which is exacerbated by walking and ill-fitting shoes and may radiate to neighboring areas.

In an anteroposterior radiograph of the foot, the diagnosis is confirmed if the angle between the first metatarsal and the big toe is larger than 10~15°.

Treatment involves wearing well-fitted, supportive shoes without pointed toes and having restraining features to prevent the toes sliding forward, reducing the load on them. Persistent bursitis may respond to a local injection.

Left untreated hallux valgus will almost always leads to osteoarthritis of the first MTP, with mechanical pain that no longer responds to simple measures.

Surgical correction, which is reserved for stubborn, incapacitating cases, usually has good results.

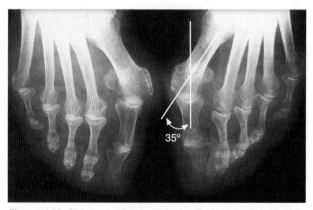

**Figure 14.18.** Clinical case "Pain in the forefoot (II)." Note the deviation of the first metatarsal bone, bilaterally. The 1st MTP joint presents features of osteoarthritis. The exostosis of the medial aspect of first metatarsal bone testifies the intensity and duration of local compression by shoes.

*What are the probable diagnoses at this stage?*

*What treatment would you recommend?*

We explained the cause of her suffering to the patient: bilateral hallux valgus, with bursitis, probable osteoarthritis and Morton's metatarsalgia on the right. Indeed, the plain film that she had with her showed osteoarthritis the hallux valgus (Figure 14.18.).

We stressed the role that her choice of footwear had played and encouraged her to change to comfortable shoes with flexible soles, low heels, malleable leather and wide at the front. The patient balked at this. We explained that if she continued to wear the same kind of shoes, she would almost certainly have continuing severe pain. She agreed to a local injection of anesthetic and a corticosteroid at the point of maximum pain between the metatarsals, followed by bed rest for 24 hours.

She came back a few months later and said that the pain was much better with the suggested changes. The paraesthetic pain in her right foot persisted, however. Our local examination was the same. We requested an ultrasound of the foot, which confirmed Morton's neurinoma. The patient opted for surgery.

## MORTON'S METATARSALGIA
### MAIN POINTS

This condition is relatively common in middle-aged and elderly women.

It is caused by the compression of the interdigital nerves of the foot, usually between the third and fourth metatarsals. In some patients there is a fibrous nodule (Morton's neuroma), which is visible on ultrasound.

This condition is responsible for intense pain in the forefoot, exacerbated by standing and ill-fitting shoes. It is sometimes dysesthetic.

Firm palpation between the metatarsals reproduces the spontaneous pain. Rarely, there may be an alteration in sensitivity to pain in the corresponding toes.

Ultrasound scan can be necessary to clarify a doubtful case or to support decisions regarding surgery.

Initial treatment is conservative and based on more appropriate footwear and achieving an ideal weight.

It stubborn cases, surgery may be considered.

## TYPICAL CASES
### 14.E. HEEL PAIN (III)

It was not really pain that she felt, but rather an ache of the right ankle, with a frequent "wobbly" feeling. The problems predominated at the end of a whole day on her feet, said this 47-year old teacher. She complained of occasional swelling in the painful ankle, mainly in the evening, which eased after a few days of partial rest. She normally wore flat shoes, not because she liked them, but because she could not tolerate high heels.

She denied any associated manifestations. Her past clinical history was not significant. When we persisted, she remembered a sprain in that foot when she was at school. She had had to rest for a few days, but had recovered fully.

Examination of the lower limbs showed the alignment to be normal. Mobility of the feet and ankles was normal. Eversion of the right foot was much more accentuated than the left. Firmly holding her heel with our fingers under the malleoluses, we found that forced eversion caused pain under the internal malleolus (Figure 14.19.). There were no other abnormalities.

*What is your diagnosis?*

*Would it be worth requesting any diagnostic tests?*

*What treatment would you suggest?*

We explained to the patient that she very likely had a chronic rupture of the ligaments in the medial side of the ankle. We suggested she wore supportive shoes and an elastic bandage to keep the heel in neutral position.

The requested ultrasound scan confirmed a rupture of the tibiocalcaneal and posterior tibiotalar ligament. The patient clearly gained relief with the suggested treatment and decided to postpone consideration of surgery.

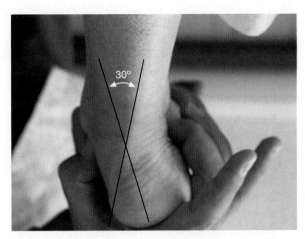

**Figure 14.19.** Clinical case "Hell pain (III)." Forced eversion of the heel.

## ANKLE SPRAIN
## AND CHRONIC INSTABILITY
### MAIN POINTS

An acute ankle sprain consists of the total or partial rupture of the articular ligaments, due to excessive force in inversion or, more rarely, eversion.

It causes acute, incapacitating pain, with subsequent swelling and/or bruising.

Mild cases can be treated with rest, icepacks, compression and elevation of the limb, with a slow return to normal activities.

Patients who cannot bear weight or present accentuated swelling, bruising or signs of instability should be referred urgently to an orthopedic surgeon.

Persistence of an untreated rupture results in chronic articular instability, with mechanical pain and recurrent flares. The ankle joint may develop osteoarthritis.

Clinical examination reveals lateral or anteroposterior instability (drawer sign).

Initial treatment of chronic instability is conservative, involving stable, well-cushioned shoes and an elastic bandage.

Stabilizing surgery may be necessary.

## TYPICAL CASES
## 14.F.  DIFFUSE MECANICAL PAIN

Dr. Manuela Fragoso, a 38-year old gastroenterologist, came to us because of pain in both feet that was making her medical work difficult. She had had the pain for a long time, since adolescence, but it had got progressively worse. It usually appeared on days when she stood or walked a lot and she sometimes had to sit down and massage her feet. The pain was diffuse but particularly affected the tarsus. She had begun to wear orthopedic sandals at work but without much relief. She had suffered a fracture of the right medial malleolus when she was 24.

Examination of the fee, with the patient lying on her back, showed no alterations other than enlargement of the forefeet and discreet, bilateral calluses under the third MTP. Palpation of the soles caused discreet discomfort along the medial edge. The anterior ends of the talus and the navicular bone were palpable on the medial edge of the foot. Articular mobility was normal and painless. Examination with the patient standing revealed flat feet, with almost all the foot in contact with the floor (Figure 14.20.). The curvature reappeared when the patient stood on tiptoe, showing flexibility of the tarsal joints.

## FLAT FEET AND CAVOVARUS FOOT
## MAIN POINTS

These are deformities of the feet with a reduction (flat foot) or heightened (cavovarus foot) arch of the foot.

Most cases are asymptomatic, but they are a common cause of pain in young adults.

Flat foot usually also involves loss of the transversal arch of the forefoot, with the formation of painful calluses.

Cavovarus foot is often associated with claw or hammer toe and with local trauma and pain.

Both may be congenital or acquired.

The diagnosis is clinical but can be confirmed by podoscopy or a lateral weight-bearing radiograph, for an exact measurement of the angle of the internal arch (Figure 14.21.).

The treatment is essentially conservative, using insoles and/or well-shaped, flexible footwear to achieve better weight distribution.

If the problems persist, consider referring the patient to a podiatrist for custom-made insoles.

Surgery is reserved for extreme, incapacitating cases that do not respond to conservative measures.

### What would you recommend to this patient?

The orthopedic sandals that she wore were well-shaped but made of hard, inflexible material.

We suggested softer, more malleable footwear, with insoles to reinforce the longitudinal arch of her feet, or comfortable, loose trainers/sneakers, possibly one size larger than normal. She would certainly have to continue alternating rest and standing. The most drastic solution involved surgical correction, which we would reassess on the basis of the results achieved with these measures.

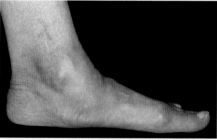

**Figure 14.20.** Clinical case "Diffuse mechanical pain." Note the loss of the antero-posterior arch of the foot, with medial and plantar displacement of the talus and navicular bones.

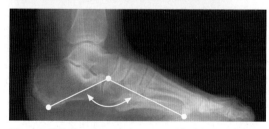

**Figure 14.21.** Pes planus and pes cavus. Radiological diagnosis based on weight-bearing radiographs: References: lowest point of the calcaneus; lowest point of the talus and lowest point of the head of the 1st metatarsal bone. Normal: 115 ~125°. (Courtesy: Prof. Caseiro Alves.)

## SPECIAL SITUATIONS

### *Rheumatoid foot*

The foot is a particularly important site of pain and disability in rheumatoid arthritis patients. The metatarsophalangeal joints are among those affected early, frequently and severely in this disease. This involvement is reflected by localized inflammatory pain, which may be a presenting feature or appear subsequently in the context of polyarthritis. Transverse squeezing of the forefeet and individual palpation of these joints causes pain and may reveal synovial inflammation. MTP joints are often the first site of bone erosions on x-rays, developing into progressive joint destruction (Figure 14.22.).

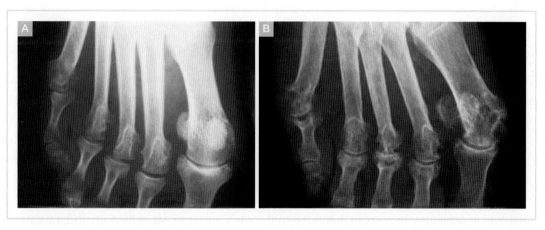

**Figure 14.22.** Radiographs of the feet in rheumatoid arthritis. **A.** Patient with symptoms for eight months. Notice the erosions in all MTP joints. **B.** Patient with disease for 5 years. Profound disorganization of the joints.

The ankle and subtalar joints are also commonly affected. The subtalar joints are particularly susceptible to early, irreversible destruction of the cartilage and bone, which may cause considerable pain and disability.

In untreated rheumatoid arthritis the feet tend to acquire a variety of deformities which are, in themselves, causes of progressive, incapacitating pain even if the inflammatory process is controlled after they are established. The most common of these deformities are calcaneus valgus (Figure 14.23A.), "triangular" forefoot with hallux valgus and crossed toes (Figure 14.23B.) and secondary

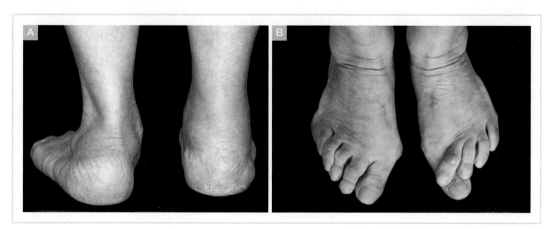

**Figure 14.23.** Common foot deformities in patients with rheumatoid arthritis. **A.** Calcaneus valgus. **B.** Triangular forefoot (hallux valgus and medial deviation of the other toes).

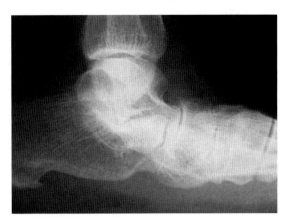

**Figure 14.24.** Rheumatoid foot. Collapse of the talonavicular joint resulting in secondary flat foot.

flat foot, with collapsed talonavicular joint and painful calluses under the third and fourth MTPs (Figure 14.24.).

Given the impact of walking on quality of life, the rheumatoid patient's feet warrant special care, based first and foremost on early, aggressive treatment of the disease, with cautious use of local injections, if necessary. Once deformities are established, we are faced with a difficult, highly incapacitating problem requiring a multidisciplinary approach, frequently with disappointing results.

### Diabetic foot

The feet of diabetic patients require very special care. Alterations caused by macro- and microvasculature changes expose patients to painful trophic skin alterations with a high risk of infection.

Polyneuropathy, which is common in these patients, may result in symptoms suggesting rheumatic disease, with diffuse pain and paresthesia. Impairment of deep sensitivity leads to disturbances of articular stability and muscle imbalance with pain and a predisposition to deformity and secondary osteoarthritis. In later stages, with accentuated loss of deep sensitivity, Charcot's arthropathy may set in, heralded in the early stages by signs of acute inflammation reminiscent of gout but with a notable absence of pain. Over time, this condition leads to total malposition of the joint and fragmentation of the bone.

Treatment should be prophylactic, based on careful control of the diabetes, comfortable shoes and regular visits to the doctor and footcare specialist or chiropodist.

### Complex regional pain syndrome (reflex sympathetic dystrophy, algodystrophy, etc.)

The foot is the most common location of this relatively rare, but interesting and potentially incapacitating condition. It results from a regional deregulation of the sympathetic nervous system that leads to persistent, chronic vasodilation. Left untreated, this conditions leads to atrophy of the bones, muscles and skin and retraction of the soft tissue.

It may affect several joints, especially the feet, knees, hands and hips (where it is sometimes called "transient osteoporosis of the hip").

It often appears after major or minor trauma. In the hands, it is a common complication of Colles' fractures or surgical procedures but may also follow myocardial infarction (Dressler's shoulder-hand syndrome).

The patient usually describes diffuse severe pain, usually unilateral, with a variable rhythm, which can go from being typically inflammatory to characteristically mechanical. The onset is insidious, with progressive deterioration that may reach total functional disability of the affected area.

In the initial stages, the affected area normally presents diffuse swelling with pitting, which extends beyond the limits of the joints. There is diffuse purplish coloring, exacerbated by a long period with the limbs dependent. There may be clear difference in temperature (warmer in the initial phases, colder in later stages) and perspiration may be more accentuated on the affected side (Figure 14.25.). Absence of these vasomotor signs makes diagnosis more difficult, particularly in deep joints.

With time, these suggestive vasomotor changes can become discreet. The diagnosis then depends on a strong clinical suspicion, the enquiry and a thorough physical examination.

Plain films may be normal, but sometimes present a typical patchy osteopenia – Figure 14.26. Tecnethium bone scanning can also be helpful. For a long

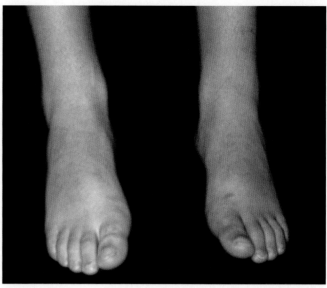

**Figure 14.25.** Algodystrophy in a 12 year old boy. Diffuse swelling of the foot which gains a purple discoloration when dependent. (Courtesy: Dr. Manuel Salgado.)

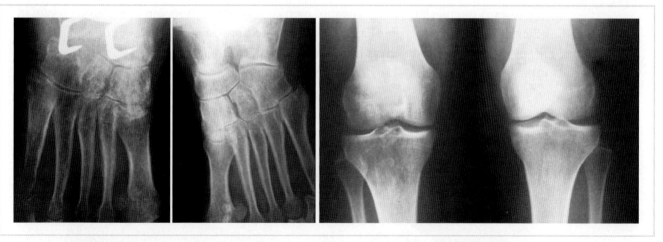

**Figure 14.26.** Algodystrophy. The right foot was affected following a surgical procedure. The patient suffering from the right knee described a minor trauma 4 months before (vd. bone scintigraphy of this patient – Figure 14.27.).

time, increased uptake of the radioligand will predominate with a diffuse appearance, extending beyond the limits of the joint (Figure 14.27.). Diffuse increased uptake in the foot is common and involves several

**Figure 14.27.** Algodystrophy of the right knee. Late phase cintigraphy images (bone phase – 2–3 hours after injection of the tracer) show increased uptake of the radiotracer. The diffuse distribution and the extension of bone activity beyond the joint suggest algodystrophy but are not specific (**A.**). Hyperfixation in the early phase (vascular phase – first few minutes after injection) is a stronger suggestion of this condition but still not specific (**B.**).

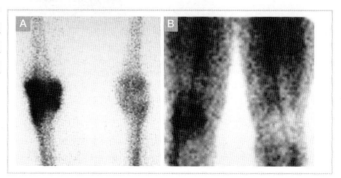

joints of the tarsus. Early scintigraphic images, in the first few minutes (the vascular phase), can reinforce the diagnosis if they show an increase in local radioactivity. Conversely, in the later stages, there may be regional decreased uptake of the radioligand. The patient's sedimentation rate remains normal.

Treatment becomes less effective over time. If not properly treated, the condition may develop into marked atrophy and retraction of the subcutaneous and muscular tissue, with total, irreversible functional disability (Sudeck's atrophy).

If the clinical picture supports a reasonable suspicion of this condition, the patient should be urgently referred to a specialist.

## TREATMENT

In general practice the vast majority of cases of pain limited to the foot will have mechanical cause. Treatment basically consists of correcting functional anomalies and relieving the load on the feet, by changing the patient's footwear and weight.

The services of qualified specialists in orthosis and podiatry are invaluable in more difficult cases. A careful choice of footwear or even custom-made shoes can be extremely useful in relieving these patients' pain (Figure 10.28.). If there are painful calluses under the heads of the metatarsals, which are very common, especially in rheumatoid patients, insoles with a retrocapital pad (Figure 10.28.) can do a lot to relieve the symptoms.

Local injections should only be administered by experienced professionals.

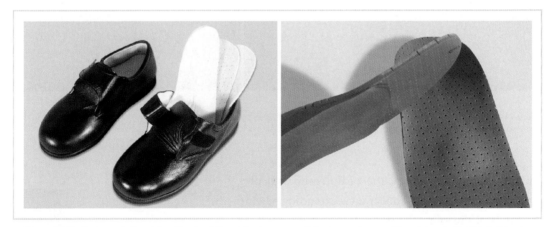

**Figure 14.28.** Patients with foot deformities should be advised to wear well-fitted, capacious, cushioned shoes with thick flexible rubbery soles Insoles with a thickened bar just behind the metatarsophalangeal joints help relieve pressure and pain in this area.

## WHEN SHOULD THE PATIENT BE REFERRED TO A SPECIALIST?

**Rheumatologist:**

- Whenever there are reasons to suspect arthritis, seronegative spondylarthropathy or algo-dystrophy;
- When there is a probable indication for local injection, if primary care physician is not qualified to perform it.

**Podiatrist or physical therapist:**

- A competent professional in this area has a lot to offer a patient with serious foot problems, especially in cases of deformity or calluses.

**Orthopedic surgeon:**

- In the case of accentuated instability of the ankle or severe deformity of the feet (hallux valgus, hallux rigidus, flat or arched feet), with functional disability resistant to conservative measures.

# ADDITIONAL PRACTICE
## REGIONAL SYNDROMES. THE FOOT AND ANKLE

# GENERALIZED PAIN SYNDROME
## FIBROMYALGIA

15.

J.A.P. da Silva, A.D. Woolf, *Rheumatology in Practice*, DOI 10.1007/978-1-84882-581-9_15,
© Springer-Verlag London Limited 2010

# 15. GENERALIZED PAIN SYNDROME FIBROMYALGIA

The main features of generalized pain syndrome have been described in Chapter 4, characterizing it as one of the first-step diagnoses. It is an extraordinarily common condition in clinical practice, affecting 2–5% of the whole population, and accounting for 2–7% of visits to GPs and 15–20% of all rheumatology consultations.

Although it only occasionally reflects a disease with any significant structural, organic impact, it is essential to recognize it not only because it is so common, but also because of the enormous disability and suffering to which it condemns patients. It can present in many different ways and, even to an experienced physician, may suggest a vast variety of diagnoses leading to a multitude of useless, if not dangerous, tests and treatments. The correct diagnosis requires diagnostic sensitivity, detailed clinical examination and patience.

Fibromyalgia accounts for the majority of cases of generalized pain.

It is a condition that, more than anything else, is diagnosed by a process of exclusion and we should only consider it when we are sure that there is no organic disease to explain the patient's complaints. Understandably, such requirements demand extreme clinical care. Behind the musculoskeletal symptoms there is often considerable psychological suffering, which is an integral part of the disease and, therefore, of the approach to treatment.

## CLINICAL PRESENTATION

### FIBROMYALGIA
The enquiry
**MAIN POINTS**

**Female patient (> 90%)**

**Pain:**

- Multifocal or generalized
- Diffuse and hard to describe
- No visible local alterations
- Migratory
- Inflammatory rhythm
- Worse after exercise

**Manifestations of anxiety:**

- Dramatic language
- Body language
- Psychopathological history

**Associated psychosomatic manifestations.**

### The enquiry

The main symptom is pain that has several suggestive characteristics. After enquiry and clinical examination, the overall picture is one of severe, incapacitating but ill-defined musculoskeletal discomfort, with no objective clinical abnormalities.

In almost all cases, the patient is a *woman*, usually aged between 30 and 50, although it can affect all age groups. Generally, the patient only goes to the doctor after many years of intermittent, diffuse pain of growing intensity and frequency. It often worsens after the menopause.

The pain affects *multiple musculoskeletal areas*, usually involving the body above and below the diaphragm bilaterally. The pain has a *pattern of distribution inconsistent* with any common joint disease. It may appear quite random. Doctors may tend to consider the possibility of multiple, successive or associated periarticular lesions.

The difficulty lies in the *migratory nature* of the pain. The patient often describes intense, incapacitating pain along, for example, one arm one day only for it to be normal the next day, and another area affected. It is not unusual, however, for a particular anatomic area to be affected more regularly. Axial pain tends to be more persistent, but this preferential location varies from one patient to another.

Usually, *the description of the symptoms is dramatic*, with words like "awful," "terrible," "excruciating," although the patient usually has great *difficulty in describing the location and nature of the pain*. Words like "tiredness" or "stiffness" are frequently used. Although the patient refers the pain to a joint, closer questioning reveals that the painful area is quite significantly larger, involving the neighboring muscle segments, if not the whole limb – *there is little or no focus on joints*. Fibromyalgic patients often point to the painful area by sliding their hands along the axis of the limb, while an arthritic patient describes a circle around the joint.

The description of the pain *generally suggests an inflammatory rhythm*. Many patients say that it is more intense during the night and in the morning and may even be accompanied by prolonged morning stiffness. They frequently wake up feeling "more tired" than when they went to bed. The pain is clearly exacerbated by exercise, particularly if it is repetitive, but with an interesting characteristic: *pain is more intense after, rather than during, the exercise*. Indeed, when asked, many patients say that the pain is particularly intense several hours after a physically demanding task.

Patients often describe fatigue and generalized weakness, with no localized deficit and no relationship with the type or quantity of "work." There is often paraesthesia, usually affecting the hands and feet, though it is usually inconsistent and variable in time.

The systematic enquiry may be totally negative, although there is often *association of manifestations of a potentially psychosomatic origin*: irritable bowel, migraines, stress headaches, tight chest, depression… Be sure to ask about symptoms suggesting hypothyroidism (sensitivity to cold, weight gain, constipation…), as this condition can also cause generalized pain. Note also that Raynaud's phenomenon is rather more frequent in these patients than in the general population. Sleep disturbances are frequent in fibromyalgia, and may consist of difficulty in getting to sleep and, especially, light, intermittent, or non-restorative sleep.

The enquiry will usually give plenty of opportunities to note *many, obvious signs of anxiety:* dramatic language, restlessness, sighs, hyperventilation. However, even when the clinical picture suggests a strong psychological component, our strategy is never to address this directly with the patient before a formal diagnosis is reached.

### The clinical examination

Clinical examination is the key to the diagnosis: it is essentially *NORMAL*.

Most patients describe *pain with almost every movement* requested in the general examination. Many are reluctant or even afraid to carry out these movements, as if they were afraid of fractures. The pain caused by movement often has odd radiations: the lumbar region hurts when we ask a patient to flex her neck, her neck hurts when we test the strength of the forearm etc. Many maneuvers testing for periarticular lesions are positive and can lead to the wrong

**FIBROMYALGIA**
Clinical examination

*MAIN POINTS*

Pain with many movements.

Atypical radiation.

No signs of inflammation.

No deformation or limitation of passive movements.

Normal neurological examination.

Typical sensitive points.

diagnosis. Note the profusion of complaints, which is the opposite of the typical regional nature of these lesions.

*The patient's **movements are not limited**, however.* Their range is normal, in spite of the pain, unless there is also another pathology. We often have to encourage the patient to carry out the whole movement, as she understandably tends to stop on experiencing pain. Always test passive mobility.

*There are no signs of inflammation, crepitus or deformity in any joint.* This means that they all have to be carefully examined.

*The summary neurological examination is normal.* Muscle strength, tested with enough authority to guarantee the patient's cooperation (fearing pain) is normal. Ask the patient to take a few steps on tiptoe and on her heels and to crouch down and get up without using the arms. The reflexes are normal or even brisk, which is often the case in anxiety. Note that the sciatic nerve stretch tests may be falsely positive!

**PLEASE NOTE**

Any clinical objective anomaly requires an explanation other than fibromyalgia.

A general clinical regional examination with these characteristics reinforces our suspicions. It is time to look for the typical sensitive points in fibromyalgia. There are 18 points arranged symmetrically, nine on each side (Table 15.1. and Figure 15.1.).

| | |
|---|---|
| Occipital | At the insertion of the occipital muscles |
| Lower cervical | On the anterior face of the spaces between the transverse processes from C5 to C7 |
| Trapezium | At the median point of its upper edge |
| Supraspinous | Above the scapular spine, near its internal limit |
| Second rib | Externally to the second chondrocostal joint, at the upper edge |
| Epicondyle | 2 cm below the epicondyles |
| Gluteus | At the anterior edge of the gluteus maximus, in the superoexternal quadrant of the buttock |
| Greater trochanter | On the posterior edge of the trochanteric eminence |
| Knee | In the internal ball of fat immediately above the joint |

**Table 15.1.** Tender points used in defining fibromyalgia.

Palpate these points with the tip of your thumb or index finger, using reasonable pressure. Look at the ungual bed of your thumb or finger. When it starts to go white, the pressure is about 4 kg/cm², which is what is required. Ask the patient if the pressure causes pain and score one "positive" point for each "yes," regardless of the intensity of the pain. Many patients will shrink away from your finger!

Move your finger slightly round the point. The pain can often be intense right next to a painless spot.

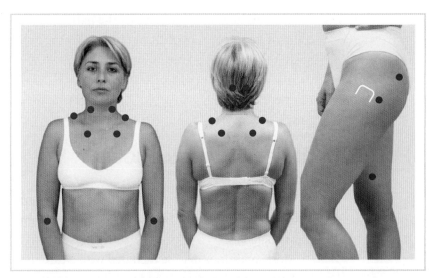

**Figure 15.1.** Tender points in fibromyalgia. (See also Table 15.1.).

Having done this, we are now ready to see whether our patient meets the American College of Rheumatology's diagnostic criteria for fibromyalgia shown in Table 15.2.

| **The patient will be classified as having fibromyalgia if she meets the following two criteria:** |
| --- |
| **1. History of widespread pain for at least 3 months** |
| Definition: Left and right-sided pain, pain above and below the waist. There should also be axial pain (along the spine or in the anterior thoracic wall). Lower back pain is considered to be below the waist for this purpose. |
| **2. Pain in 11 or more tender points (Figure 15.1.) on digital palpation** |
| Definition: Digital palpation should be done with a pressure of about 4 kg/cm². For a point to be "positive," the patient must describe pain and not just discomfort. |

Table 15.2.
Criteria for the classification of fibromyalgia, according to the American College of Rheumatology.[1]

[1]Wolfe F, Smythe HA, Yunus MB, et al. The American College of Rheumatology 1990 criteria for the classification of fibromyalgia: Report of the Multicenter Criteria Committee. *Artrhitis and Rheumatism*, 1990; 33: 160–172.

In terms of diagnostic criteria, the patient is considered to have fibromyalgia if she has a count of 11 or more out of 18, but in a highly suggestive clinical context do not exclude the diagnosis if the count is a little lower.

## DIFFERENTIAL DIAGNOSIS

As we can see in Table 15.2., the diagnosis of fibromyalgia is purely clinical. There are, however, other rheumatic and metabolic conditions that involve widespread pain above and below the waist bilaterally.

Most conditions may be excluded with a careful enquiry and clinical examination: generalized osteoarthritis, rheumatoid arthritis, psoriatic arthritis, and progressive systemic sclerosis.

Our systemic enquiry and clinical examination are decisive in eliminating other potential causes: polymyalgia rheumatica, systemic lupus erythematosus, dermatomyositis, Sjögren's syndrome, debilitating infectious diseases like tuberculosis or AIDS, etc.

Others require tests.

> We suggest that you perform the following investigations on all patients with suspected fibromyalgia:
>
> - Full blood count;
> - Serum calcium, phosphorus and magnesium;
> - Electrophoretic protein strip;
> - Free T4 and TSH;
> - Erythrocyte sedimentation rate.

These tests enable us to screen for diseases of the connective tissue, rheumatic polymyalgia, multiple myeloma and chronic infections (anemia, leuko and thrombocytopenia, hypergammaglobulinemia, and elevated SR), hypothyroidism (T4 and TSH), hypo-parathyroidism (calcium corrected for albumin, phosphorus, and magnesium).

We can add other tests to this list depending on the characteristics of each case:

- CPK and aldolase – if the muscles are very painful and the test of proximal muscle strength is doubtful;

- X-rays – of areas with any localized, persistent pain (special attention to the pelvis – seronegative spondyloarthropathy);

- Antinuclear antibodies – if we suspect a disease of the connective tissue;
- Etc.

**FIBROMYALGIA**
*Differential diagnosis*

| | |
|---|---|
| Rheumatoid arthritis | Polymyositis |
| Systemic lupus erythematosus | Hypothyroidism |
| Sjögren's syndrome | Hypoparathyroidism |
| Polymyalgia rheumatica | Polyneuropathy |
| Ankylosing spondylitis | Debilitating systemic diseases |

In fibromyalgia, all these tests should be normal or near-normal. Any changes need some other explanation.

Our aim is to be absolutely sure that there is no organic or metabolic cause of the pain syndrome. Note, however, that the existence of another disease does not exclude a diagnosis of fibromyalgia, provided that it alone cannot account for the widespread pain. The high prevalence of fibromyalgia in the general population makes the coexistence of two conditions very common likely, which makes matters more difficult for the physician. According to some studies, about 12% of patients with rheumatoid arthritis also have fibromyalgia, while the percentage is 22% in systemic lupus erythematosus.

*TYPICAL CASES*
**15.A. INFLAMMATORY BACK PAIN**

According to this 42-year old university lecturer, it all seemed to have started 8 months before, when she spent a long time working on her doctorate. She attributed the lumbar pain to sitting in the same position for long periods. The pain persisted and even got worse, however, extending progressively to the thoracic region. The pain, described as "violent, as if everything was being ground up inside," was clearly more intense at night and in the early morning. It was accompanied by marked morning stiffness (more than an hour) and improved with back exercises. She had noticed a progressive reduction in the mobility of her spine and growing difficulties at the gym. She had tried several anti-inflammatories in appropriate doses and even an intramuscular injection of glucocorticoid with no response.

In the systematic enquiry she described recurrent episodes of diarrhea, only during the day, with no blood or fever. She denied any other problems.

She had a spinal x-ray, which showed no changes. However, a bone scan dhad apparently shown the presence of sacroiliitis. Furthermore she was found to be HLA-B27 positive!

"My doctor says that I've got spondylitis and I'm terrified…"

*Consider the diagnosis indicated.*

*What information from the clinical examination should we assess in our diagnosis?*

Our general rheumatologic examination did not reveal limitations to active or passive mobility. The patient complained of pain elsewhere on mobilization of the cervical spine, however (it hurt in the thoracic and lumbar region), the shoulders (pain in her arms) and the lumbar spine (local pain). Schobber's test showed a distension of 10 → 16 cm. Palpation of the lumbosacral spine caused pain in the vertebrae from L2 to S1. Springing of the sacroiliac joints triggered pain under the examiners hands but not in the sacral region. The summary neurological examination was normal.

*Reconsider your diagnosis.*

*What information, if any, seems incompatible with the initial possibility?*

*What other possibilities would you suggest?*

Palpation of the typical points of fibromyalgia caused pain in 9 of the 18 sites.

*What is your diagnosis?*

When asked again in more detail, the patient described occasional, migratory, transient pain in several locations – hips, arms, thighs, and cervical region for more than 7 years, to which she had not paid much attention. She admitted having been treated several times for depression…

The diagnosis now seemed clear… We asked for some laboratory tests and scheduled a long talk for when we had the results.

But… what about the scintigraphy and the HLA-B27? Look at Chapter 24.

## TYPICAL CASES
## 15.B. OSTEOPOROSIS AND PAIN

The patient, a 42-year old secretary, had come for treatment of her osteoporosis, detected in a recent bone densitometry scan. When asked why the scan had been requested, she said that it was to investigate the pain that she had "all over her body," for which no explanation had been found, although she had been to several doctors and had countless tests – all of which had been normal.

She described highly intense, almost permanent pain with intermittent flares that had confined her to bed on several occasions. As for its location, the patient pointed dramatically to many areas, always diffusely located. She described particular intensity in the lumbar region, but the other areas were affected for periods varying from hours to several days. She described swelling in her hands and feet, which were not related to the worst periods of local pain. She denied any deformities or limitations to movement except those due to pain. The pain was exacerbated by exercise, but mainly the following day.

She denied any relevant personal history. Her mother had osteoporosis, with fractures of the spine and femur. Her elder sister also had osteoporosis.

*Give a brief summary of the patient's complaints.*[2]

*Had the densitometry finally revealed the cause of this patient's pain?*

*What other possibilities are there? How would you explain them? How would you study them?*

Clinical examination revealed an anxious patient who found it very hard to relax when we tested her passive movements. Almost all the movements were "intensely" painful, especially in the cervical and lumbar regions. There was no articular swelling, crepitus or deformation of any kind. The range of passive movements, when possible, was normal. Neurological examination was also normal.

Palpation revealed pain in 16 of the 18 tender points of fibromyalgia.

*What is the probable diagnosis?*

*Would you request any tests?*

*How would you assess the presence of osteoporosis?*

*What treatment would you suggest for this patient?*

The (countless) test results that the patient had with her were completely normal, including a protein strip, erythrocyte sedimentation rate, calcium and phosphorus, CPK, and thyroid hormones. Her T score was –2.7 in the lumbar densitometry. The spinal x-ray excluded any significant pathology including osteoporotic fractures.

We explained that her osteoporosis, probably of genetic origin, had nothing to do with the pain. Our diagnosis of fibromyalgia was categorical and we addressed the psychological connotations of this syndrome. The patient recognized that her pain increased at times of stress and improved with a hot bath. She had had a difficult childhood and her current family environment seemed to be disastrous…

There was plenty of time to treat the osteoporosis.

## *Physiopathological interpretation*

Can we consider a condition involving only subjective symptoms, with no visible alterations in the clinical examination and laboratory tests, to be an "illness"?

In fact, in spite of intense research into the origin of fibromyalgic pain, nothing decisive has yet been found. Some abnormalities have been observed in muscle energy reserve, but they do not reach a pathological level and are more compatible with poor muscle condition. Quality of sleep has been extensively evaluated and there can be no doubt that patients' sleep is of poor quality, with significant alterations in REM and NREM sleep. But is this a causal disturbance or just a reflection of their anxiety? Studies of the hypothalamic–adrenal axis have also detected slight, though inconclusive alterations.

---

[2]Widespread, diffuse, migratory pain, not centerd on joints, in a middle-aged woman, no deformities, worse after exercise, poor response to treatment, family history of osteoporosis.

More recent research with positron emission tomography and functional MRI has shown that the central nervous system processes pain abnormally in fibromyalgia. But is this a cause or a consequence of the pain and the emotive temperament of these patients?

In view of these difficulties, even today, many authors still question the actual existence of "fibromyalgia" as a disease. In our opinion, this is just a matter of semantics. Even if we doubt the existence of fibromyalgia, it is hard to doubt the existence of patients with these characteristics and the clinical independence of this condition. At the very least, the definition of this syndrome is extremely useful in identifying a group of patients whose symptoms defy their integration in any other category of disease.

On the other hand, we have to recognize that the clinical definition of fibromyalgia is just as good as that of other pathological conditions like depression, manic-depressive psychosis or even headache.

The important thing in our opinion is that these characteristics identify patients who experience great suffering, whatever its origin, and therefore need medical help and guidance!

Even if we think that most of the symptoms are of psychological origin, there is still suffering and it is just as deserving of medical attention whether its cause is physical or psychological. At most, we may argue about what kind of doctor is the most qualified to treat the condition.

From all the literature and our own experience, we would like to suggest two ways of interpreting fibromyalgia.

The first is more practical and interprets the muscle pain as a consequence of continuous muscular tension caused by the permanent psychological stress that these patients clearly show.

Note that the ACR criteria make no reference to psychological characteristics. Most of the literature actually says that there is no "fibromyalgic personality." On the basis of countless interviews and profound psychological debate with many patients, we are convinced that these patients have psychological traits in common: excessive worry, a somewhat obsessive personality, perfectionism, inability to relax, dissatisfaction, and the dominance of obligation over satisfaction and a sense of duty over a sense of pleasure. With rare exceptions, these traits leave these patients in a permanent, inescapable state of dissatisfaction, anxiety and unhappiness. Fibromyalgia could, from this point of view, be interpreted as a widespread stress headache.

This model is the basis for our own personal approach to treating these patients.

Another model, with a more scientific and physiopathological approach, is based on the recognition that the same biological mediators that modulate our state of mind and temperament – serotonin, adrenalin, noradrenalin, corticotrophin releasing factor, etc. – intervene in the perception and processing of pain. Psychological processes do not occur in a biological vacuum!

It is perfectly plausible that small variations in the fine control of the mediators, determined by genetic polymorphisms and the impact of past experience, can also affect the psychological and biological sphere. Generalized pain is therefore not a consequence of "mere" psychological disturbances, but only the other side of the same "neurobiological climate."

# TREATMENT

Even today, the treatment of fibromyalgia is still difficult and often unsatisfactory. Each doctor has his or her own strategy, exploiting the doctor-patient relationship and the psychological and social facets of the problem to a greater or lesser extent. In terms of evidence-based medicine, only tricyclic antidepressants and some muscle relaxants have been shown to have significant impact. My opinion is that a more profound approach, based on the relationship between psychological stress and pain, is more rewarding, not only for the patient, but also for the physician. It is a question of dealing with the whole patient, rather than the disease.

Admittedly, our suggestion is a mixture of scientific evidence and personal conviction based on experience, but it has proved highly satisfactory.

- Complete the study, make a clear, conclusive diagnosis of fibromyalgia, and establish the basis for the conclusion: type of pain, distribution, migratory nature, lack of clinical alterations, tests normal.

- Reassure the patient as to the functional and life prognosis.

- Explain that the disease has no organic component and there is no need for any further tests.

- Address this question. If there is no pathology, why does it hurt so much?
  We feel that it is productive to assure the patient that, in fibromyalgia, there is a close relationship with a *certain temperament*. Describe it without referring to the patient, asking her to say whether this psychological profile is similar to her own. The answer is almost always a definite yes. This little trick helps the patient to focus on the psychological dimensions that are the main cause of her physical and general suffering. It also helps her to believe that we are not trying to back out on possible psychological grounds.

- What can psychological profile have to do with pain? Explore the relationship: psychological tension → muscular tension → pain, in terms that the patient can understand. A tensed hand will begin to hurt, even if it does not move!

- Ask the patient whether she has not found that the pain fluctuates with her degree of anxiety or worry. Make it clear that you are not saying that the pain is merely psychological. The pain is real and intense; it is just a matter of understanding its cause.

- Suggest a regular program of treatment based on:
  - *Psychological relaxation* – leading a quieter life, settling conflicts, adapting her work to her capacities, paying more attention to herself, pursuing personal fulfillment, and greater tolerance. Make it clear that this is the mainstay of the treatment (although few patients manage the "transformation"). In any case, it is absolutely essential to get the patient to commit to her own treatment.
  - *Gymnastics* twice a day – non-strenuous stretching exercises. Gymnastics in a heated pool is particularly effective.
  - *Hot baths* – The patient will already have noticed that hot baths relieve her pain. If she is able to say why, it means that she has understood your explanations. Suggest that she

takes a hot bath whenever the pain is really bad. Exercises at the end of the day followed by a hot bath will help her to sleep, thus making a fundamental contribution to an improvement.

- *Regularizing sleep* – we should tell the patient how to try to improve her sleep as much as possible: having a regular bedtime, avoiding daytime sleeps, keeping the bedroom dark and quiet, avoiding stimulants (like coffee or tea) in the evening, or even sleeping in separate beds if her partner is a restless sleeper.

• **Medication** – low doses of tricyclic antidepressants or SSRIs (fluoxetine, paroxetine) can do a lot to help these patients, not only because they modulate the pain, but also because they facilitate sleep, calmness and muscle relaxation. Duloxetin, a selective, serotonin, and norepinephrine reuptake inhibitor (SSNRI) has also demonstrated efficacy in fibromyalgia. Explain to the patient that the idea is only to help her achieve a different psychological balance. Pregabalin, an antiseizure and atinociceptive agent, has been shown to offer more benefit than placebo in trials of fibroamyalgia treatment.

Muscle relaxants (especially cyclobenzaprine), analgesics and anti-inflammatories may be useful during flares to control more intense pain. If they are used regularly, the benefit tends to wear off after a time.

Spa treatments may be useful in more difficult cases.

• If the intensity of the psychological condition suggests psychopathology, consider referring the patient to a psychologist or psychiatrist with experience in these fields.

This approach obviously requires time and patience. Nevertheless, in patients capable of understanding and assimilating the information, we have achieved very encouraging results not only in terms of relieving the pain but also and especially in improving their quality of life, which is our primary goal.

## ADDITIONAL PRACTICE
### GENERALIZED PAIN SYNDROMES. FIBROMYALGIA

25.E. RAYNAUD'S AND GENERALIZED PAIN                    PAGE 25.32

# OSTEOARTHRITIS

**16.**

J.A.P. da Silva, A.D. Woolf, *Rheumatology in Practice*, DOI 10.1007/978-1-84882-581-9_16,
© Springer-Verlag London Limited 2010

# 16. OSTEOARTHRITIS

Osteoarthritis is caused by a degenerative process that takes place in the articular cartilage and subchondral bone. It involves deterioration of the articular cartilage, with an early alteration in its biomechanical properties followed by a progressive loss of thickness. The cartilage becomes rugose, and in time the subchondral bone may even become exposed. Clinically, these structural lesions manifest themselves by the presence of crepitus. The thickness of the cartilage may be assessed radiologically by the width of the joint space. The loss of cartilage is thought to be more accentuated at the sites where mechanical pressure is greatest and hence results in radiographs as an **asymmetrical** narrowing of the joint space.

The subchondral bone is exposed to a substantial increase in pressure, to which it reacts with increased mineralization (presenting as subchondral sclerosis) and a disorganized attempt to enlarge the supporting area by forming exostoses at the edge of the articular surfaces. These are osteophytes, which are palpable as irregular bony excrescences and which are also visible on plain film (Figure 16.1.).

From a pathophysiological point of view, the process is not just a consequence of wear and tear or the effect of ageing, although it is age-related. There is an inflammatory process which generates cytokines, growth factors and proteolytic enzymes, which lead to the destruction of tissue and exostotic reaction. Occasionally, the inflammatory process becomes more obvious clinically, producing signs and symptoms of inflammation. There may be synovial swelling, with or without effusion, and the pain may become more "inflammatory," i.e. persisting during the night and accompanied by longer periods of morning stiffness.

Osteoarthritis is extremely prevalent in the general population. Its frequency increases considerably with age and it becomes widespread after the age of 70. It is found mostly in the weight-bearing joints and in the hands. If the disease appears earlier than 45 years of age or affects other joints, the physician must consider traumatic, inflammatory or metabolic factors that may contribute to osteoarthritis.

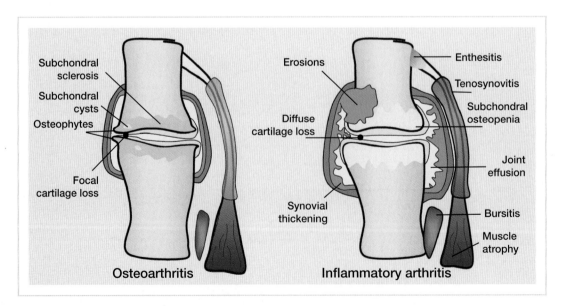

**Figure 16.1.** Schematic representation of degenerative and inflammatory arthopathies.

## When can we say a patient has osteoarthritis?

**The pain is articular in origin:**

- The patient complains of pain in the joints with possible regional radiation.
- A physical examination confirms the origin.

**The pain is typically "mechanical" (it may also have slight inflammatory characteristics during acute exacerbations).**

**Slow progressive worsening over months or years.**

**The physical examination is typical.**

- Crepitus
- Osteophytes (palpated as localized sprouts of bony consistency).
- Limited active and passive mobility (in the more advanced stages).
- Usual absence of signs of inflammation (there may be mild signs during acute exacerbations).

**Radiographs confirm the diagnosis (Figure 16.2.).**

- Asymmetrical loss of joint space – as opposed to a uniform loss of joint space, which suggests inflammatory arthritides.
- Subchondral sclerosis – an increase in bone density near the joints, as opposed to the typical subchondral osteopenia of other types of arthritis.
- Subchondral cysts and geodes – areas of hypodensity within the subchondral sclerosis.
- Osteophytes – bony spurs at the edges of the joints.

**Acute-phase reaction protein levels are normal.**

**Table 16.1.**
Typical features of osteoarthritis.

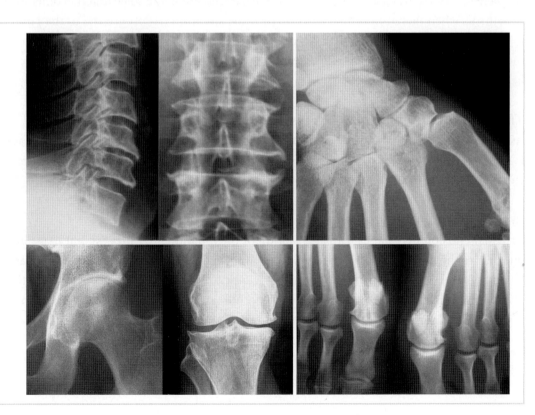

**Figure 16.2.**
Radiological features typical of osteoarthritis (early stage).

## PRACTICAL POINTS

Some of the clinical aspects mentioned above are worth further discussion.

### Age and time of onset

Primary or idiopathic osteoarthritis usually appears in middle-aged or elderly people and gets worse over time. Therefore, when a younger patient's enquiry suggests osteoarthritis (articular pathology with mechanical pain), we have to characterize the pain very carefully and consider the possibility of osteoarthritis secondary to a prior or associated disease – arthritis, trauma, aseptic necrosis, etc. It is also necessary to consider these options if the onset of the apparent osteoarthritic condition was fast, over days or weeks.

### Affected joints

Primary or idiopathic osteoarthritis usually affects two types of joint:

- **Weight-bearing joints** – the spine, hips, knees and first metatarsophalangeal joints.

- **The hands** – first carpometacarpal joint and/or proximal and distal interphalangeal joints ("nodal" osteoarthritis).

If any other joints are affected by osteoarthritis, consideration must be given to underlying causes, which may justify special treatment.

### Crepitus and effusion

The presence of crepitus on moving and palpating the joint indicates that the articular surface is irregular. This is particularly suggestive of osteoarthritis, but may also be found in other forms of arthritis when there is minimal effusion or if the situation has progressed to the point of inflammatory deterioration of the cartilage. On the other hand, when there is articular effusion, the crepitus may be less perceptible because the surplus synovial fluid alleviates the friction between the articular surfaces.

### There are usually minimal signs of inflammation in osteoarthritis

As we have seen, they may, however, appear during acute exacerbations. When inflammation **is** present, its signs are distinct and are seen as mild synovial swelling (of a rubbery consistency), slight local heat, and tenderness along the joint line.

### Articular effusion is quite common in advanced osteoarthritis

Articular effusion may indicate an aggravation of the inflammatory process, but may also be due only to the mechanical disturbance of the joint. On the other hand, effusion accompanied by very obvious signs of inflammation suggests septic or microcrystalline arthritis, in addition to osteoarthritis. If in doubt, conduct an arthrocentesis to collect and analyze a sample of the synovial fluid. In osteoarthritis, the synovial fluid is usually transparent, maintains its viscosity and has a leukocyte count of less than $2{,}000/mm^3$.

### *Association with periarthritis*

Osteoarthritis, especially of the hip or the knee, is often associated with inflammation of the adjacent periarticular structures: tendinitis, ligamentitis or bursitis. Tendinitis of the adductors, and trochanteric bursitis/tendinitis are particularly frequent in the hip. In the knee, pes anserine bursitis/tendinitis often accompanies osteoarthritis.

These lesions may constitute the main cause of pain and disability. Always consider this possibility, as simple treatment of periarticular soft tissue inflammation can be extremely rewarding.

### *Instability*

Articular instability is a problem that arises particularly in the knee and ankle joints. Instability in the knee may be the cause or consequence of osteoarthritis. In the ankle, it is generally the cause. In either case, its existence is a decisive factor in the progression of osteoarthritis, as the joint is subject to much greater pressure and friction. Compensating this instability with elastic supports, muscle strengthening, orthoses or even surgery is an essential part of treatment. Always take articular stability into consideration.

### *Radiological and clinical examinations*

Statistically, there is a correlation between the radiological appearance and the intensity of the symptoms in osteoarthritis: more advanced osteoarthritis has more severe radiological signs and tends to be more incapacitating. There may, however, be considerable disparity between the radiological and the clinical examination in individual patients. This aspect is particularly obvious in the spine, but can be seen at any site. It is the patient's clinical condition and degree of disability, and not the radiological aspect of the joint that should take priority in the choice of treatment, especially when considering surgery.

## CLINICAL SUBTYPES

When faced with a case of osteoarthritis, it may be useful to consider whether the patient falls into one of two patterns:

### *1. Typical osteoarthritis*

This develops progressively in middle-aged or elderly patients and involves one or more commonly affected joints:

a) Spine, hip, knee and the first metatarsophalangeal joint;

b) The first carpometacarpal and proximal and distal interphalangeal joints of the hands.

As a rule there is polyarticular involvement, which is very often symmetrical. This type of osteoarthritis is most likely to be primary and related to age, exercise, and genetic predisposition. Excess weight is particularly associated with the development of patellofemoral osteoarthritis, though its relationship with osteoarthritis at other sites remains controversial. Some occupations constitute a risk factor for osteoarthritis of the hip (miners, agricultural workers) or of the knee (pavers and mechanics).

Its clinical characteristics and basic treatments are described in the chapters about each anatomical region. Nodal osteoarthritis of the hands is also discussed later in this chapter.

## 2. Atypical osteoarthritis

Osteoarthritis may be called "atypical" when it appears in young people (aged under 45), develops rapidly, or affects less usual sites such as the shoulders, elbows, wrists, metacarpophalangeal joints or ankles.

This type of osteoarthritis is almost always secondary to some other cause (Table 16.2.).

| |
|---|
| Fracture involving the articular surface |
| Meniscectomy |
| Axis deviations |
| Articular instability |
| Intra-articular foreign bodies |
| Osteochondritis dissecans |
| Particularly demanding occupations |
| Aseptic necrosis |
| Preexisting arthritis |
| Chondrocalcinosis |

Table 16.2.
Most common causes of secondary osteoarthritis.

Some of these causes can be detected by standard enquiry. Others may become apparent only after more specific questioning.

Hemochromatosis is one of the causes of early atypical osteoarthritis and it should be suspected in face of coexisting systemic manifestations typical of this condition, such as diabetes, skin hyperpigmentation, liver disease, heart failure, etc. There may be a family history of a similar condition. The involvement of the metacarpophalangeal joints is an important clue.

A history of thyroidectomy can also put us on the track of hypoparathyroidism, which is one of the causes of chondrocalcinosis. Other conditions will require additional clinical tests. Aseptic necrosis and chondrocalcinosis are discussed in detail in Chapters 12 and 18 respectively.

Whenever appropriate, osteoarthritis therapy should be associated with treatment of the underlying disease.

## TYPICAL CASES
## 16.A. HIP PAIN

Maria de Lurdes was 62 and enjoyed life to the full, except for the pain in her right hip, for which she went to see her family doctor. The pain had started about 6 years before and had worsened very slowly. She only had pain when she walked or got up after sitting for a long time. She was fine at rest and did not wake up with any pain at night (except when she moved in bed). She denied any significant morning stiffness but described brief stiffness after being at rest for any length of time. There was no radiation of the pain.

When asked if she had any other complaints, she described mechanical knee pain, particularly when going up and down stairs. She was being treated for high blood pressure and angina pectoris and was taking anti-inflammatories when the pain got worse.

The pain was limiting her everyday activities considerably, although she was still independent. She could manage to walk for about an hour before she had to stop.

A clinical examination showed an obese woman (weight 62 kg, height 1.47 m), without any significant abnormalities in her general examination or in her spine or arms.

She walked with a limp, taking small steps with her right leg and tipping her pelvis. Range of movement in her right hip joint was reduced, with 10° internal rotation and zero external rotation. Flexion was about 100°, but there was a visible limitation in extension during forced flexion of the left hip joint. Adduction and abduction were also limited. There was pain on forced passive movements. Her left hip joint also presented limited range in several directions, though it was less marked. An examination of the knees revealed patello-femoral crepitus without any limitations in range of movement. There were no periarticular lesions in the hips or knees.

*Summarize the main problems.*[1]

*Consider your diagnosis, any further investigation and choice of treatment.*

A plain film of the pelvis and knees is shown in Figure 16.3.

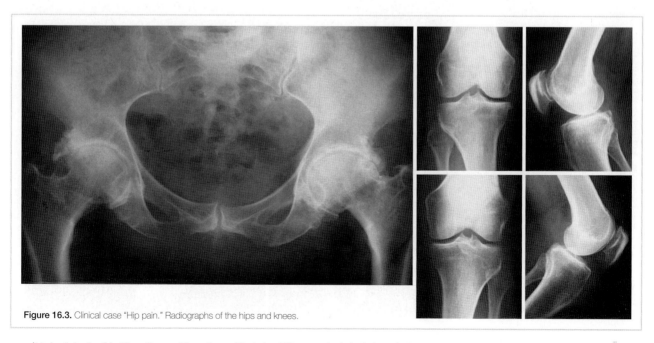

**Figure 16.3.** Clinical case "Hip pain." Radiographs of the hips and knees.

[1]Mechanical pain of the hip and knees with crepitus and limited mobility, no periarticular lesions, obesity.

We explained the situation to the patient and suggested the treatment described at the end of this chapter.

The pain was reduced significantly in the following months. Nevertheless, her function continued to deteriorate as the years went by. At 70 the patient was practically housebound and she found lying on her right side very difficult. We suggested a total hip replacement, with excellent results.

## TYPICAL CASES
## 16.B. DEFORMITY AND PAIN IN THE HANDS (I)

It was difficult to define the rhythm of the pain affecting the joints in the patient's hands. Exercise aggravated the pain and it was worse at the end of the day, though the patient also said that she had pain during the night and prolonged morning stiffness. Occasionally she noticed oedema or even redness over some joints but most of the time there were no signs of inflammation. The pain was not particularly intense or incapacitating. What worried her most was the progressive deformity that she had noticed observed and the fear that this was similar to her mother's condition, which had severely deformed her hands.

The patient, a 53 year-old teacher, said that the problem had started with very mild pain about 5 years before but had become much worse in the last 2 years, as a result, she thought, of the menopause.

Otherwise she was in very good health. She denied any personal or family history of skin lesions.

Looking at her hands, we noticed the nodular aspect of some joints. We asked her to point out which ones were painful. She indicated all the distal interphalangeal and some of the proximal interphalangeal joints. She also suffered pain at the base of her right thumb. Local palpation showed that these nodes had a bony consistency. There was no fluctuation on bidigital palpation of any of the joints. Flexion was slightly reduced. The wrists and metacarpophalangeal joints were normal on physical examination.

*Look at the patient's hands in Figure 16.4.*

*What do you think is the probable diagnosis?*

*Are any additional tests necessary? Which ones?*

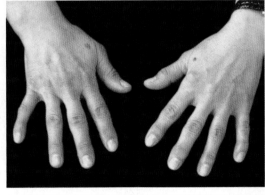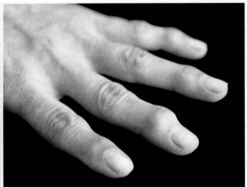

**Figure 16.4.**
Clinical case "Deformity and pain in the hands (I)." Note the focal nodular deformities around the distal interphalangeal joints. There is no diffuse swelling or redness of the joints.

The diagnosis was made.

Figure 16.5. shows the x-ray of this patient's hands. Please note that this it was not indispensable for diagnosis.

We told the patient that she had nodal osteoarthritis. We explained that the prognosis for nodal osteoarthritis is quite good and that the pain tends to remain mild, except for short episodes of exacerbation. Function will, generally speaking, be maintained even in very deformed hands (Figure 16.6.), which was, in fact, what had happened with her mother. We mentioned that this kind of osteoarthritis tends to have a strong family association and that it usually gets worse after the menopause.

We told the patient that, unfortunately, we can only treat the symptoms and relieve the pain, as there are no proven treatments to prevent the progression of this type of osteoarthritis. We encouraged the patient to remain active and do regular mobility exercises with her fingers. We prescribed the treatment described later in this chapter.

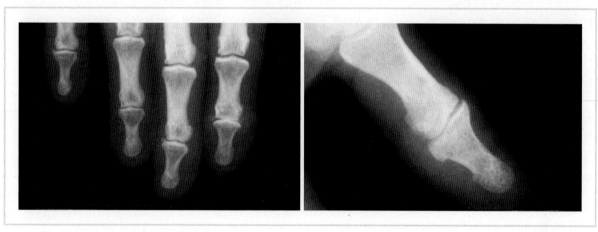

**Figure 16.5.** Clinical case "Deformity and pain in the hands (I)." Detail of the hand X-rays. Please identify the features of osteoarthritis.

As for the osteoarthritis of the first carpometacarpal joint – Figure 16.7., the prognosis is rather different. This lesion can, in fact, be extremely incapacitating. Anti-inflammatories relieve the pain but not always completely. We advised the patient to reduce more demanding activities involving the thumb and to wear an immobilizing splint around the first metacarpal, which still allows some function (see Chapter 10). In acute phases, we could use local injections. The other alternative is prosthetic surgery, which we prefer to postpone for a few years, if possible.[2]

[2]Why do we take the trouble to exclude skin lesions? Of course! It could be psoriatic arthritis.

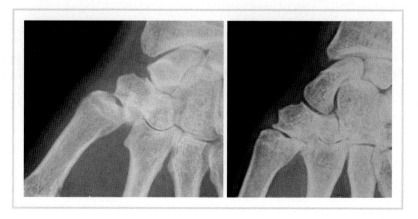

**Figure 16.6.**
Osteoarthritis of the first carpo-metacarpal joint – radiographs in different stages of progression.

## NODAL OSTEOARTHRITIS OF THE HANDS
### *MAIN POINTS*

This is a very common condition, especially in middle-aged and elderly women.

The first carpometacarpal, the distal interphalangeal and the proximal interphalangeal joints (nodal osteoarthritis) are often the site of osteoarthritis in the hands.

Osteoarthritis at other sites (e.g. the wrist or metacarpo-phalangeal joints) suggests an underlying cause (traumatic? metabolic?).

Nodal osteoarthritis is hereditable.

It may appear alone or with polyarticular osteoarthritis.

The pain may have a mixed rhythm with inflammatory flares.

The patient's enquiry and physical examination strongly suggest the diagnosis:

- Bony swelling in the vicinity of the proximal (Bouchard's nodes) and/or distal interphalangeal joints (Heberden's nodes);
- Absence of synovial swelling;
- In the initial stages, there may be signs of inflammation with thinning of the skin and leakage of articular fluid (mucous cysts).

It demands a differential diagnosis including rheumatoid arthritis and psoriatic arthritis (note the absence of synovitis, the hard consistency of the swelling and the normal levels of the acute-phase reaction proteins).

Radiological abnormalities are typical of osteoarthritis (see Chapter 10). Rarely, erosions may occur (Erosive osteoarthritis – Figure 16.8.).

Treatment is essentially symptomatic.

In spite of the tendency towards progressive deformation, the patient maintains good functional capacity.

## OSTEOARTHRITIS OF THE FIRST CARPOMETACARPAL JOINT
### *MAIN POINTS*

Osteoarthritis of the first carpometacarpal joint is common.

It may appear alone or in conjunction with nodal or generalized osteoarthritis.

It is a very common in middle-aged and elderly women.

It is associated with demanding, repetitive, manual work.

It causes mechanical pain in the base of the thumb and there may be episodes of inflammation. Visible deformation may occur (Figure 10.17.).

Physical examination will detect tenderness on palpation of the joint, with or without crepitus. It is important to exclude de Quervain's tenosynovitis.

X-rays confirm the diagnosis.

Treatment is symptomatic and conservative.

Immobilizing the thumb with a splint can be very useful (Figure 29.2.).

In incapacitating situations, temporary relief can be achieved with local steroid injections or surgery may be indicated. (See also Chapter 10.).

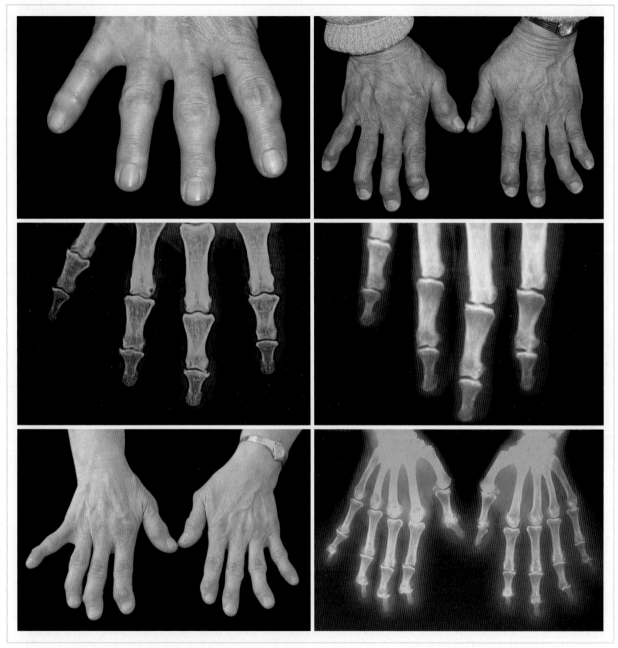

**Figure 16.7.** Nodal osteoarthritis of the hands in more advanced stages: despite deformity, pain is usually tolerable and function satisfactory.

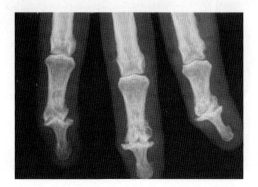

**Figure 16.8.**
Erosive nodal osteoarthritis. Although rarely, nodal osteoarthritis can cause erosions in association with the typical features of osteoarthritis. Differential diagnosis with psoriatic arthritis is more difficult.

*TYPICAL CASES*
## 16.C. POLYARTICULAR PAIN (I)

João Silvestre, a 63 year-old farmer with two children, began to experience mechanical pain in the joints of his hands at the age of 34, particularly in the second and third metacarpophalangeal joints. The pain persisted, accompanied by progressive deformation of these joints and functional limitations. In a few years, the joint pain spread to his elbows, knees, ankles and lumbar spine, with similar characteristics. He described occasional episodes with distinct signs of inflammation. He denied any extra-articular symptoms. He took anti-inflammatories to relieve the pain. At the age of 51 he retired due to incapacity caused by his joint disease.

*Summarize the patient's problems.*[3]

*Consider the possible diagnoses.*

*What additional information would you try to obtain?*

Our clinical examination revealed firm swelling and moderate tenderness of the second and third metacarpophalangeal joints of both hands, which showed very limited flexion mobility (Figure 16.9.). Several interphalangeal joints in both hands presented Bouchard's and Heberden's nodes. Bony swelling was felt in both elbows associated with limited extension (−30° on the right and −15° on the left). The other joints were normal. Our general physical examination showed no anomalies in any other systems.

*Reconsider your diagnosis on the basis of this information.*

*What would you expect to find in an x-ray?*

X-rays of the hands and wrists showed major bilateral structural alterations in the second and third metacarpophalangeal joints with a reduction in the intra-articular space, bone cysts, subchondral sclerosis and, especially, exuberant hook-shaped osteophytes at the radial edge of the distal extremity of the metacarpals (Figure 16.10.). More discrete alterations of the same type were found in other metacarpophalangeal joints. The proximal and distal interphalangeal joints showed typical degenerative changes. The x-rays of his elbows showed bilateral osteo-

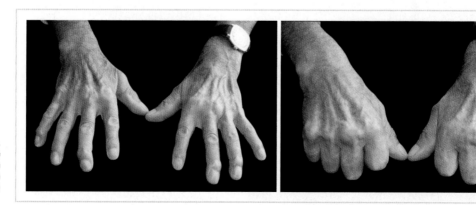

**Figure 16.9.**
Clinical case "polyarticular pain (I)." (Vd. description in the text.)

[3]Deforming, degenerative polyarthropathy at a young age, involvement of metacarpophalangeal joints, intercurrent inflammatory episodes.

phytes in the distal humerus and olecranon (Figure 16.10.). There were no signs of calcification of the cartilage (chondrocalcinosis).

*What is your diagnosis?*

*Would you conduct any etiological investigation?*

The clinical and radiological aspects of this joint disease pointed to polyarticular **osteoarthritis with atypical characteristics**: site, age at onset, and rapid development.

The principle etiological possibility was hereditary hemochromatosis (HH). We requested a number of additional tests on the basis of this hypothesis. Serum transferrin saturation was 78.4% and serum ferritin over 1,500 mg/l. A histopathological examination of a fragment of liver biopsy showed massive deposits of hemosiderin located mostly in the hepatocytes and moderate portal fibrosis (non-cirrhotic phase). His hepatic iron index was 3.82. A genetic study showed that the patient was a homozygous carrier of the mutation that is most frequently responsible for hereditary hemochromatosis (C282Y in the HFE gene).

We confirmed the diagnosis of HH in this patient and then screened his five living direct family members by measuring both serum ferritin and transferrin saturation. A second case of HH was detected.

The treatment of hemochromatosis (phlebotomy) does not alter the course of the joint disease but it does prevent the progression of hepatic lesions and the development of other extra-articular manifestations.

Was any additional rheumatologic concern justified?[4]

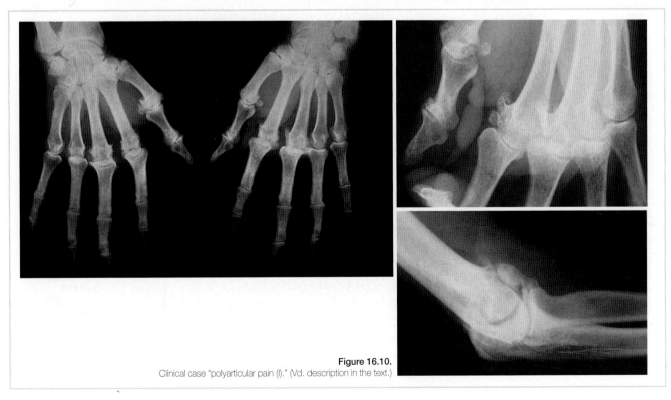

**Figure 16.10.**
Clinical case "polyarticular pain (I)." (Vd. description in the text.)

[4]Yes, with the possibility of osteoporosis. Hypogonadism, a frequent manifestation of hemochromatosis, is one of the main causes of male osteoporosis.

*TYPICAL CASES*
## 16.D. ANKLE PAIN

Abel was a stoical 72 year-old farmer. He had had a very hard life but had borne up well and remained active. He had been suffering from pain for a long time but he "managed" with the help of his pain-killers. Recently, however, he had ceased to be able to do the farm work that he loved so much because the pain in his right ankle was much worse, leaving him hardly able to walk. It was typical mechanical pain. It soon stopped completely when at rest and got much worse during any attempt at weight bearing.

He did not have any other significant complaints and a general examination revealed no other problems. He categorically denied any relevant history such as trauma or local infections.

An examination of his ankles showed greatly reduced and painful mobility in the right ankle joint. The subtalar joint was normal. There was no swelling or articular instability and there were no signs of periarticular lesions.

*What could be causing this condition?*

*How would you investigate the causes?*

An x-ray of his ankle showed indisputable advanced osteoarthritis in the right tibio-tarsal joint.

In view of his degree of incapacitation we told the patient that the only way to achieve any significant improvement would be arthrodesis (surgical fusion of the joint). He would lose the little movement that he had left but should no longer have such severe pain.

The patient said that he would talk it over with his wife. At his next appointment, he agreed to the surgery and mentioned that this wife had reminded him of a fall onto his feet that he had suffered when he was about 30, which had forced him to spend about 3 weeks in bed.

*TYPICAL CASES*
## 16.E. KNEE PAIN OF SUDDEN ONSET

Arlete, a 32 year-old nurse, was attending the chest clinic because of her bronchial asthma, which was difficult to control, and was being treated with bronchodilators and glucocorticoids (inhaled or oral).

She was referred to us because of progressive incapacitating pain in her left knee that had appeared about 4 months previously. The pain was marked while standing or walking but disappeared almost completely at rest. She experienced brief morning stiffness. She had noticed some swelling of the knee at the beginning but it had subsided in the meantime. She denied any other musculoskeletal complaints.

A general examination revealed slightly Cushingoid facies, with no other findings. On examination of the knee, we found it to be painful on forced flexion, without any limitations in range of movement. There were no signs of inflammation or effusion. Palpation of the medial aspect of the joint line was tender, particularly over the tibial plateau. Clinical examination of the meniscus was inconclusive and there was no articular instability.

*Consider the possible explanations and any additional tests.*

We requested plain films of the knees (2 planes, weight-bearing) – (Figure 16.11.).

The medial tibial plateau showed increased bone density and the articular surface was depressed in relation to the lateral tibial plateau. These characteristics strongly suggested aseptic necrosis at this site, probably related to the asthma and corticosteroid treatment.

We explained the situation to the patient, stressing the limited choice of conservative treatment when bone deformity has already set in. The situation would definitely lead to early-onset osteoarthritis of the knee in a few years and she would probably need a knee prosthesis. In view of the limited lifespan of these prostheses, however, we let the patient consider the possibility of postponing surgery till later, depending on the intensity of the pain and her degree of functional disability. We referred the patient to a prosthetics expert to consider the best design for an orthosis to offload the medial plateau.

## ATYPICAL OSTEOARTHRITIS
### MAIN POINTS

The identification of atypical features in osteoarthritis suggests the existence of an underlying cause.

The following aspects are relevant:

- Early onset (before the age of 50);
- Uncommon locations: metacarpophalangeal joints, wrists, elbows, shoulders, etc.;
- Recurring inflammatory episodes;
- Rapid, progressive development;
- Calcification of the articular cartilage in x-rays (see Chapter 18).

Possible causes:

- Trauma, previous local inflammation, aseptic necrosis, etc.;
- Articular instability or deviation;
- Hemochromatosis, ochronosis, hypophosphatasia, etc.

Guidelines:

- Investigation of these causes is mandatory in any case of atypical osteoarthritis;
- The threat of subsequent osteoarthritis justifies early, intensive treatment of these conditions in all cases;
- The treatment of established osteoarthritis follows the general principles applicable to osteoarthritis of any cause.

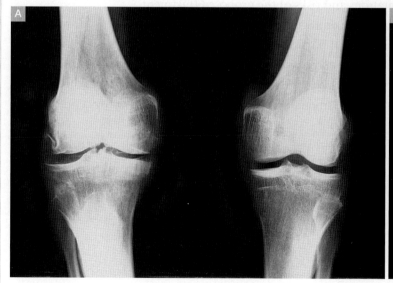 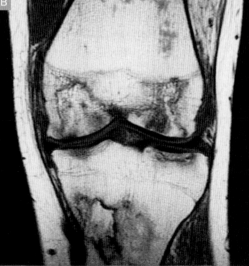

**Figure 16.11.** Clinical case "Knee pain of sudden onset." **A.** Standard weigh-bearing X-rays. **B.** Magnetic resonance imaging of the left knee.

## ADDITIONAL TESTS

The only diagnostic tests that are justified in osteoarthritis, other than standard films, are those used to investigate an underlying cause, if appropriate. In the case of a difficult diagnosis, additional tests may be important, including acute-phase reaction proteins, for example.

## TREATMENT OF OSTEOARTHRITIS

### Objectives of the treatment

Relief of the pain and other symptoms, such as stiffness of the joints and anxiety, with minimal iatrogenic risk.

Maintaining function and minimizing the impact of the disease on the patient's quality of life.
Retarding the progression of the disease by making the degenerative process less aggressive.

### Educating the patient

Educating the patient plays a fundamental role in achieving these objectives. We should inform the patient of the nature of his or her condition, while explaining the benign nature of the prognosis: if the worst comes to the worst, there is still surgery, which is usually highly effective. We should make the patient aware of factors that may aggravate the disease, such as high-impact exercise and any sports involving physical contact or intensive use of the joints.

In common cases of osteoarthritis of the hip, knee or spine, loss of weight in the obese patient relieves the symptoms and protects the joints. The patient's diet and target weight should be clearly established, with the help of specialists in the case of extreme obesity. The patient should be informed of the scope, limitations and risks of the proposed treatment.

Osteoarthritis patients should be encouraged to remain active and to strengthen the muscles around the affected joint. This aspect is particularly important in osteoarthritis of the knee. Patients should be taught to do regular exercises at home to strengthen their quadriceps. Clear instructions (Figure 16.12.), the doctor's commitment and regular follow-up visits will ensure the patient's compliance with this fundamental aspect. A visit to a physiotherapy centre is an ideal opportunity for this type of teaching.

Continued support from the physician and other professionals plays a decisive role in the patient's compliance with treatment and in maintaining function and quality of life in the future.

## KNEES. Exercise prescription.

Perform these exercises each morning and evening. Initially, do each exercise three times in each session and increase the number of repeats progressively until each exercise is done ten times, twice daily. Do not force yourself too much and avoid pain. Increased swelling, pain arising while you exercise or on the following day suggest that the amount of effort is excessive for you: consult with your doctor.

Perform your exercises regularly: stopping if pain subsides will probably bring it back!

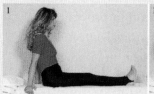 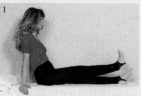

**1.** Sit down (on the floor or on the bed) with your legs stretched. Bend you foot up (towards you) and raise your leg, keeping your knee straight, until the heel is about 15 cm above the floor. Count until five. Rest and repeat.

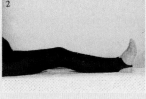 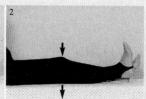

**2.** Sit down (on the floor or on the bed) with your legs stretched. Bend you foot up (towards you) and force your knee against the floor. Count until five. Rest and repeat.

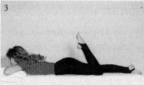 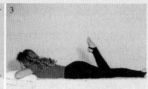

**3.** Lie face down. Bend and stretch one knee at a time, as completely as possible. Rest and repeat.

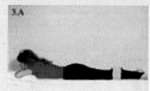 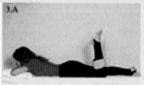

**3.A.** Once you feel able to do it, attach some weight to your leg as shown and repeat the exercise. Increase the added weight progressively up to one kilo.

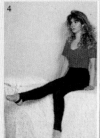 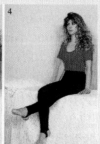

**4.** Sit on a bed or tall chair, with your legs hanging. Stretch your knee completely. Count until five. Rest and repeat.

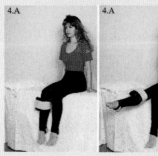

**4.A.** Once you feel able to do it, perform the same exercise with some extra weight attached to your leg (as in exercise 3.A.).

**Please note:** ask you doctor if exercises 3 and 4 are adequate for you.

### More advice to protect and improve your knees.

**1. Adaptations to your environment.** Some daily activities place considerable burden on your knees. This is especially the case with sitting and rising from low chairs; going up and down-stairs, kneeling down or entering the bath. With a little imagination these efforts can be reduced:
- Choose higher chairs or have your chairs raised;
- Avoid, if you can, using the stairs. While climbing stairs, use first your best leg and go step by step. When going downstairs let the worst leg go first. It may be worthwhile having an additional handrail installed;
- Avoid kneeling down. Often you can avoid needing to reach down low by rearranging things at home or by using a longhandle grip;
- If getting out of the bath is a problem, consider having some handles installed or changing to a sitting bath or shower.

**2. Do not sleep with cushions under your knees.** This can make you comfortable but, with time, it will make bending your knees more difficult.

**3. Canes.** A well-fitted walking stick can reduce the burden on your knees to about half. Ideally the stick's handle will be at the height of you wrist, when you are standing with your arms pending. Use on the less affected side. Keep the stick's tip in a good state to guarantee adherence to the floor.

**4. Body weight.** Excess body weight is major cause of knee osteoarthritis. Keeping an ideal weight represents a valuable relief for your knees while improving your general health. Loosing weight may not be an easy thing to do but it can be the best help you can give your knees and back. Take advice from your physician.
(As a general rule, body weight in kilos should be similar to the number of centimetres your height is above one meter. Example. Height: 1,56 m – target weight: 56 kilos.)

**5. Resting your knees is important.** Programme not only your activities but also your periods of rest. The application of local heat (hot water bag) or cold (ice pack) can help relieve pain: most patients prefer cold applications if the knee is swollen or inflamed and heat in chronic phases.

*Do your exercises regularly. Help yourself!*

**Figure 16.12.** Example of a patient leaflet explaining adequate exercises for patients with knee osteoarthritis. This advice should be considered as a "prescription." (Developed in cooperation with Prof. Páscoa Pinheiro.)

## TREATING OSTEOARTHRITIS
### MAIN POINTS

Educating the patient:

- Basic understanding of the disease and its treatment;
- Normal range body weight;
- Walking aids;
- Appropriate footwear;
- Appropriate physical exercise.

Drugs:

- Ordinary analgesics;
- Non-steroidal anti-inflammatories;
- Topical anti-inflammatories;
- Glucosamine sulfate and chondroitin sulfate.

Intra-articular injections:

- Glucocorticoids in acute phases;
- Hyaluronic acid (?).

Treatment of associated periarticular lesions

Surgery:

- Arthroscopic cleaning;
- Osteotomy;
- Partial or total prosthesis.

## Drugs

Ordinary analgesics (like paracetamol (acetaminophen), up to 1 g 4 times a day) are the first step. Many patients will achieve adequate pain relief with a minimum of risk. If this medication proves to be insufficient, careful use of non-steroidal anti-inflammatories is justified. We should bear in mind, however, that patients with osteoarthritis are highly likely to be at risk of side effects from these drugs, as a result of their age, a history of gastric problems, polypharmacy, heart failure, hypertension, etc. (see Chapter 30).

The local application of heat-producing rubefacients or topical anti-inflammatories provides relief to many patients with osteoarthritis of the superficial joints.

Glucosamine sulfate and chondroitin sulfate may result in significant relief of symptoms in moderate osteoarthritis. The former has been mentioned in some studies as being able to retard the radiological progression of osteoarthritis of the knee, but this remains controversial.

## Intra-articular injections

Intra-articular injections of corticosteroids usually have a short-term effect on osteoarthritis. However, in inflammatory phases involving effusion, nocturnal pain and increased stiffness, they can be extremely useful. More recently, intra-articular injections of hyaluronic acid polymers have been proposed. The aim of their effect is to improve articular lubrication. Their therapeutic value is controversial, however.

Advanced osteoarthritis of the knee can benefit substantially from articular washouts performed by specialists, usually.

## Treatment of associated periarticular lesions

It is essential to bear in mind that, in many patients, osteoarthritis is accompanied by periarticular lesions that may be the main cause of pain and incapacitation. Before these patients can be properly treated, we must first make an accurate diagnosis of the cause of the pain. Identifying and treating associated tendinitis, bursitis or ligamentitis and compensating for joint instability are important aspects of the treatment of osteoarthritis, especially of the knee and hip.

### *Walking aids*

The use of well-cushioned footwear can do a lot to help reduce the pain in patients with osteoarthritis of the lower limbs, as it reduces the mechanical impact of walking. In more advanced stages, using a stick or crutch on the opposite side from the dominant disease can be very useful. Patients with accentuated instability of the knee may benefit from elastic knee supports or, better still, from articulated orthoses, which are available on prescription.

Some corrective measures at home, such as ramps, a shower instead of a bathtub and handles in the bathroom can be extremely useful and may be provided by an occupational therapist.

### *Surgery*

In moderate to advanced stages of osteoarthritis arthroscopic washout of intra-articular detritus may be highly beneficial, especially in the knee. Closed lavage followed by infiltration also brings relief to many patients.

The criteria for surgery in osteoarthritis are not well defined. Generally speaking, a patient who has considerable difficulty sleeping, walking or working because of osteoarthritis which is not responding to oral medication is suitable for orthopedic consideration. In younger patients (< 60), osteotomy to correct deviations in the case of unicompartmental osteoarthritis of the knee may be highly effective in terms of symptoms and function, and postpones the need for a total knee prosthesis. The results of a prosthesis, a final resort that is sometimes inevitable, are better before accentuated instability, deviation or muscle wasting have set in. Obesity may also compromise the success of surgery.

## WHEN SHOULD THE PATIENT BE REFERRED TO A SPECIALIST?

Unfortunately, at the moment there are no "specialized secrets" in the treatment of osteoarthritis. A general practitioner should be able to make a definite diagnosis. A careful clinical examination will also make it possible to identify factors that aggravate the condition and identify associated periarticular lesions, which may also be amenable to treatment.

Referring the patient to a rheumatologist may be justified if there are doubts as to the diagnosis, or if a basic treatment program has not achieved satisfactory results in a patient for whom surgery is not indicated. Today, osteoarthritis is the subject of very active biological and therapeutic research and such efforts may change the panorama outlook for this condition in the relatively near future.

Physiotherapy can do a lot for arthritic patients with intense pain and incapacitation. More intensive or specific plans of physical exercise or the design of special orthoses are indicated for these kinds of patient.

Orthopedic surgery should be considered when the pain prevents the patient from sleeping, walking or going about his or her everyday activities.

## ADDITIONAL PRACTICE
### OSTEOARTHRITIS

# INFLAMMATORY ARTHRITIDES

## DIAGNOSTIC STRATEGIES

17.

J.A.P. da Silva, A.D. Woolf, *Rheumatology in Practice*, DOI 10.1007/978-1-84882-581-9_17,
© Springer-Verlag London Limited 2010

# 17. INFLAMMATORY ARTHRITIDES DIAGNOSTIC STRATEGIES

## INTRODUCTION

By "arthritis" we mean an inflammatory process in a joint. It can be caused by infectious agents lodged in the joint (septic arthritis), microcrystals that lead to the degranulation of neutrophils (microcrystalline arthritis), by an immunological reaction to remote infectious agents (reactive arthritis), or it can be of unknown cause, as is the case in most inflammatory joint diseases.

Whatever its nature, the inflammatory process results in the local production of large quantities of inflammatory mediators, which have a great potential for damaging articular cartilage, bone and periarticular soft tissue. Proinflammatory cytokines, especially interleukin 1 (IL-1) and tumor necrosis factor-alpha (TNFα), stimulate bone and cartilage cells to destroy their own matrices and inhibit their reconstruction, resulting in progressive tissue damage. Proteolytic enzymes released into the synovial fluid by activated leucocytes and synoviocytes contribute directly to tissue destruction. Depending on its nature and duration, the inflammatory process may result in the total destruction of the joint (Figure 17.1.), which can be irreversibly established in days or weeks, in the case of septic arthritis.

These pathophysiological mechanisms help explain the clinical and radiological characteristics of arthritis. Sensitized by inflammatory mediators, the periarticular nociceptive nerve endings cause *pain* at the smallest movement or pressure. The inflammatory vascular reaction explains the *heat and redness* found in many forms of arthritis. The engorged synovium and excess synovial fluid distend the capsule, causing *diffuse swelling* around the joint, with an elastic consistency and fluctuance (when there is significant articular effusion).

The destruction of the cartilage, induced by catabolic factors present in the synovial fluid, occurs homogeneously all over the articular surface at a pace that varies according to the type of arthritis and from patient to patient. This results in a *diffuse, symmetrical loss of joint space* in x-rays, as opposed to the more focal, asymmetric loss seen in osteoarthritis. The subchondral bone loses calcium in response to the same inflammatory mediators. This shows in x-rays as *periarticular osteopenia*, unlike the subchondral sclerosis typical of osteoarthritis.

Muscles, ligaments and the capsule are also influenced by these catabolic effects, becoming atrophied (*muscular atrophy*) and lax (*articular instability, subluxations, and articular deviations*). Bursae, tendons and ligaments may be involved in the inflammatory process, causing *periarthritis or peripheral nerve compression syndromes.*

In some types of joint disease, the inflammatory synovial tissue has invasive properties, leading to the focal destruction of bone in the synovial insertion areas – this is reflected radiologically by *erosions*, commonly seen in rheumatoid or psoriatic arthritis.

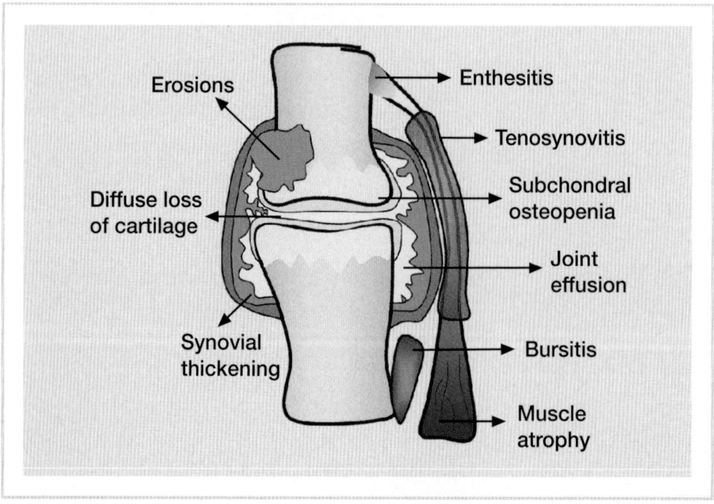

**Figure 17.1.** Schematic representation of inflammatory arthropathies.

Erosions, joint space loss and other structural changes of the joint are essentially irreversible.

The immunological reaction may cause *systemic manifestations*, consisting of fever, weight loss, lymphadenopathy and fatigue. In laboratory tests, this systemic reaction is reflected by *elevated acute-phase reactants.* Finally, inflammatory arthritis can be part of *multisystem diseases* that may involve virtually all organs and systems, as exemplified by systemic lupus erythematosus and systemic vasculitis.

Many types of arthritis have a devastating effect on the quality of life and on the survival of patients. They therefore require careful diagnosis and appropriate early treatment.

---

### When can we say that a patient has arthritis?

**The pain is articular in origin:**

- The patient locates the pain in the joints, with possible regional radiation;
- The clinical examination confirms the articular origin of the pain;
- The pain has an inflammatory rhythm (variable over time and particularly after treatment).

**The clinical examination shows articular inflammation:**

- Firm, rubbery swelling reflecting an engorged synovium in the joints accessible to palpation;
- Usual presence of signs of inflammation (local heat and swelling. Redness is relatively rare and appears most commonly in the small peripheral joints);
- Painful limitation of active and passive joint motion (in more advanced stages).

**Acute-phase reactants are usually elevated.**

**Radiographs:**

- Normal in the initial stages;
- Swelling of soft tissues;
- Periarticular osteopenia;
- Uniform loss of joint space;          Varying with the type of arthritis
- Periarticular erosions;
- Joint deformity.

**Table 17.1.**
Basis for the diagnosis of inflammatory arthritis.

---

NB: The description of signs of inflammation by the patient but not confirmed by the physician should be considered as an indication, but not proof, of an inflammatory process.

The diagnosis of arthritis is essentially clinical. In fact, some patients have no significant elevation of acute-phase reactants. If the clinical enquiry and examination are highly suggestive of arthritis, normal acute phase reactants raise questions but do not exclude the diagnosis.

## RADIOLOGY

In the ***initial stages of arthritis***, radiological aspects are nonspecific or absent. If the clinical examination suggests the diagnosis, a normal x-ray certainly does not rule it out (Figure 17.2.).

Arthritis is a potentially very serious condition requiring appropriate, timely intervention, ideally before permanent structural alteration sets in so that this can be prevented. By the time radiological changes are obvious we have missed the ideal timing for therapy.

We therefore suggest that,

> Any patient with a clinical diagnosis of arthritis persisting for more than six weeks, should be referred to a specialist as soon as possible.

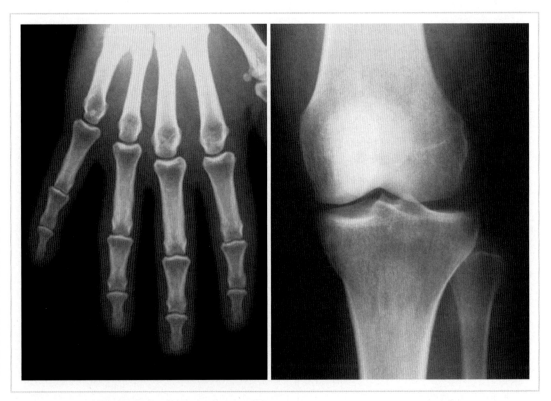

**Figure 17.2.**
Radiological features of inflammatory arthritis – early phases. The x-ray of the hands shows periarticular osteopenia, which is really only of significance in combination with the clinical signs. Joint space width is preserved. The plain radiograph can be considered "normal."

In ***more advanced stages of arthritis***, radiology may show (Figure 17.3.):

- **Symmetrical loss of joint space** – as opposed to the asymmetrical loss in osteoarthritis;
- **Bone erosions** – typical of rheumatoid and psoriatic arthritis but not usually found in other types of chronic arthritis;
- **Periarticular lytic lesions** (may appear in gout);
- Almost total **destruction of the epiphyses** (e.g. in untreated septic arthritis);
- **Deviations** in axis and subluxations in deforming arthropathies;
- **Features of osteoarthritis** (secondary in this case) may appear in advanced stages of the disease, even after the inflammatory process has been under control.

Note that many types of arthritis are typically neither erosive nor deforming. This is the case with systemic lupus erythematosus and other connective tissue diseases (excluding rheumatoid arthritis), short-term reactive arthritis, post-viral arthritis and arthritis related to inflammatory bowel diseases. In these cases, we will not find the late radiological characteristics, but timely treatment is still important, not only to avoid unnecessary suffering but also because the inflammatory process may lead to marked laxity of the ligaments, with resulting instability, subluxations and loss of function.

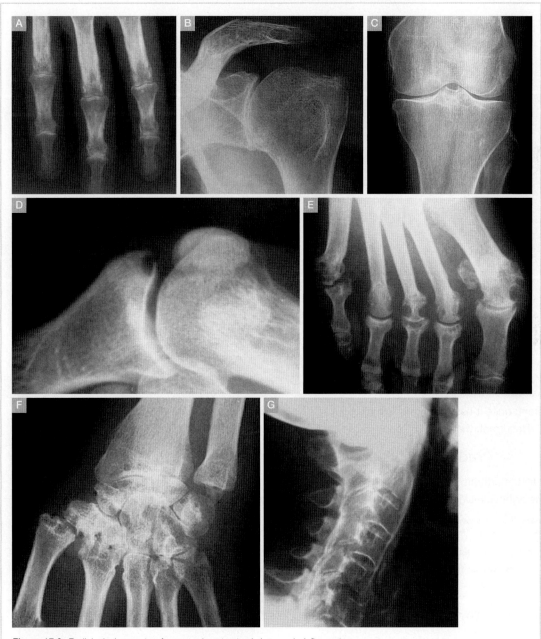

**Figure 17.3.** Radiological aspects of progressive structural damage in inflammatory arthritis. These lesions are essentially irreversible. **A**, **B** and **C** – Uniform loss of joint space and periarticular osteopenia. **D** and **E** – Erosions. **F** and **G** – Total loss of joint space, joint disorganization, ankylosis.

# DIAGNOSTIC STRATEGY IN INFLAMMATORY ARTHRITIS

Having taken the first step in the diagnosis, i.e. establishing that it is an "inflammatory articular syndrome, i.e. arthritis" (see Chapter 4), how can we approach the second step, to identify the type of arthritis and make the final diagnosis?

We suggest that you do the following:

1. Ascertain exactly **which joints are affected and hence their pattern of distribution**, through directed enquiry and complete clinical examination;

2. Find out if the patient also has **back pain**. If so, determine exactly whether it is inflammatory or mechanical in rhythm;

3. Find out **how the condition began and how it developed** over time;

4. Investigate any **accompanying extra-articular manifestations**.

Once you have this information, classify the arthritis, according to the following parameters:

## Mono *versus* Oligo *versus* Polyarthritis

Monoarthritis: only one joint affected
Oligoarthritis: 2 to 4 joints affected
Polyarthritis: 5 or more joints affected

## Acute *versus* Chronic

Acute: onset in hours or days
Chronic: onset over weeks or months

## Additive *versus* Migratory

Additive: the affected joints are added progressively
Migratory: the inflammatory process flits from one joint to another

## Persistent *versus* Recurrent

Persistent: once it has set in, the arthritis persists over time, albeit with flare-ups and partial remissions
Recurrent: there are episodes or crises of arthritis, separated by symptom-free intervals

## Predominantly proximal *versus* Predominantly distal

Proximal: the arthritis mainly involves large joints, i.e. proximal to the wrist or ankle or the axial skeleton.
Distal: the arthritis mainly involves the small joints of the hands and feet, with or without the wrist and ankle

## Symmetrical *versus* Asymmetrical

Symmetrical: the inflammatory process affects approximately the same joints on each side of the body.
Asymmetrical: there is no relationship between the joints involved on either side of the body
(e.g. right knee, 3rd right PIP, 5th left DIP)

## With inflammatory low back pain *versus* Without inflammatory low back pain

## With systemic manifestations *versus* Without systemic manifestations

Consider the systemic manifestations commonly associated with arthritis.

**Table 17.2.** Clinical descriptors for the characterization of inflammatory arthritis.

The appropriate use of the wording in Table 17.2. represents the most important step in the differential diagnosis of arthritis, as subtypes usually adhere to reasonably reliable clinical patterns.

We suggest that you try to describe actual cases using only these terms, e.g.:

a)  Chronic monoarthritis;

b)  Acute, recurrent, migratory monoarthritis;

c)  Inflammatory back pain;

d)  Asymmetrical proximal oligoarthritis;

e)  Chronic, additive, symmetrical, peripheral polyarthritis;

f)  Etc.

This will make the final diagnosis a lot easier and reliable. The most common patterns (Figure 17.4.) are described briefly below to provide a structured overview. They are dealt with in more detail in the following chapters.

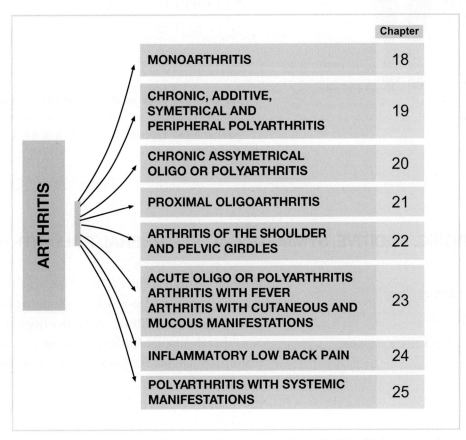

| | Chapter |
|---|---|
| MONOARTHRITIS | 18 |
| CHRONIC, ADDITIVE, SYMETRICAL AND PERIPHERAL POLYARTHRITIS | 19 |
| CHRONIC ASSYMETRICAL OLIGO OR POLYARTHRITIS | 20 |
| PROXIMAL OLIGOARTHRITIS | 21 |
| ARTHRITIS OF THE SHOULDER AND PELVIC GIRDLES | 22 |
| ACUTE OLIGO OR POLYARTHRITIS ARTHRITIS WITH FEVER ARTHRITIS WITH CUTANEOUS AND MUCOUS MANIFESTATIONS | 23 |
| INFLAMMATORY LOW BACK PAIN | 24 |
| POLYARTHRITIS WITH SYSTEMIC MANIFESTATIONS | 25 |

ARTHRITIS

**Figure 17.4.** Having established the diagnosis of "inflammatory arthritis" try to identify its clinical pattern in each case.

## MONOARTHRITIS

| *Most probable causes* |
| --- |
| SEPTIC ARTHRITIS (until proved otherwise) |
| Gout |
| Pseudo-gout |
| Reactive arthritis |
| Juvenile idiopathic arthritis (monoarticular form) |
| Sarcoidosis |

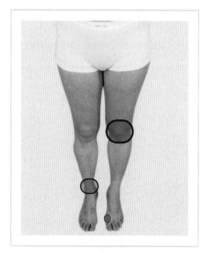

**Figure 17.5.** Monoarthritis. Most common locations. Relevant extra-articular manifestations: fever, infected wounds, recent infections, kidney stones.

The most commonly affected joints in monoarthritis and relevant associated extraarticular manifestations are presented in Figure 17.5.

Even though gout and pseudo-gout are more common, monoarthritis should be considered to be due to infection until proven otherwise, because this situation is rapidly destructive and can endanger the patient's life if not properly treated.

It is important to look for fever, history of recent infection and any previous episodes that may suggest gout or pseudo-gout. Note that, in 50% of cases, the initial episode of gout is located in the first metatarsophalangeal joint. However, it is the same to say that in 50% of cases the initial episode of gout occurs elsewhere, although it still predominates in the lower extremities.

See Chapter 18.

> **All patients with acute, initial monoarthritis should undergo an urgent arthrocentesis to examine the synovial fluid, which is the key to the diagnosis.**

## CHRONIC, ADDITIVE, SYMMETRICAL, PERIPHERAL POLYARTHRITIS

| *Most probable causes* |
| --- |
| RHEUMATOID ARTHRITIS |
| Arthritis of other connective tissue diseases |
| Psoriatic arthritis (pseudo-rheumatoid form) |
| Polyarticular gout? |
| Pseudo-gout? |

With this pattern (Figure 17.6.), it is essential to look systematically for extra-articular manifestations suggesting psoriasis or diffuse connective tissue diseases. Note that rheumatoid arthritis can cause extra-articular manifestations, but joint symptoms and signs are largely predominant. Gout can, over time and also in females, become polyarticular, unlike its typical pattern of recurrent monoarthritis. A careful enquiry, however, almost always identifies an initial phase with the usual pattern.

Additional initial investigations may include routine tests, x-rays, rheumatoid factor and antinuclear antibodies by immunofluorescence. The interpretation of these tests is discussed in other chapters. In any case, if the clinical diagnosis of arthritis is conclusive, referral to a specialist should already be underway. This pattern is discussed in more detail in Chapter 19.

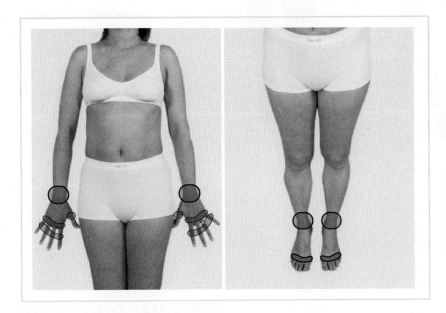

**Figure 17.6.**
Chronic, additive, symmetrical and peripheral polyarthritis. Typical pattern of distribution. Relevant extra-articular manifestations: subcutaneous nodules, dry eyes, dry mouth, muscle weakness, psoriasis, photosensitivity and other manifestations associated with systemic lupus.

## CHRONIC, ASYMMETRICAL OLIGO- OR POLYARTHRITIS

The most characteristic form of psoriatic arthritis is asymmetrical oligo- or polyarthritis. The affected joints may be proximal or distal. Dactylitis or the involvement of the distal interphalangeal joints is also highly suggestive of this diagnosis (Figure 17.7). The joints affected in psoriatic arthritis usually show clear signs of inflammation with intense, fusiform swelling and a suggestive purple tinge to the overlying skin. A personal or family history of psoriasis, if present, will provide strong support for this diagnosis.

Reactive arthritis and arthritis associated with inflammatory bowel disease may also show this pattern, but when distal joints are affected they usually adopt a symmetrical distribution. Rheumatoid arthritis may be asymmetrical at the beginning, but

| Most likely causes |
| --- |
| PSORIATIC ARTHRITIS |
| Some other seronegative spondyloarthropathy |
| Incipient rheumatoid arthritis |
| Juvenile idiopathic arthritis |
| Polyarticular gout? |
| Pseudo-gout? |
| Behçet's disease? |

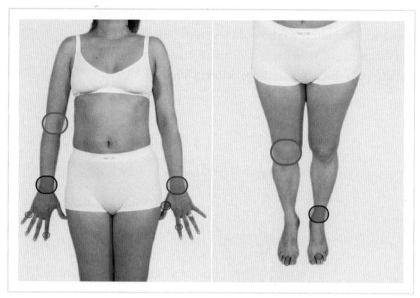

**Figure 17.7.** Chronic, asymmetrical oligo- or polyarthritis. Common patterns (different colors). Relevant extra-articular manifestations: psoriasis, inflammatory bowel disease.

has a strong tendency to develop into its typical pattern in weeks or months. Polyarticular gout may also imitate this pattern, but there will almost always be a period of recurrent monoarthritis at the outset. Pseudo-gout and Behçet's disease are rare conditions suggested by other clinical aspects.

See Chapter 20 for a more detailed study.

---

### Most likely causes

SERONEGATIVE SPONDYLOARTHROPATHY

- Reactive arthritis

- Psoriatic arthritis (asymmetrical oligoarticular form)

- Arthritis of inflammatory bowel disease

Unclassified oligoarthritis

Behçet's disease

Juvenile idiopathic arthritis

Incipient rheumatoid arthritis

---

## PROXIMAL OLIGOARTHRITIS

Patients may present with arthritis involving only some of the proximal joints (Figure 17.8.). This pattern makes it especially important to find out whether there is also inflammatory low back pain. The clinical enquiry must also explore psoriasis, intestinal symptoms suggesting inflammatory bowel or celiac disease as well as infections in the two or three weeks before the onset of arthritis. Recurrent severe oral and/or vaginal ulceration suggests Behçet's disease or systemic lupus. In rare cases, rheumatoid arthritis may start in the proximal joints.

Diagnostic tests will be selected to address the hypotheses suggested by the enquiry and clinical examination. Tests for possible triggering infectious agents in reactive arthritis are not very productive if the clinical signs of infection have already disappeared. With the exception of urethral infection by *Chlamydia*, the treatment will not be affected by the exact diagnosis. In many cases, even an intensive bacteriological and serological study in a highly suggestive clinical context fails to identify a potential causal agent. In this case, the condition should be described as "unclassified oligoarthritis."

In any case, if the arthritis persists for more than six weeks, the patient should be referred to a specialist.

Learn more about this syndrome in Chapter 21.

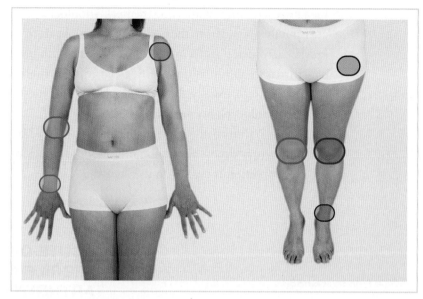

**Figure 17.8.** Proximal oligoarthritis. Common patterns (different colors).

## ARTHRITIS OF LIMB GIRDLES

**Concept:** inflammatory pain with marked stiffness, affecting the hip and shoulder girdles.

The clinical picture of polymyalgia rheumatica is highly suggestive: the patient, usually an elderly person, presents with insidious onset of pain accompa-

| *Most probable causes* |
| --- |
| POLYMYALGIA RHEUMATICA |
| Seronegative spondyloarthropathy |
| Incipient rheumatoid arthritis |

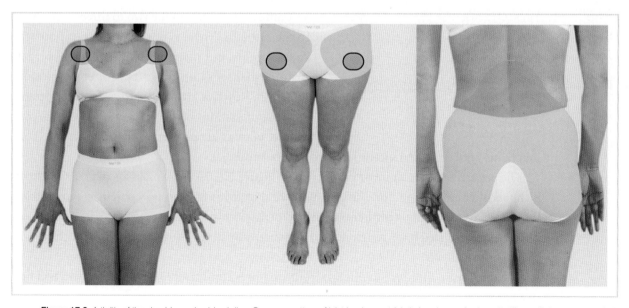

**Figure 17.9.** Arthritis of the shoulder and pelvic girdles. Common pattern of joint involvement (*circles*) and area of pain and stiffness. Relevant extra-articular manifestations: fever, weight loss, temporal headache, jaw claudication, sudden blindness, inflammatory low back pain, psoriasis, ....

nied by severe stiffness affecting the neck, shoulder and hip girdles (Figure 17.9.). Pain may radiate from the shoulders to the neck and proximal part of the arms or thighs. Imaging reveals bilateral subacromial bursitis in almost all patients with polymyalgia rheumatica and glenohumeral arthritis in about half of them. Occasionally, there is mild synovitis of peripheral joints. Routine lab tests usually show very high erythrocyte sedimentation rate, frequently accompanied by normocytic normochromic anemia.

Spondyloarthropathy may have a similar pattern. These cases are predominantly young people and there is almost always inflammatory low back pain.

This condition is dealt with in Chapter 22.

### Most likely causes:

REACTIVE ARTHRITIS

- Post-dysenteric
- Post-sexually acquired disease
- Post-streptococcal

Viral arthritis

Stills Disease

- Systemic juvenile idiopathic arthritis
- Adult Still's disease

Gonococcal arthritis

Behçet's disease

Systemic lupus erythematosus

Dermatomyositis

Rheumatoid arthritis

# ACUTE OLIGO- OR POLYARTHRITIS FEBRILE ARTHRITIS ARTHRITIS WITH MANIFESTATIONS OF THE SKIN AND MUCOUS MEMBRANES

**Concept:** rapid onset of oligo- or polyarthritis, often associated with a recent infection, fever or changes in skin and mucosus membranes. Predominates in young people.

Acute onset oligo- or polyarthritis (hours or days) suggests the possibility of reactive arthritis. In these cases, the patient is most often a young adult male. The enquiry should try to identify the occurrence of a significant infection in the two to three weeks prior to the arthritis. There is a wide variety of potential causal agents, but most frequently this will be gastrointestinal, genitourinary or upper respiratory infection. Reactive arthritis is frequently associated with manifestations in the skin (rash, erythema, pyoderma, plantar keratoderma...) and mucosae (conjunctivitis, oral or genital ulceration, circinate balanitis...).

The pattern of articular involvement varies (Figure 17.10.). Proximal oligoarticular arthritis is the most common, but, for example, post-viral arthritis is often polyarticular, symmetrical and distal. Systemic lupus erythematosus and dermatomyositis may have an acute or subacute onset, with associated fever, weight loss or lymphadenopathy, a situation which is much rarer in rheumatoid arthritis.

The diagnostic approach to this syndrome requires considerable detail, which you will find in Chapter 23.

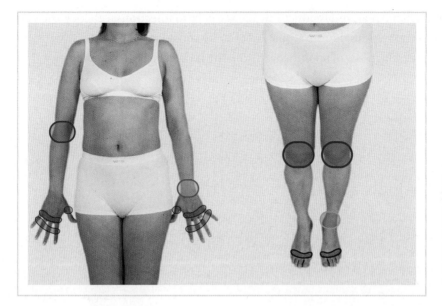

**Figure 17.10.**
Acute oligo- or polyarthritis. Arthritis with fever. Arthritis with cutaneous and mucous manifestations. Common patterns (different colors). Relevant extra-articular manifestations: fever, recent infections, rash, mucous lesions (aphthae, conjunctivitis, urethritis, …), lymphadenopathy, serositis, ….

# INFLAMMATORY LOW BACK PAIN

*Concept:* inflammatory low back pain, with or without arthritis of the appendicular skeleton.

Sacroiliitis is a paramount manifestation of a large group of arthritides called seronegative spondylarthropathies (axial involvement, no rheumatoid factor). The main complaint is inflammatory low back pain (Figure 17.11.). If the clinical examination confirms the involvement of the sacroiliac joints, this is the most likely diagnosis. When the condition is strictly limited to the spine, ankylosing spondylitis becomes the most probable diagnosis. If peripheral joints are also involved, the pattern of distribution and the associated systemic manifestations are the key to the final diagnosis. In this context, young adult males predominate.

The association of fever, weight loss and localized pain on palpation of the lumbar spine or unilateral sacroiliitis is suggestive of infectious discitis or sacroiliitis (see Chapter 11). It can appear at any age.

An anteroposterior radiograph of the sacroiliac joints is the most important test in these circumstances. Radiology of the lumbar spine is also indicated to look for syndesmophytes or signs of discitis. The erythrocyte sedimentation rate is usually mildly elevated in spondyloarthropa-

---

**Most probable causes**

SERONEGATIVE SPONDYLOARTHROPATHY

- Ankylosing spondylitis
- Psoriatic arthritis (spondylitic form)
- Reiter's syndrome
- Spondylitis of inflammatory bowel disease

Behçet's disease

Infectious or aseptic discitis

thy but is often normal, and is noticeably higher in local infections. Leucocytosis suggests infection, but it is not essential for this possibility to be considered.

Differential diagnosis of spondyloarthropathy is dealt with in Chapter 24.

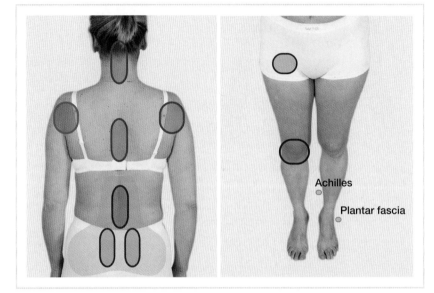

**Figure 17.11.**
Inflammatory low back pain. Common patterns of joint involvement and pain distribution (*blue color* – occasional involvement). Relevant extra-articular manifestations: fever, weight loss, psoriasis, inflammatory bowel disease, oral or genital ulcers, conjunctivitis and enthesitis.

Achilles

Plantar fascia

# POLYARTHRITIS WITH SYSTEMIC MANIFESTATIONS

**Most likely causes:**

SYSTEMIC LUPUS ERYTHEMATOSUS

Other diffuse diseases of the connective tissue

Adult or childhood Still's disease

Systemic vasculitis

Rheumatoid arthritis

Reactive arthritis

Viral arthritis

**Concept:** Polyarthritis with clear manifestations or strong suggestion of compatible systemic involvement.

Polyarthritis may predominate in the clinical presentation of these diseases and lead the differential diagnosis (Figure 17.12.). However, many of these patients present with a multisystem syndrome, of which the polyarthritis is only one aspect. Articular manifestations may even be absent. For this reason, connective tissue diseases and their differential diagnosis are dealt with in a dedicated chapter: systemic syndromes (Chapter 25).

If polyarthritis is the predominant symptom, systematic enquiry is the key to the diagnosis. Table 5.2. shows the most important systemic manifestations in this clinical context.

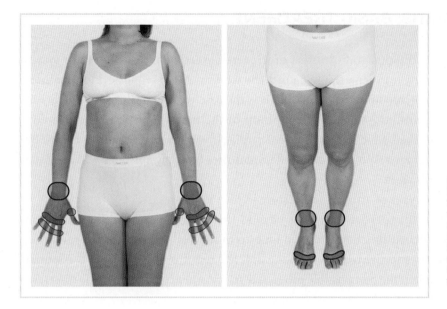

**Figure 17.12.**
Polyarthritis with systemic manifestations. Typical pattern of joint involvement. Relevant extra-articular manifestations: dry eyes, dry mouth, muscle weakness, Raynaud's phenomenon, lower limb oedema, serositis, photosensitivity and other manifestations associated with systemic lupus.

## *Migratory arthritis*

We have deliberately not mentioned any pattern of migratory arthritis. Typical migratory arthritis used to be found mainly in rheumatic fever, which is now very rare in the developed world. This is a reactive arthritis that otherwise follows all the patterns mentioned for this type of pathology: history of throat infection, preference for large joints, subacute onset, with associated changes in the skin and mucous membranes, affecting mainly young people. Other forms of reactive arthritis may occasionally follow a migratory pattern. Gout clearly tends to migrate from one joint to another. It is, however, recurrent, with symptom-free periods at least in its early stages.

Rarely, spondyloarthropathies may present as enthesopathy (inflammation of the entheses, i.e. tendon and ligament insertions), that is recurrent or unresponsive to treatment. The need to look for inflammatory back pain in this situation has already been emphasized.

When seemingly inflammatory pain moves rapidly from one joint to another, without appreciable signs of inflammation, don't forget to consider fibromyalgia!

---

### *MAIN POINTS*

Inflammatory arthritis may present with different patterns of joint involvement.

This can be unclear at the onset.

It is often wiser to wait rather than leap straight in to making an uncertain diagnosis and treatment.

Consider referral to a specialist center before prescribing potentially toxic medication which may mask a later diagnosis (such as glucocorticoids).

## ARTHRITIS: BASIC TREATMENT

Arthritis devoid of significant risk of irreversible articular destruction or systemic involvement is usually transient, resolving in a few weeks with no sequelae after treatment with nonsteroidal anti-inflammatory drugs. This is the case with typical reactive arthritis. It does not respond to antibiotics once the symptoms of the causal infection have cleared up, with the exception of rheumatic fever (to prevent cardiac involvement) or arthritis caused by *Chlamydia*. A gout flare may respond to anti-inflammatories but new episodes will almost always make the diagnosis clear.

All these types of arthritis will resolve in four to six weeks.

Arthritis that persists or recurs beyond this period has the potentially to influence the patient's articular function and even long-term survival. In the case of psoriatic and rheumatoid arthritis, effective treatment in the first few months of the disease is essential if we are to offer the patient the best possible prognosis. In the other connective tissue diseases, the patient's life may be at stake, in the short or medium term.

Because of these considerations, for non-specialist physicians faced with arthritis we recommend the approach shown in Table 17.3.

1. Is it highly likely that the diagnosis is inflammatory arthritis?

2. Have you characterized it clinically?

3. Begin treatment with an anti-inflammatory that is appropriate to your patient's condition. Avoid using corticosteroids in the absence of a definite diagnosis. A patient who urgently needs corticosteroids also needs an urgent appointment with a specialist. Hasty corticosteroids will only delay the final diagnosis and the proper treatment, and may even have serious consequences in the case of infection.

4. Request the lab tests appropriate to the clinical context, always including full blood count, acute phase reactants (don't forget to ask for C reactive protein), liver and kidney tests. Consider an x-ray of the affected joints.

5. **Promptly request an appointment at a rheumatology center, whenever your clinical evaluation does not strongly suggest gout.**

**Table 17.3.** Practical immediate approach to inflammatory arthritis.

# MONOARTHRITIS

J.A.P. da Silva, A.D. Woolf, *Rheumatology in Practice*, DOI 10.1007/978-1-84882-581-9_18,
© Springer-Verlag London Limited 2010

# 18. Monoarthritis

Many patients who go to the doctor because of musculoskeletal complaints have symptoms limited to one area. The first task of the physician is to find out whether the pain is articular, periarticular (most commonly), neurogenic or referred. The clinical basis for this distinction is described in Chapter 4. Specific local and regional syndromes are dealt with in Chapters 8–14.

Table 17.1. shows the foundations for a diagnosis of "arthritis." *Monoarthritis* (first diagnostic step) means that there is inflammation in a single joint.

## Monoarthritis: second diagnostic step

What is our second step in the diagnosis, i.e. how can we identify the cause of this monoarthritis?

First of all, it is important to consider for how long it has been developing. All types of polyarthritis can, naturally, begin in only one joint before evolving into their typical pattern. Some persist as monoarthritis.

## Acute monoarthritis

The potential causes for acute monoarthritis (clear inflammatory signs installed in a few hours or days) are limited to a small number of conditions.

---

### ACUTE MONOARTHRITIS

**Most likely causes**

Arthritis induced by microcrystals

- Gouty arthritis (monosodium urate crystals)
- Arthritis induced by calcium pyrophosphate crystals

Infectious arthritis

Posttraumatic synovitis

---

### MAIN POINTS

**In cases of acute monoarthritis of unknown cause:**

- Septic arthritis should be considered the most likely cause until excluded and requires urgent action.
- An analysis of the synovial fluid is essential and should be performed as soon as possible.

---

### Chronic monoarthritis

**Chronic monoarthritis** is characterized by its progressive onset and slow development, with usually mild inflammatory signs. It has a number of causes, including infection with on tuberculosis and, in some countries, brucellosis. The clinical features of villonodular synovitis, a benign tumoral process, are similar. Idiopathic monoarthritis is common in children. Seronegative spondyloarthropathy (e.g. psoriatic arthritis) may assume this pattern in its initial phases. The examination of the synovial fluid is mandatory and may establish the diagnosis of infection. A negative bacteriological test of the fluid does not, however, exclude infection with absolute certainty. The key to diagnosis in these cases is a synovial biopsy with histological and bacteriological examination.

In many cases, however, the actual cause of arthritis remains elusive.

---

**CHRONIC MONOARTHRITIS**

**Most probable causes**

Chronic infectious arthritis

- Arthritis caused by mycobacteria
- Brucella arthritis
- Other infectious agents

Villonodular synovitis

Juvenile idiopathic arthritis

Seronegative spondyloarthropathy

Persistent reactive arthritis

Recurrent hydroarthrosis

Idiopathic monoarthritis

Sarcoidosis

---

## SEPTIC ARTHRITIS

---

### TYPICAL CASES
### 18.A. ACUTE MONOARTHRITIS (I)

João Rodrigues, a 43-year old man, had had pain in his ankle for four weeks when he was finally sent to our emergency department. The onset of the pain was rapid (over a few days), with no apparent cause. His ankle had been swollen, hot and red from the start. He described a low-grade fever in the first few days, which had settled following treatment with an anti-inflammatory and allopurinol prescribed by his GP, who had diagnosed acute gout. It was his first episode. The articular swelling and redness had not changed, however. He still experienced intense pain when he put weight on the joint and was unable to walk.

On examination, the right ankle joint was swollen, red and extremely painful on any attempt at mobilization (Figure 18.1.). The range of movement was markedly reduced. There were no extra-articular abnormalities and no suggestion of infection elsewhere.

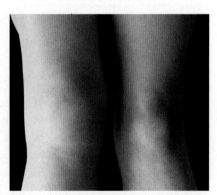

**Figure 18.1.** Clinical case "Acute monoarthritis (I)".

*Summarize the main points of the case.*[1]

*What diagnoses would you consider?*

*Comment on the original diagnosis made by the GP.*

*What would you do?*

[1]Acute-onset febrile monoarthritis.

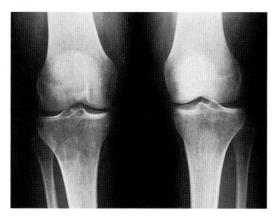

**Figure 18.2.** Clinical case "Acute monoarthritis (I)".

## SEPTIC ARTHRITIS
### MAIN POINTS

This is an articular infection caused by bacteria, mycobacteria, fungi or parasites.

It almost always presents as acute monoarthritis, usually in the knee, shoulder or hip.

The most common agents are Staphylococcus aureus, followed by Hemophilus influenza (in children) and gonococcus (in young adults).

There may be fever, rigors and a general feeling of malaise, but they are inconstant.

Diabetes, sickle-cell anemia, chronic arthritis (e.g. rheumatoid arthritis), joint prosthesis, skin or intestinal infections, invasive articular procedures, intravenous drugs and immunosuppression are all risk factors.

Without appropriate treatment, it causes rapid destruction of the joint.

Analysis of the synovial fluid is the key to the diagnosis.

Treatment involves intravenous antibiotics (following microscopy, culture and sensitivities of synovial fluid), repeated articular lavage, followed by physical therapy.

Surgical lavage may be necessary in some cases.

X-rays showed a marked reduction of the articular space and accentuated periarticular osteopenia (Figure 18.2.). Full blood count revealed leukocytosis (14.5 g/l) with neutrophilia. His sedimentation rate was 42 mm in the first hour. We aspirated synovial fluid which was cloudy, with low viscosity. The fluid was sent for cytological and bacteriological tests and screening for crystals and intravenous antibiotic treatment was immediately started. The microbiological examination showed a high number of gram-positive cocci but no crystals. In the next few days we conducted repeated articular lavage. The bacteriological culture revealed Staphylococcus aureus, with antibiotic sensitivities that obliged us to change the treatment.

The infection was finally treated. Unfortunately, the patient was left with incapacitating mechanical pain, limited mobility and articular instability. A few months later he underwent arthrodesis of the ankle joint.

Acute septic arthritis leads to a fast destruction of the joint. It is a rheumatologic emergency.

If left untreated, it can lead to the total lysis of the articular cartilage, erosion of the adjacent bone and instability of the joint. There is also a substantial risk of the infection spreading.

Most cases of septic arthritis present as acute monoarthritis, with frank signs of inflammation. Infections caused by mycobacteria, fungi or parasites may present with a more insidious course and become chronic.

The infected joint, usually only one, is painful, swollen and red. Note that these signs may be absent in the case of deep joints. In most cases, the patient has a fever, but this may be low-grade in the elderly and settle with anti-inflammatory medications prescribed to relieve pain. Many patients have an infected lesion in another location, in the skin for example, which is the site of entry for the organism. This original source of infection is not always apparent, however.

In addition to common monoarticular conditions, the possibility of gonococcal arthritis should be considered in a young patient presenting with febrile polyarthritis, tenosynovitis and skin rash. Gonococcemia is suggested by the association of arthritis, fever, rash and neurological changes. In endemic areas, Lyme's disease (borreliosis) should be considered in a patient with arthritis and the typical rash (called erythema migrans).

Lab tests usually show leukocytosis and elevated sedimentation rate.

If in doubt, assume the diagnosis is septic arthritis until proven otherwise. Request a bacteriological study of the articular fluid as soon as possible.

Timely, appropriate treatment is essential to achieve full recovery without sequelae.

# GOUT

*TYPICAL CASES*
## 18.B. ACUTE MONOARTHRITIS (II)

João Albino, a 42-year old waiter, came to emergency at 6 a.m. having woken up with excruciating pain in his right big toe. He had been fine when he went to bed around 11 p.m. the night before, after dinner with friends. Nothing like this had ever happened to him before! He was usually healthy, although he consumed a lot of alcohol. He was not taking any regular medication. He denied any episodes of renal colic. His father had "gout."

Clinical examination revealed an obese man, who was extremely upset with the pain. The first metatarsophalangeal joint was markedly swollen and red and highly sensitive to touch (Figure 18.3.). Blood pressure was 170/90 mmHg. He had no fever and the clinical examination showed no other alterations.

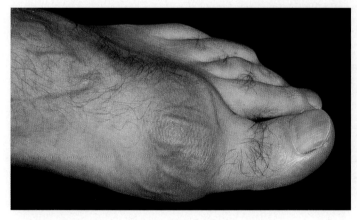

**Figure 18.3.** Clinical case "Acute monoarthritis (II). The first metatarso-phalangeal joint was hot, red and extremely tender.

*What is the most likely diagnosis?*

*How would you investigate this?*

*What would you do immediately?*

The patient was given indomethacin, 25–50 mg every 6 hours, until the flare was over. Meanwhile, he would have to rest his foot and put ice packs on the painful joint. He was advised to come back if the condition did not clear up in one or 2 days and to see his doctor after the crisis was over.

The patient was seen again 2 weeks later. The crisis had passed in about 24 hours. His doctor requested serum uric acid, liver enzymes and serum lipids and recommended total abstinence from alcohol. These and subsequent tests showed hyperuricemia of 9–11 mg/dl, associated with hypertriglyceridemia, even though the patient denied taking any alcohol. Gama-GT levels were high. The doctor insisted on total abstinence from alcohol. After about 7 months, he came back with another crisis. This episode was treated with an anti-inflammatory followed by increasing doses of allopurinol to be taken continually, beginning a few days after the crisis had subsided. He was given a regular dose of colchicine, 0.5 mg, twice a day.

The patient has been well since then.

## TYPICAL CASES
## 18.C. ACUTE POLYARTHRITIS

Arnaldo Marques, a 46-year old man, was sent to the emergency department because of wide-spread articular pain and swelling. His wrists, several proximal metacarpophalangeal and inter-phalangeal joints, knees, ankle and metatarsophalangeal joints were clearly swollen and very painful. Mobilization of the shoulders was extremely painful. His axillary temperature was 37.8°C.

These symptoms had started in just a few hours, 2 days before. He denied any recent infections. He had been to a party the night before, which he considered significant, as he had already had similar pain after a "night on the tiles."

Detailed questioning revealed that patient had suffered recurring crises of acute monoarthritis since the age of 27. They had started in his feet and progressively involved other joints. The first episodes had been monoarticular and fairly infrequent. More recently he had noticed that two or three joints could be affected at the same time and that flare-ups were becoming more frequent.

Previous episodes subsided after 24–48 hours on antiinflammatory drugs. This crisis had not responded, however.

*What is the most probable cause of this condition?*

*How could we investigate it?*

The patient was hospitalized. An examination of his synovial fluid revealed a large number of monosodium urate crystals. His hyperuricemia during the episode was 8.7 mg/dl. He also had mixed hyperlipidemia and elevated AST and γ-GT.

The polyarthritis persisted after full dose non-steroidal anti-inflammatories and it was necessary to use glucocorticoids. While he was in hospital, we began appropriate preventive treatment and took the opportunity to try to educate the patient.

## TYPICAL CASES
## 18.D. CHRONIC DEFORMING ARTHRITIS

Ulisses Gameiro was sent to our clinic with a diagnosis of tophaceous gout. There could be no doubt as to the diagnosis: there were multiple articular deformations with large tophi affecting various joints of the hands and feet and the olecranon area (Figure 18.4.).

His doctor had diagnosed gout more than 15 years ago, on the basis of the typical symptoms of recurring monoarthritis that became increasingly chronic and deforming. He had had two episodes of renal colic. He took furosemide regularly for peripheral oedema and hypertension. Tests had repeatedly shown hyperuricemia. He had been advised on diet and had been pre-scribed anti-inflammatories and allopurinol.

His diet consisted of avoiding fried food and too much meat. He swore that nothing had been said about alcohol. He was taking 300 mg of allopurinol per day, irregularly, as he only remem-bered the medication during flares and stopped taking it after a few weeks. Anti-inflammatories were taken more regularly because the pain was now continuous, mechanical and interspersed with flares. His latest serum uric acid when not in crisis was 12 mg/dl. He also had ongoing hypertension and hypercholesterolemia.

A recent x-ray of the affected joints showed multiple periarticular lytic lesions, with the typical appearance of "corkscrew lesions."

*Comment on the patient's treatment.*

*Would you suggest any changes?*

We insisted on the need to take allopuri-nol regularly without stopping, even dur-ing acute episodes. He was advised to continue with his usual anti-inflammatory in regular doses and to stop furosemide. We advised the patient to lose weight, give up alcohol completely and reduce salt intake.  Two months later his serum uric acid had reduced to 8.4 mg/dl. We increased the dose of allopurinol to 600 mg/day, insisting that he continued to be careful with his diet. Four months later, his serum uric acid was 6 mg/dl. We maintained the treatment.

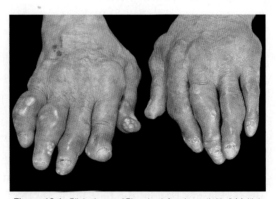

**Figure 18.4.** Clinical case "Chronic deforming arthritis." Multiple nodules with whitish areas. On palpation these nodules were firm and some showed crepitus. Gouty tophy.

Gout comprises articular or periarticular inflammation induced by monosodium urate crys-tals. For them to form, patients usually have longstanding hyperuricemia This is not enough, however, as most people with hyperuricemia do not develop gout.

Once the solution capacity of the organic fluids is saturated, the surplus uric acid precipitates in the form of crystals that can form large deposits – gouty tophi.

Joints are the main sites for these deposits. Occasionally, crystals are phagocytosed by neutrophils in the joints. This process causes the degranulation of these cells, resulting in the release of proteolytic enzymes and triggering the inflammatory process – gouty arthritis or acute gout.

Deposits of uric acid are also found in the kidneys and ureters. There may be diffuse deposits in the renal parenchyma (urate nephropathy) or form kidney stones, which cause recurring episodes of renal colic. The kidneys must therefore be studied carefully in all gout patients.

Hyperuricemia may be caused by excess production of uric acid resulting from the metabolism of purines or, more commonly, deficient renal excretion. Many patients have a family history of gout. In most cases, this is a polygenic condition that only manifests itself in adulthood and is limited to articular and renal problems. Overproduction of uric acid is often part of the so-called metabolic syndrome characterized by obesity, abnormal glucose tolerance, hyperlipidemia and hypertension. For this reason, patients with gout have a higher cardiovascular risk to which we must pay attention.

There are some rare hereditary causes of gout, but they should only be considered if the disease appears in very young patients or is particularly severe and resistant to treatment.

Some non-genetic factors contribute to hyperuricemia: obesity, alcoholism, renal insufficiency, diuretics and low-dose aspirin. Severe acute hyperuricemia may also be caused by antineoplastic treatment, though it is more commonly reflected by urate nephropathy than by gout. High alcohol intake is an important risk factor for gout and should therefore be systematically assessed.

### The clinical examination

Gout usually appears in middle-aged men. It is rare in post-menopausal and exceptional in premenopausal women.

The disease almost always begins with recurring episodes of acute monoarthritis. The "attack" sets in suddenly (in a matter of hours), reaching its height in less than 24 hours. The affected joint is swollen, painful and extremely tender. Intense redness is common in superficial joints.

The first metatarsophalangeal joint is the site of the first episode of gout in about 50% of cases. Crises at this location are often called "podagra" (Figure 18.3.). This preference is worth noting, but it also means that the initial location is elsewhere in the other 50% of cases. The most affected joints, besides the first MTP, are the tarsal joints, ankle and knee. In the first months or years, the affected joints are mainly in the lower extremities. If untreated, the attacks will occur more and more often and will begin to affect the upper limbs as well.

The attack clears up spontaneously or with medication after a few days or weeks, leaving the patient asymptomatic. New episodes will recur at varying intervals affecting the same or other joints – normally one at a time, at the beginning. Later, two or more joints may be affected at the same time (Figure 18.5.) and it may even become polyarticular and persistent, with no symptom-free intervals. Occasionally, the patient presents with polyarthritis that may suggest other diagnoses. Careful questioning will, in most cases, find a typical initial phase. In some patients, the soft tissues may be involved, sometimes in the form of cellulitis.

A small number of patients will develop chronic, tophaceous gout, which can be highly destructive (Figure 18.4.). The deposits of monosodium urate crystals cause erosions around the joints (Figure 18.6.) and may form large masses that can mechanically block articular movement. Some of these deposits are palpable: they are called tophi. They are more commonly located over the extensor surface of the elbow, hand and tarsal joints or in the ear helix (Figures 18.4. and 18.5.). Tophi have a firm consistency and whitish surface. Compression can produce a characteristic crepitus. When tophi burst, a granular, whitish fluid comes out. Superinfection is then common and very difficult to overcome (see the clinical case *"ELBOW PAIN (II),"* Page 9.10).

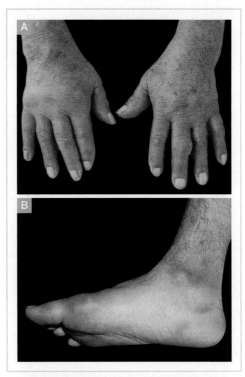

**Figure 18.5.** With time gouty attacks can become oligo- or even polyarticular. **A.** Acute arthritis of the 3rd,4th and 5th right MCPs and of the left wrist. Tofaceous deformity of the 3rd left PIP. **B.** Acute gout affecting the right ankle, midfoot and 1st MTP joint.

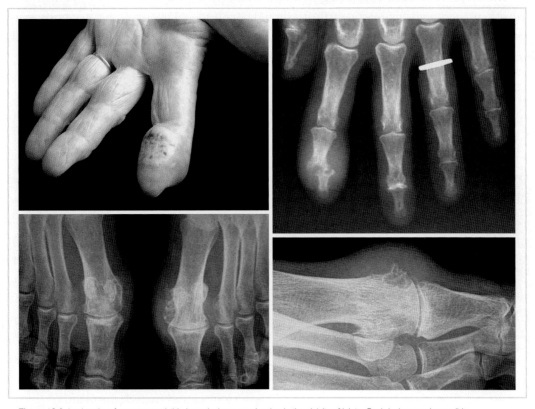

**Figure 18.6.** In chronic tofaceous gout lythic bone lesions can develop in the vicinity of joints. Such lesions are irreversible.

## CLINICAL ASPECTS OF GOUT
### MAIN POINTS

It is a common cause of arthritis, especially in middle-aged and elderly men.

It is caused by an inflammatory reaction to monosodium urate crystals that can form in patients with hyperuricemia.

The initial stages are characterized by recurring episodes of acute monoarthritis, with asymptomatic intervals.

With time, the episodes become more frequent and possibly continuous. The chronic form is associated with the formation of tophi and the destruction of bone and joints.

The most affected joints are the first MTP, followed by the tarsus, tibiotarsal and knee.

Gout is often associated with obesity, alcoholism, hypertension, hyperlipidemia, renal impairment and the use of diuretics.

The risk of recurrence of the attacks and of the progression into the chronic form depends on the degree and persistence of hyperuricemia.

### Diagnosis

The clinical pattern of acute recurring attacks is extremely suggestive and almost specific. Septic arthritis, pseudo-gout and reactive arthritis should be considered in differential diagnosis. When episodes occur repeatedly with a typical course and good response to anti-inflammatories, the probability of gout is very high even without lab tests.

**A definite diagnosis of gout requires the demonstration of intra-articular monosodium urate crystals, phagocytosed by neurophils cells.**

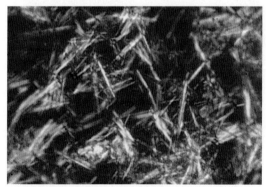

**Figure 18.7.** Monosodium urate crystals (polarized light, 400X, *red compensator*). Under polarized light, monosodium urate crystals are *spindle shaped* and strongly birefringent. (Courtesy: Prof. Eliseo Pascual. Alicante, Spain.)

For this reason, even if the clinical examination is suggestive, it is important to conduct at least one examination of the synovial fluid, preferably before beginning treatment. Examined fresh under a polarized light microscope, monosodium urate crystals are needle-shaped with characteristic bifrefringence (Figure 18.7.). During a gout attack, the synovial fluid has extremely high counts of neutrophils (often > 20.000/ l), making it look cloudy or even purulent.

Most patients with gout have high serum uric acid levels. This reinforces the diagnosis, but is not enough to confirm it on its own, as most people with hyperuricemia never develop arthritis. Note that serum uric acid levels may go down to normal during an acute gout attack. If this test is only performed when the patient is suffering a flare-up, hyperuricemia may be underestimated or even missed. On the other hand, given that the prevalence of hyperuricemia is high, we may misdiagnose another type of arthritis as gout if we do not examine the synovial fluid.

If doubt as to the diagnosis persists and it is not possible to examine the synovial fluid, it is worth testing the efficacy of colchicine in the regime described below for acute attacks. A frank response to this drug reinforces the diagnosis, even if it does not completely confirm it.

It is good practice to study the kidneys and assess the cardiovascular risk factors in all patients with gout.

Differential diagnosis of acute gout should consider the possibilities of septic arthritis, other types of arthritis caused by microcrystals like pseudo-gout, acute periarthritis and trauma.

Please note: Gout is almost exclusive to adult and middle-aged men. It is exceptional in pre-menopausal women and very rare in post-menopausal women, usually associated with kidney disease or the use of diuretics. Whenever you consider diagnosing gout in a woman, think twice!

---

**DIAGNOSING GOUT**
*MAIN POINTS*

The clinical manifestations can be highly suggestive but they do not establish a definite diagnosis.

The final diagnosis requires the presence of tophi or demonstration of phagocytosed monosodium urate crystals in the synovial fluid.

Most patients with gout have hyperuricemia.

Serum uric acid levels tend to go down during acute attacks.

Most people with hyperuricemia never develop gout.

Patients with gout should be assessed for kidney stones and cardiovascular risk factors.

---

## Treatment

The treatment of gout is usually extremely satisfactory. When followed strictly and applied opportunely, it almost always results in total prevention of further attacks.

---

*PLEASE NOTE.*

**GOUT HAS NO CURE. TREATMENT IS LIFELONG!**

---

For this reason, do not start preventive treatment unless you are absolutely sure about the diagnosis (or the mistake will become chronic). Attacks usually respond well to anti-inflammatories and irreversible damage only occurs after many repeated episodes. There is time to confirm the diagnosis and start prevention.

If you suspect gout, we therefore suggest the following approach.

### Make sure that it is gout

a) Assess the clinical features carefully. Exclude septic arthritis.

b) Examine the synovial fluid as soon as possible.

c) Measure serum uric acid and 24-hour uricosuria.

### Treatment of the acute attack

a) Rest the joint (possible application of ice packs)

b) Full doses of an anti-inflammatory, e.g. indomethacin 25–50 mg every 6 hours or naproxen 500 mg bid, until the pain goes. The patient should start taking the medication as soon as the pain begins.

c) If you are still in doubt as to the diagnosis, try colchicine: 0.5–1 mg every 4–6 hours until the pain goes or diarrhea occurs.

d) High doses of colchicine almost always cause diarrhea. Anti-inflammatories are at least just as effective. Therefore, colchicine is not usually recommended during an attack except as a therapeutic test.

e) In stubborn cases or if anti-inflammatories are contraindicated, consider a short course (2–3 days) of oral glucocorticoid or an intra-articular steroid injection.

### Preventing attacks: basic treatment

a) **Diet**. It is absolutely essential to reduce alcohol intake to the minimum. Alcohol increases the frequency of attacks, reduces the level necessary to induce an acute episode, reduces urinary excretion of uric acid and antagonizes the effect of allopurinol. This is the main point in the patient's diet.

In addition, we should try to correct obesity and advise against excessive intake of purines, found mainly in red meat, sausage, seafood and canned meat or fish.

b) Assess **associated medication** to identify agents that can contribute to hyperuricemia, such as furosemide or pyrazinamide, and correct it if possible.

c) **Allopurinol**. This agent is a xanthine oxidase inhibitor and thus reduces the synthesis of uric acid. It is the cornerstone of the pharmaceutical treatment of gout when the above measures prove insufficient

Begin with a dose of 100 mg/day and progressively increase it to 300–600 mg/day, over 3–4 weeks. The required dose is determined by the level of serum uric acid. The therapeutic goal is a concentration of less than 6 mg/dl (0.36 mmol/l). The saturation point of monosodium urate solutions is 6.4 mg/dl. Higher values may prevent attacks but will not free the organism of accumulated excess uric acid. If necessary, increase the dose while controlling toxicity.

**Never begin allopurinol during a flare-up.** It tends to prolong it.

Once started, however, do not interrupt the treatment, even during subsequent attacks.

d) **Uricosurics**. These include agents like probenecid and sulfinpyrazone, which increase renal excretion of urate. They are indicated in cases of low urinary excretion of urates (<600 mg/24 hours) or intolerance of allopurinol (hepatic or cutaneous). These agents are not very effective if the glomerular filtration rate is less than 60 ml/minutes. They are contraindicated if the patient has kidney stones and should always be accompanied by good water intake.

e) **Colchicine/regular anti-inflammatories**. The first 6 months of allopurinol or uricosurics are associated with an increased risk of acute attacks. For this reason,

**regular colchicine (0.5–0.6 mg, twice a day) should always be associated for 6–9 months after achieving normal uricemia,** then gradually discontinued.

A regular dose of an anti-inflammatory is a good alternative in case of intolerance.

**TREATING GOUT**
*MAIN POINTS*

Make sure of your diagnosis before beginning preventive treatment.

**Acute attacks**

- Rest, local ice
- Early, full dose of anti-inflammatory
- Colchicine as a therapeutic test

**Preventing attacks**

- Diet (alcohol, purines, obesity)
- Allopurinol (continuously, forever), and/or
- Uricosurics
- Anti-inflammatory or colchicine in the first 6–9 months
- Check associated medication

**Correction of associated cardiovascular risk factors**

### *Asymptomatic hyperuricemia*

Hyperuricemia is extremely common in the general population and only a minority will ever develop gout. This means that there is a great risk of misdiagnosis if we assume that every patient with joint pain and hyperuricemia has gout.

Hyperuricemia does not constitute a risk for anything other than gout, renal stones and (exceptionally) urate nephropathy. There is therefore no point in requesting this test if there are no signs or symptoms of any of these pathologies. If the joint pain is mechanical, for example, hyperuricemia is irrelevant.

What should be done if a patients has high serum uric acid levels?

a) Advise the patient about diet and especially alcohol intake.

b) Check kidney function and the cardiovascular risk factors and correct them.

c) Find out whether the patient is taking any medication that might be responsible for this alteration and change it, if possible.

d) **Do not prescribe pharmaceutical treatment** unless there are signs of gout or renal disease caused by uric acid. The risk of side effects is much greater than the risk of an initial attack of gout![2]

---

**GOUT**

*DONT'S*

Do not begin uric acid lowering drugs if you are not absolutely sure of the diagnosis.

Do not begin uric acid lowering drugs during an acute gout attack.

Do not stop uric acid lowering drugs during an acute gout attack.

Do not begin uric acid lowering drugs without associating regular colchicine or anti-inflammatory in the first few months.

---

Gouty tophi tend to get smaller in time with the right treatment. Surgical removal is not advisable, unless they are causing significant mechanical problems. Superinfection of ulcerated tophi requires intravenous antibiotics and often surgical cleansing.

---

**GOUT**

*WHEN SHOULD THE PATIENT BE REFERRED TO A SPECIALIST?*

Uncertain diagnosis

Recurring attacks that do not respond to the appropriate treatment

Uncontrolled tophaceous gout

Gout associated with renal impairment

Intolerance to allopurinol

---

[2]Some authors recommend prophylactic treatment of asymptomatic hyperuricemia, when its values are persistently above 11.5 mg/dl (0.7 mmol/l) or in cases of renal impairment.

# PSEUDO-GOUT, CHONDROCALCINOSIS

**The most suggestive clinical features**

- Clinical features of gout in an elderly patient, especially a woman

- Symptoms suggesting gout with atypical development or response to treatment

- Atypical osteoarthritis (especially if onset was early and it involves recurring, acute inflammatory episodes)

- Clinical pattern suggestive of rheumatoid arthritis starting in older age

## *TYPICAL CASES*
## 18.E. RECURRENT MONOARTHRITIS

Jorge Lambeiro, a 44-year old economist, sought our help because of recurring episodes of migratory monoarthritis over the last 15 years. The first MTP, tarsus, ankles, right fourth PIP and third MCP, elbows, knees and wrists had already been affected. He had asymptomatic periods, initially lasting for 18–24 months and recently no more than 3–4 months. He now had discreet mechanical pain between attacks.

There was evidence of hyperuricemia (about 8 mg/dl) in some tests. His doctor had diagnosed gout and begun treatment with allopurinol (continuous, 300 mg/day) and anti-inflammatories, when required. He had complied with the treatment for about 10 years, though without apparent benefit.

On physical examination we found painful periarticular inflammation of the knee and firm subcutaneous masses in the external face of the right knee and tarsus as well as over the above two joints of the hands, which we assumed were tophi.

The dose of allopurinol was increased in order to lower serum urate to less than 6 mg/dl. He gave up alcohol. The attacks continued, however, and showed little response to the anti-inflammatories.

*What aspects, if any, do not seem typical of gout?*

*What would you do?*

In view of this lack of response to treatment, we conducted a more detailed study.

Figure 18.8. shows the x-rays. We took the opportunity of a flare-up in the knee to take some synovial fluid. Examination under polarized light showed monosodium urate and calcium pyrophosphate crystals. A detailed laboratory study showed slight elevation of corrected calcium and a corresponding high value of parathyroid hormone in two measurements.

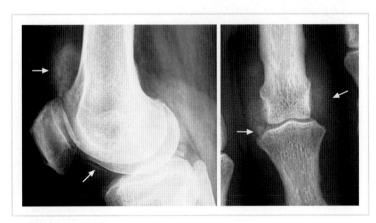

**Figure 18.8.** Clinical case "Recurrent monoarthritis." Note the calcification of articular cartilage and soft tissues.

An ultrasound scan of the cervical region revealed a nodule in one of the parathyroid glands, which was later removed. The attacks cleared after a few months. The patient is currently without treatment, while continuing to watch his diet.

## TYPICAL CASES
## 18.F. DIFFICULT OSTEOARTHRITIS

52-year old Isabel Matias was sent to us by her GP because of intense, incapacitating pol-yarticular pain that was unresponsive to medication. The condition had set in at the age of 42 and consisted of typically mechanical pain that, over the years, had progressively spread to the knees, lumbar spine, hips, shoulders, wrists and several metacarpophalangeal joints. The patient also described repeated episodes of articular pain (intense), swelling and redness that kept her awake at night.

She had been treated with different non-steroidal anti-inflammatories, which she said were inef-fective. Allopurinol had not worked either. She got some relief from colchicine during attacks.

She denied any significant extra-articular symptoms. Her father had had similar symptoms since he was 40.

Clinical examination revealed bony swelling, coarse crepitus and limited mobility in the knees, MCPs and shoulders. There were no signs of inflammation or tophi.

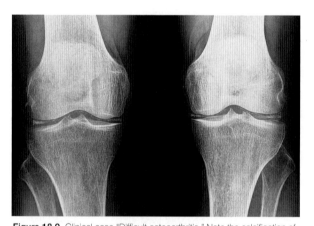

**Figure 18.9.** Clinical case "Difficult osteoarthritis." Note the calcification of articular cartilage and meniscus.

*Give a brief description of this condition.* [3]

*What is your interpretation?*

*Consider the possibility of gout.*

An x-ray of her knees is shown in Figure 18.9.

The diagnosis of chondrocalcinosis was evident and entirely compatible with the symptoms of early degenerative joint diseases with acute inflammato-ry flares.

Unfortunately, laboratory tests for causes of chondrocalcinosis were negative.

### Clinical forms
### Pseudo-gout

Pseudo-gout is the most common form of acute arthritis in the elderly. It is induced by an inflammatory reaction to calcium pyrophosphate crystals in the joint (microcrystalline arthri-tis).

In typical pseudo-gout, the patient describes recurring episodes of acute mono- or oligoarthritis that sets in over 2–3 days. Physical examination may show signs of local inflam-mation, sometimes with associated effusion. There may be a low-grade fever. The joint most commonly affected is the knee, though it may appear in other locations, such as the elbows, wrists, MCPs and tibiotarsal joints.

The differential diagnosis should include gout and septic arthritis. It may be quite difficult to distinguish between them, as pseudo-gout is often accompanied by intense local inflamma-

[3]Recurrent monoarthritis in a context of atypical osteoarthritis.

tory signs and systemic manifestations, including fever. In some cases, the pyrophosphate deposits may be extra-articular and acquire a pseudo-tumoral appearance, simulating tophi.

Ideally, synovial fluid should be collected for observation under a polarized light microscope and bacteriological tests.

The synovial fluid is often bloody. Under polarized light, calcium pyrophosphate crystals are rhomboid in shape and have low refraction (Figure 18.10.). Note that, as in this case, gout and pseudo-gout can coexist.

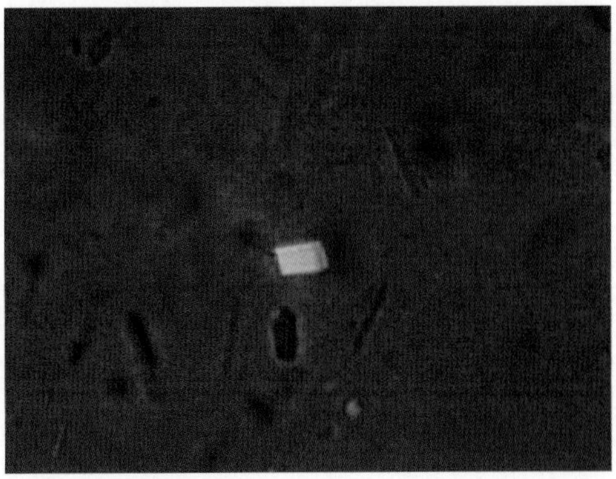

**Figure 18.10.** Calcium pyrophosphate dihydrate crystals (CPPD – polarized light, 400X, *red compensator*). Under polarized light, CPPD crystals are romboid or *needle shaped* and weakly birefringent. (Courtesy: Prof. Eliseo Pascual. Alicante, Spain.)

### Chondrocalcinosis

In most cases, the acute episodes described above are superimposed on mechanical polyarticular pain that sometimes begins at a relatively early age (chronic joint disease induced by pyrophosphate – "atypical osteoarthritis" – see Chapter 16). This situation has a differential diagnosis of osteoarthritis or, depending on the preferential location, rheumatoid arthritis or polymyalgia rheumatica.

X-rays of the joints may show signs of chondrocalcinosis – calcification of the articular cartilage, disks or menisci (Figure 18.11.). This radiographic findings makes the diagnosis. X-rays of the wrists (carpal meniscus), knees, pelvis (pubic symphysis) and spine (intervertebral

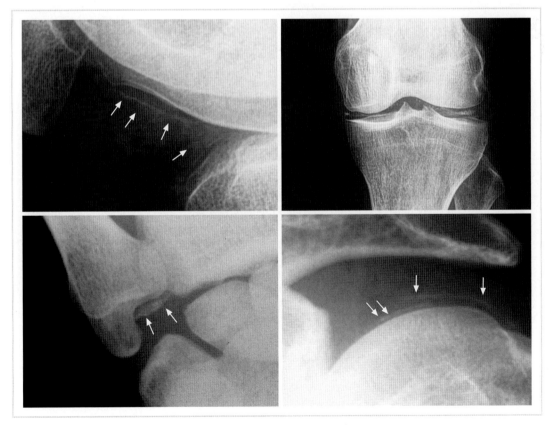

**Figure 18.11.**
Typical radiological features of chondrocalcinosis.

| |
|---|
| Hemochromatosis |
| Hyperparathyroidism |
| Hypophosphatasia |
| Hypomagnesemia |
| Gout |

**Table 18.1.** Metabolic diseases predisposing to pseudo-gout/chondrocalcinosis.

disks) are the most productive. In some cases, there are calcified periarticular deposits. In chondrocalcinosis, associated osteoarthritis tends to be frankly exostotic ("hypertrophic osteoarthritis") with large osteophytes. Osteoarthritic involvement of atypical locations is particularly suggestive of this diagnosis.

It is important to bear in mind that several metabolic diseases can contribute to chondrocalcinosis. If the diagnosis is made early, before irreversible articular damage, progression can usually be prevented (Table 18.1.). There is a strong family tendency. Older age and a history of osteoarthritis are important risk factors.

### Treatment

Exacerbations are treated as described for gout. There is more often a need to administer intra-articular injections of corticosteroids, after excluding the possibility of infection. The joint should be mobilized as soon as possible to prevent contracture, which is common in the elderly.

Treatment of the chronic form is much the same as for osteoarthritis, associated with correction of any metabolic factors identified. Flares require frequent use of local therapy, such as joint aspiration, short-term rest, and intra-articular injection of corticosteroids or radioisotopes.

## CHRONIC MONOARTHRITIS

### TYPICAL CASES
### 18.G. CHRONIC MONOARTHRITIS

We had been following Eduardo Monteiro, a 32-year old mechanic, for about 5 years and we had only recently reached an accurate diagnosis. When we first saw him, he was suffering from typical, unquestionable arthritis of the left knee, which had set in about 4 months before. Its onset had been progressive and had not been preceded by any type of infection. Systematic enquiry and general examination did not find any additional alterations. Examination of the sacroiliac joints was normal.

Lab tests, including serological screening for infections and rheumatoid factor, were entirely normal. His initial sedimentation rate was 32 mm in the first hour. Tests for Chlamydia and gonococci in the urethral exudate were negative. Examination of the synovial fluid showed 8.000 cells/ l (80% neutrophils). The search for crystals and the bacteriological examination were negative. We finally performed a synovial biopsy, which showed "chronic, non-specific synovitis." The bacteriological culture of the synovial tissue, including mycobacteria, was negative.

*What possible diagnosis and additional investigation would you suggest?*

*What would you do in this particular case?*

We explained the situation to the patient, and told him of our uncertainty as to the diagnosis. We suggested a local injection of glucocorticoids, which completely cleared up the signs and symptoms… for about a year. In 5 years, there were three recurrences. All clinical examinations and lab tests were still negative. We classified the condition as "chronic, undifferentiated monoarthritis." We continued the same treatment.

On our last examination, we found a small, scaly lesion in his right ear. It was psoriasis…

Occasionally patients present with a single chronically inflamed joint. Many of these cases of arthritis are only slowly erosive, though they can cause significant functional problems. The knee, ankle or hip are most often involved.

Onset is often insidious, hampering and delaying the diagnosis.

It is obviously possible that diseases which are typically polyarticular may be limited to a single joint, at least for some time. Seronegative spondyloarthropathies are often oligoarticular. While the process is limited to one joint, however, it may be impossible to establish the diagnosis, especially if there are no suggestive extra-articular manifestations.

It is important to bear in mind the possibility of chronic septic arthritis, usually caused by mycobacteria, brucella, fungi (histoplasma, blastomyces, etc.) or, rarely, parasites or protozoa. Chronic septic arthritis leads to slowly progressive articular destruction and can be complicated by osteomyelitis (Figure 18.12.). Villonodular synovitis, a benign neoplastic process of the synovium, is clinically indistinguishable.

In chronic monoarthritis, synovial biopsy with histological and bacteriological examination, is the main route to diagnosis. It clearly establishes the diagnosis of chronic septic arthritis and villonodular synovitis. In cases of chronic monoarticular gout the histology of a synovial fragment fixed in alcohol may show monosodium urate crystals not present in the fluid.

Nevertheless, in many cases no definite etiological diagnosis can be made. It is not possible to exclude the possibility of persistent reactive arthritis, but it is impossible to confirm it with existing techniques. In some patients, new inflamed joints appear with time, eventually leading to a more typical pattern.

Treatment is etiological when possible. In other cases, anti-inflammatories are the mainstay of treatment. In stubborn cases, intra-articular corticosteroids or arthroscopic synovectomy may be necessary.

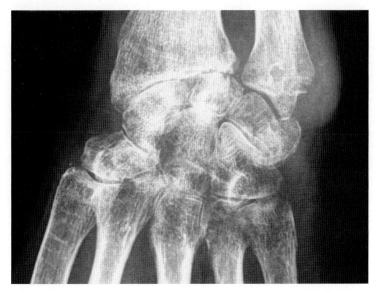

**Figure 18.12.** Septic arthritis (mycobacterium tuberculosis) of the left wrist.

## ADDITIONAL PRACTICE
### MONOARTHRITIS

# CHRONIC, ADDITIVE, SYMMETRICAL, PERIPHERAL POLYARTHRITIS

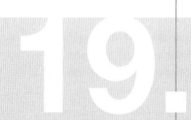

J.A.P. da Silva, A.D. Woolf, *Rheumatology in Practice*, DOI 10.1007/978-1-84882-581-9_19,
© Springer-Verlag London Limited 2010

# 19. CHRONIC, ADDITIVE, SYMMETRICAL, PERIPHERAL POLYARTHRITIS

This concept requires the presence of articular inflammation (arthritis[1]) affecting five or more joints (polyarthritis) that is persistent (>6 weeks), additive (rather than migratory or recurrent), and approximately symmetrical (the same joints or articular areas affected on each side of the body), with preferential involvement of the wrists, hands, ankle joints and feet.

Identifying this syndrome is the first diagnostic step.

## Second diagnostic step

Rheumatoid arthritis (R.A.) is the predominant cause of this syndrome, not only because it is the most common, but also because the other situations that can cause it are almost always accompanied by additional suggestive signs: systemic manifestations, psoriasis or a history of monoarticular gout, which place them in other clinical patterns or syndromes.

The differential diagnosis is essentially clinical but several tests can be useful in establishing the diagnosis and assessing the disease activity and prognosis.

---

### TYPICAL CASES
### 19.A. POLYARTHRALGIA

Isabel Marinho, a 32-year old businesswoman, was sent to our clinic urgently by her doctor because of a history of 2 months of inflammatory, symmetrical joint pain mainly affecting the wrists, MCPs, PIPs and forefeet. She described morning stiffness that lasted for several hours. The patient had recently complained of nocturnal paresthesia in her hands. She denied any extra-articular manifestations, apart from fatigue.

The painful joints were swollen and tender, with signs of articular effusion (fluctuance). The overlying skin looked normal but there was a perceptible increase in the local temperature. Flexion of the fingers was markedly limited, which was partly positive bilaterally in the carpal tunnel. The general examination found no other changes, including skin lesions.

---

*Give a brief description of this clinical condition.[2]*

*What is the most probable diagnosis and why?*

*What tests would you request?*

[1]To review the clinical concept of "arthritis" see Table 17.1.

[2]Chronic, additive, symmetrical, dominantly peripheral polyarthritis, with no axial symptoms or systemic manifestations in a young woman. Carpal tunnel syndrome.

The patient had test results with her which showed a high rheumatoid factor titer (1:1280), a sedimentation rate of 66 mm in the first hour and mild normocytic normochromic anemia. The immunofluorescence antinuclear antibody test was negative. Liver and kidney tests were normal.

There were no alterations in the x-rays of her feet and hands except for soft tissue swelling and mild periarticular osteopenia in the MCPs and PIPs (Figure 19.1.).

*What is your diagnosis?*

*What treatment would you suggest?*

Our diagnosis, in view of the clinical data, was **rheumatoid arthritis**, complicated by **bilateral carpal tunnel syndrome**. We noted the points suggesting a poor prognosis: acute polyarticular onset, highly positive rheumatoid factor and high sedimentation rate. We opted for aggressive treatment under close supervision. The clinical response was very good, but we were obliged to adapt the medication several times over the years. Although she still requires combined treatment involving several drugs, the patient is well 6 years after the onset of her condition. Her functional capacity is excellent and x-rays show only discreet loss of articular space in some MCPs and MTPs. Two of these joints show erosions.

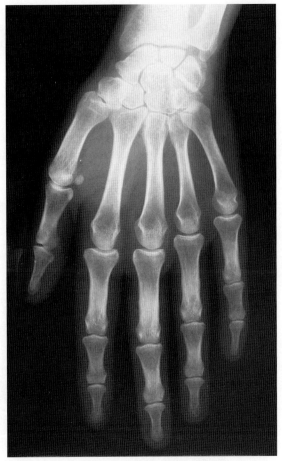

**Figure 19.1.** Clinical case "Polyarthralgia". Hand X-rays show periarticular osteopenia and no other changes.

## TYPICAL CASES
## 19.B. DEFORMING ARTHRITIS

Maria de Jesus, a 52 year old housewife, said that her disease had started 7 years before. The manifestations in the first few years were highly suggestive of rheumatoid arthritis: inflammatory joint pain and swelling. There were even subcutaneous nodules, which she still had.

When we examined her for the first time there could, unfortunately, be no doubt as to the diagnosis. The deformities in her hands and feet were typical (Figure 19.2.). Mobility in her wrists, hands and knees was significantly limited. Her left elbow was limited to −40° extension. She had moderate signs of inflammation in many of her joints.

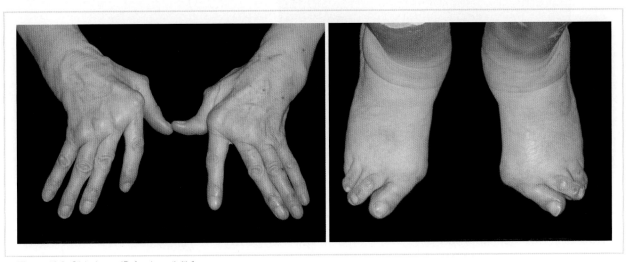

**Figure 19.2.** Clinical case "Deforming arthritis".

Some years before, she had been admitted urgently to the local hospital for sudden, incapacitating dorsal and lumbar pain. Cutaneous atrophy and Cushingoid facies testified to the lengthy glucocorticoid therapy that she had undergone. Her dorsal kyphosis suggested fracturing osteoporosis, which was confirmed by an x-ray. She described a frequent burning sensation in her eyes with some recurring, painful episodes of red eye. X-rays showed extensive destruction of several joints (Figure 19.3.). Lab tests revealed anemia, a high sedimentation rate and hyperglycemia.

We took over the treatment of this patient, seriously regretting that we had not seen her six or 7 years earlier. The impact of our treatment would now leave a lot to be desired.

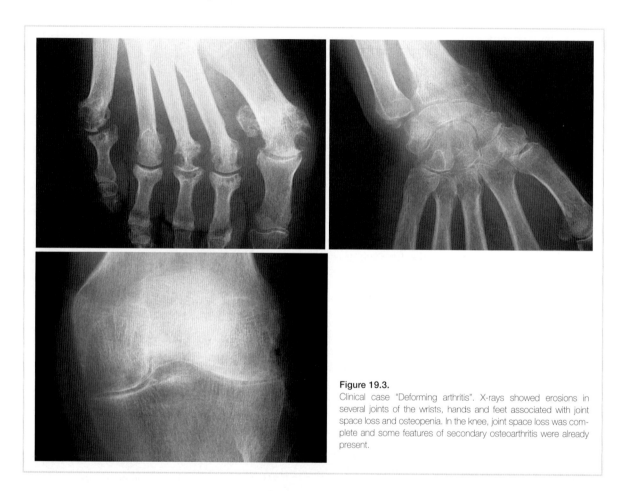

**Figure 19.3.**
Clinical case "Deforming arthritis". X-rays showed erosions in several joints of the wrists, hands and feet associated with joint space loss and osteopenia. In the knee, joint space loss was complete and some features of secondary osteoarthritis were already present.

## RHEUMATOID ARTHRITIS

Rheumatoid arthritis is a systemic inflammatory disease of unknown cause that mainly affects the joints. Its main feature consists of chronic inflammation of the synovium, which may, in time, lead to massive articular destruction and accentuated disability. There may be involvement of multiple organs and extra-articular systems, though articular manifestations are the dominant symptoms.

Its prevalence is 0.5–1% of the population, depending on the country. Women are affected more frequently than men, in a proportion of two to one. This difference is greater at reproductive age, and less marked in the elderly. The disease starts most often between the ages of 35 and 50, but it can appear at any age.

## Practical implications of the pathogenesis

The inflammatory process is primarily located in the synovium and can affect many joints at the same time. Synovial inflammation explains the **signs of articular inflammation, pain** and elevated **acute-phase reactants**, reflected by a high sedimentation rate and C-reactive protein, for example.

The synovium releases inflammatory mediators, such as TNF and IL-1 that induce the **progressive destruction of the articular cartilage**. This results in loss of articular mobility and a typically uniform loss of joint space in x-rays, a common feature in arthritis. The inflamed synovial tissue becomes invasive, causing **erosion of the bone** around the joint (visible in x-rays). The inflammatory process also directly or indirectly involves subchondral bone (causing periarticular osteopenia) and periarticular soft tissue, often resulting in bursitis, ligamentitis and tenosynovitis. Tendons and ligaments become weakened and loose, with the resulting **tendency towards subluxation and articular deviation**. These aspects contribute to **pain** and **limited mobility**.

Functional compromise at any given time depends on the inflammatory activity of the disease (which explains pain, swelling, stiffness and limited mobility) and accumulated structural damage.

> **Structural damage (erosion, loss of cartilage, etc.) begins during the first months of rheumatoid disease.**

As a rule, structural damage is irreversible. Once it has started, it creates favorable conditions for the development of secondary osteoarthritis, even if the inflammatory process subsides. Severe rheumatoid arthritis also has important vascular and visceral repercussions. Overall, the mortality associated with this condition is comparable to that of Hodgkin's disease and triple coronary disease!

Recognition of this and recent evidence from clinical trials has led to a profound change in the treatment of rheumatoid arthritis over recent years.

> **Adequate treatment of rheumatoid arthritis must begin as early as possible, i.e. as soon as the diagnosis has been confirmed!**

To do this, it is vital that GPs, to whom almost all these patients turn first, are able to make an early diagnosis, before any irreversible damage takes place, and promote timely referral to physicians experienced in this disease.

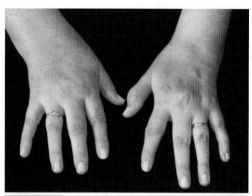

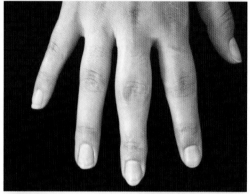

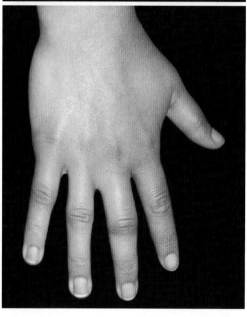

**Figure 19.4.** Clinical aspect of the hands in patients with early rheumatoid arthritis. Notice the fusiform swelling around the proximal interphalangeal joints and the absence of rubour. Palpation is essential to demonstrate the presence of synovial inflammation.

For this reason, this chapter focuses on the early stages of rheumatoid arthritis and only mentions later aspects to illustrate the type of suffering and functional disability that we want to and can avoid.

## EARLY SYMPTOMS

In the vast majority of cases, rheumatoid arthritis presents as chronic, additive, symmetrical, peripheral polyarthritis. It may also be accompanied by extra-articular and radiological manifestations.

### Polyarthritis

This is reflected by inflammatory joint pain, associated with clear signs of articular inflammation: heat, elastic swelling or articular fluctuation. There is pain on palpation and on mobilization (active and passive), with possible limitation of (active and passive) mobility. Confirmation of these aspects requires careful, competent examination of all the affected articular areas (see Chapters 6–14). Elevated sedimentation rate and C-reactive protein reinforce the conviction that we are dealing with a significant inflammatory process.

The process affects five or more joints (**poly**arthritis). This aspect makes RA different from other types of arthritis that normally affect only one (monoarthritis – gout, septic arthritis, etc.) or a few joints (oligoarthritis – some forms of seronegative spondyloarthropathy, reactive arthritis, etc.). It does not exclude other types of polyarthritis, such as those associated with lupus and other diseases of the connective tissue as well as certain forms of psoriatic and reactive arthritis (Figure 19.4.).

### Chronic

Rheumatoid arthritis typically has a progressive onset (in weeks) and a chronic course (>6 weeks). Some types of reactive arthritis, such as post-viral forms, can be very similar to RA. Their onset is usually abrupt, however, and most of them clear up, spontaneously or in response to treatment, in less than 6 weeks. On the other hand, RA may start by affecting only one or a few joints, taking several weeks to acquire its typical polyarticular pattern. Polyarthritis must therefore be chronic, i.e. persist for more than 6 weeks, before this diagnosis can be confirmed.

### Additive

This characteristic makes rheumatoid arthritis different from certain other types, which can affect multiple joints successively or migrate from one to another, with (like gout) or without disease-free intervals, as is the case in rheumatic fever and other forms of reactive arthritis. In these cases, no more than one or two joints are affected at any given time.

Articular involvement is also typically additive in lupus, psoriatic arthritis, and other types of seronegative spondyloarthropathy.

### Symmetrical

Rheumatoid arthritis tends to be markedly symmetrical. This symmetry is sometimes remarkable, even when we consider individual MCP or PIP joints on either side, though it is almost constant if we consider only the articular areas: MCPs on both sides, and PIPs or wrist on both sides. This aspect helps to distinguish it from seronegative spondyloarthropathy in general and from psoriatic arthritis in particular, as they are generally asymmetrical. Symmetry is also common in the arthritis of lupus and other diseases of the connective tissue.

### Peripheral

Rheumatoid arthritis can affect practically all the joints in the skeleton, with the exception of the thoracic and lumbar spine. In its initial stages, however, it has a strong preference for MCPs, PIPs and metatarsophalangeal joints. The wrists and ankle joints follow in frequency. Proximal joints, like elbows, shoulders, knees and hips are usually affected later.

Conversely, psoriatic arthritis and seronegative spondyloarthropathy, including most types of reactive arthritis, preferentially involve the more proximal joints and even the sacroiliac joints and lumbar spine. RA often involves the upper cervical spine but not the thoracic or lumbar joints.

Arthritis in lupus and other connective tissue diseases is normally peripheral. Psoriatic arthritis may misleadingly present in a similar way to rheumatoid arthritis (pseudo-rheumatoid form). Note that RA in the hands rarely involves the distal interphalangeal joints which are a common location for psoriatic arthritis. In some patients the onset of rheumatoid arthritis may be dominated by tenosynovitis of the flexor tendons in the fingers/hands[3], with relatively discreet articular signs – always suspect RA in these circumstances.

### Systemic manifestations

The initial stages of rheumatoid arthritis, especially in its severe forms, with abrupt, polyarticular onset *ab initio,* may be accompanied by fever, weight loss or lymphadenopathy. When these manifestations are predominant, other diagnoses are definitely worth considering, including, in this case, the possibility of paraneoplastic arthritis, in the right age group. Rheumatoid nodules, described below, may be present from the initial stages, thus further reinforcing the diagnosis.

Other extra-articular manifestations of this disease normally appear in more advanced stages and will be addressed later.

---

[3]See Chapter 10 and the clinical case "*PAIN IN THE HANDS (III)*", Page 10.25.

## DIFFERENTIAL DIAGNOSIS

The clinical characterization described above obviously requires a thorough, sensitive enquiry and clinical examination. Nevertheless, if these features can be confirmed, the differential diagnosis is basically limited to five possibilities:

- **Rheumatoid arthritis.**

    Please Note: rheumatoid arthritis, with identical features, can appear in childhood (juvenile rheumatoid arthritis).

- **Systemic lupus erythematosus and other connective tissue diseases** – arthritis will almost always be accompanied by suggestive systemic manifestations, such as malar erythema, photosensitivity and other skin alterations, mouth ulcers, serositis, Raynaud's phenomenon, proximal muscle weakness, etc. Dryness of the eyes and mouth, suggesting Sjögren's syndrome, is more difficult to value, as this syndrome is often associated with RA. The arthritis is usually more discreet than in RA.

    When in doubt some lab tests will help in the diagnosis: alterations in the hemogram and renal function, antinuclear antibodies, Schirmer's test, electromyography, etc.

- **Pseudo-rheumatoid psoriatic arthritis** – most patients have psoriasis. In those who do not, a family history of psoriasis suggests this diagnosis. Their rheumatoid factor is normally negative, but this is also true of 25% of RA patients. Differential diagnosis may be difficult but it is reassuring to know that the treatment of the two conditions is very similar.

- **Nodal osteoarthritis** – a thorough clinical examination is usually enough to distinguish between the two conditions. In nodal osteoarthritis, the rhythm of the pain may be mixed and suggest and inflammatory process. Onset is slow and progressive. On palpation, there is a predominance of hard, bony nodes (rather than fusiform swelling and elastic fluctuation), which affect not only the PIPs, but also almost always the DIPs (Figure 19.5.). Occasionally there may be misleading signs of inflammation, although they are generally limited to one or two joints. It usually appears after the menopause.

- **Chondrocalcinosis** – The clinical pattern may be very similar to RA. In most cases, however, there will be a longstanding story of mechanical joint pain with recurring inflammatory episodes. It is more common in the elderly.

    In view of these possibilities what diagnostic tests are justified?

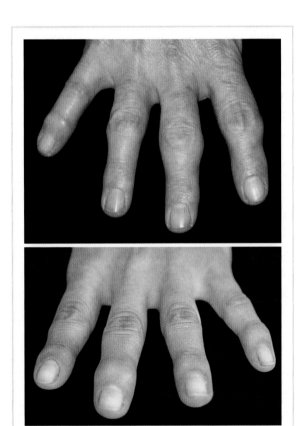

**Figure 19.5.** Nodal osteoarthritis of the hands. The aspect of the hands may suggest rheumatoid arthritis at first sight. Note, however, that the swelling is more nodular and distal interphalangeal joints are almost always involved. These nodules are hard and bony on palpation.

## Diagnostic tests

### Laboratory

Table 19.1. shows the most useful lab tests when we suspect rheumatoid arthritis and the most suggestive abnormality for each differential diagnosis.

| | Rheumatoid arthritis | Other CTDs | Psoriatic arthritis | Nodal osteoarthritis |
|---|---|---|---|---|
| Hemoglobin and red cell indices | Normocytic normochromic anemia | Hemolytic anemia | Normocytic normochromic anemia | Normal |
| White cell count | Normal. Leukocytosis | Leucopenia Lymphopenia | Normal | Normal |
| Platelets | Thrombocytosis | Thrombocytopenia | Normal or ↑ | Normal |
| Erythrocyte sedimentation rate and C-reactive protein | Elevated | Raised ESR CRP may be normal | Elevated | Normal |
| Rheumatoid factor | High | Negative or low | Negative | Negative |
| Antinuclear antibodies | May be positive | Usually positive | Negative | Negative |
| Liver enzymes | Normal | Normal | Normal | Normal |
| Serum creatinine | Normal | Normal or elevated | Normal | Normal |
| Urine | Normal | Proteinuria Cylindruria | Normal | Normal |

Table 19.1. Most common laboratory abnormalities in diseases that may present as symmetrical, peripheral polyarthritis. (CTD: Connective tissue diseases).

When faced with the clinical possibility of rheumatoid arthritis, it is worth requesting a full blood count, inflammatory markers, liver enzymes, serum creatinine and electrolytes and urinalysis. Although these tests are usually normal in the initial phase of the disease, they will serve as a basis for assessing any side effect of subsequent treatment. Some changes may strongly influence the diagnosis (Table 19.1.).

In the initial stages of rheumatoid arthritis, it is also important to test for antinuclear antibodies (by immunofluorescence) to exclude other connective tissue diseases, which, like lupus, can present with very similar polyarthritis. Note, however, that about 15% of RA patients have circulating antinuclear antibodies.

### Rheumatoid factor

Rheumatoid factor is an autoantibody. It is an immunoglobulin with anti-IgG reactivity. The usual tests for it, RA test, Waaler-Rose and nephelometry, only detect the IgM subtype, but they can also be of subtype IgA or IgG. The pathogenetic role of rheumatoid factor is still controversial, but its presence is associated with a worse functional and structural prognosis.

They are present in 75–80% of patients with rheumatoid arthritis. The percentage of negative results is much greater in the initial phase of the disease, as many patients will develop rheumatoid factor in time.

Please keep in mind that rheumatoid factor is not specific to rheumatoid arthritis. It may be present in a wide variety of situations, including systemic lupus erythematosus (Table 19.2.). It is actually found in about 5% of the normal population and this percentage increases with age. In most situations, however, the rheumatoid factor level is much lower than in RA: the higher the concentration, the greater the probability of rheumatoid arthritis.

| Disease | Percentage with rheumatoid factor |
|---|---|
| Rheumatoid arthritis | 75–80% |
| Sjögren's syndrome | |
| Systemic lupus erythematosus | |
| Bacterial endocarditis | 25–50% |
| Chronic hepatitis | |
| Idiopathic pulmonary fibrosis | 10–24% |
| Tuberculosis | |
| Osteoarthritis | |
| Psoriatic arthritis | 5–10% |
| Rheumatic fever | |
| Gout | |
| Normal | <5% (higher after the age of 70) |

**Table 19.2.** Examples of conditions accompanied by rheumatoid factor.

Some practical lessons can be learned from this information:

1. Rheumatoid factor must be quantified (not just qualified as positive or negative).

2. The presence of rheumatoid factor does not allow the diagnosis of rheumatoid arthritis, unless there are compatible symptoms.

3. The absence of rheumatoid factor does not rule out the diagnosis, if the symptoms are compatible.

### Radiology

In this context, we should always request x-rays of the hands, feet and any other affected joints.

Ideally these x-rays will be normal, which means we have reached a diagnosis before the onset of irreversible lesions. Common anomalies in the initial phase include soft tissue swelling (which is assessable clinically) and periarticular osteopenia (Figure 19.1.). Loss of articular space is a later manifestation and something we want to avoid. In the initial stages, it may be difficult to assess. Try comparing the other joints in the same area and joints on the other side (Figure 19.6.).

Erosions are lytic lesions affecting the bone cortex around the joint. They tend to appear first in the metacarpophalangeal joints, styloid process of the ulna and metatarsophalangeal joints (Figure 19.7.). Erosions frequently develop in the first months of the disease, but they should be considered as late manifestation, in that it means we have missed the best opportunity for treatment.

All radiological lesions tend to have a very symmetrical distribution.

When present, these radiological changes support differential diagnosis: arthritis associated with the other connective tissue diseases does not usually cause erosions or joint space loss. In psoriatic arthritis there may be erosions and loss of articular space, but the distribution is usually asymmetrical and DIP joints may be involved. In nodal osteoarthritis, the loss of space is asymmetrical in each joint and osteophytes develop, instead of erosions. Osteopenia is replaced by subchondral sclerosis and involvement of the DIPs is almost universal (see Figures 10.36.–10.41.).

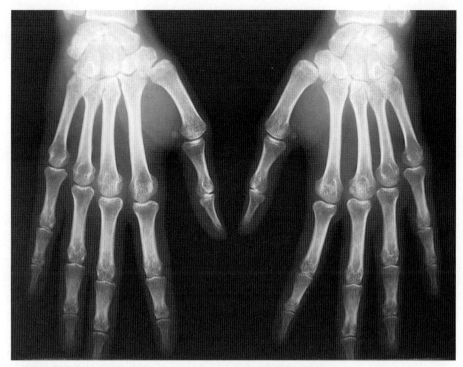

**Figure 19.6.** Early rheumatoid arthritis. Joint space loss may be difficult to assess in the early stages. This picture shows loss of joint space affecting the 3rd left and right MCPs and all the PIPs. This patient had had disease manifestations for 4 months.

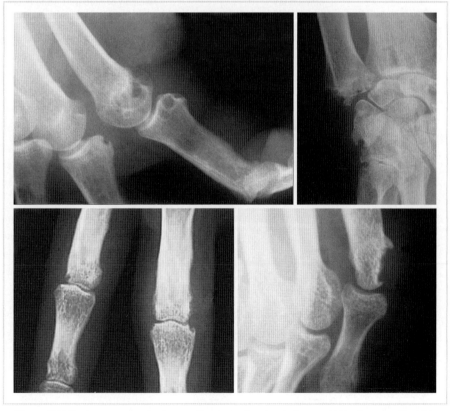

**Figure 19.7.** Erosions present as focal areas of bone resorption close to the synovial insertion around the joint. Metatarsophalangeal, metacarpophalangeal and proximal interphalangeal joints, as well as the styloid process of the ulna are preferred locations.

## Bone scintigraphy

There is no point in requesting a scintigraphy in patients with chronic symmetrical peripheral polyarthritis. The results will add nothing to clinical examination, as it does not distinguish between inflammatory and degenerative lesions and the affected joints are easily accessible. Indeed, this scan is often misleading and suggests increased uptake of the radioligand in perfectly normal joints.

## Criteria for the classification of rheumatoid arthritis

Having performed the assessment described above, the physician can check whether criteria for classification of rheumatoid arthritis have been satisfied. The classification criteria proposed by the American Rheumatism Association (now the American College of Rheumatology) have gathered remarkable consensus over the years (Table 19.3.). These criteria should, however, be considered as guidelines only and not as essential conditions for the diagnosis, as they were not created for diagnosing the disease in each individual patient but rather to harmonize research in population and family studies. Furthermore, they have low sensitivity for identification of very early disease. Alternative criteria are currently being developed by international organizations.

| | |
|---|---|
| 1. Morning stiffness | Morning stiffness in and around the joints lasting at least 1 hour before maximal improvement at any time in the disease course. |
| 2. Arthritis of three or more joint areas* | At least three joint areas simultaneously have had soft tissue swelling or fluid (not bone overgrowth alone) observed by a physician. |
| 3. Arthritis of hand joints | At least one area swollen (as described above) in a wrist, MCP or PIP joint. |
| 4. Symmetric arthritis | Simultaneous involvement of the same joint areas* on both sides of the body. (Bilateral involvement of MCPs, PIPs or MTPs is acceptable without absolute symmetry.) |
| 5. Rheumatoid nodules | Subcutaneous nodules, over bony prominences, or extensor surfaces, or in juxtaarticular regions, observed by a physician. |
| 6. Serum rheumatoid factor | Demonstration of abnormal amounts of serum rheumatoid factor by any method for which the result has been positive in <5% of normal control subjects. |
| 7. Radiographic alterations | Radiographic changes typical of rheumatoid arthritis on posteroanterior hand and wrist radiographs, which must include erosions or unequivocal bony decalcification localized in or most marked adjacent to the involved joints. Osteoarthritis changes alone do not qualify. |
| Criteria 1–4 must be present for at least 6 weeks. To be classified as having rheumatoid arthritis, the patient must satisfy at least four of the criteria. The association of other diseases does not rule out the diagnosis. | |

*The 14 possible joint areas are the left or right: MCP, PIP, wrist, elbow, knee, ankle and MTP joints.

**Table 19.3** Criteria for the classification of rheumatoid arthritis. American Rheumatism Association, 1987.[4]

[4]Arnett FC et al. The American Rheumatism Association 1987 revised criteria for the classification of rheumatoid arthritis. *Arthritis and Rheumatism* 1988; 31: 315– 324.

## TREATMENT

The most appropriate measure that a GP can take in a probable or confirmed case of rheumatoid arthritis is to

**send the patient to a specialist as soon as possible**

and avoid all treatment other than non-steroidal anti-inflammatories.

## LATER STAGES

With time, rheumatoid arthritis can involve almost all the joints, either simultaneously or successively, including the temporomandibular and sternoclavicular joints and the cervical spine. In some patients more than others, the persistence of the inflammatory process will lead to the accumulation of structural damage with erosions increasing in size and number in more and more joints (Figure 19.8.).

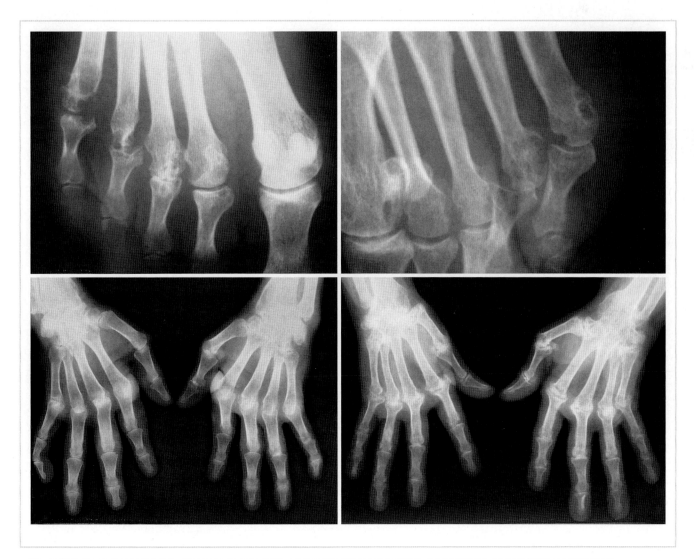

**Figure 19.8.** Progression of joint destruction in rheumatoid arthritis: erosions (larger in size and number), bone resorption, ankylosis (wrist) and subluxations.

The hips, shoulders and knees can also be seriously damaged causing severe functional limitation, sometimes imposing the need for a prosthesis (Figure 19.9.).

The elbow, wrist and subtalar joints are particularly vulnerable to inflammation and therefore merit special attention and adjuvant intra-articular treatment, if necessary.

The wrists frequently suffer palmar subluxation, acquiring a "fork back" shape. The extensor tendons of the fingers can undergo early subluxation at the level of the MCP joints, due to loosening or rupture loss of their attachment to the bones. Abnormal traction leads to deformities: ulnar deviation of the fingers, buttonhole deformity, swan-neck deformity, Z-shaped thumb, etc. (Figure 19.10.). The use of custom-made splints is important in preventing these bone deviations (Figure 29.4.). The extensor tendons, especially those of the ring and little fingers, can tear at the wrist as a result of the inflammatory process and friction with the bony excrescences. Synovitis and deformity of the wrist is often complicated by carpal tunnel syndrome. Patients with pain and limited mobility in the wrist may also benefit from wearing splints (Figure 29.3.).

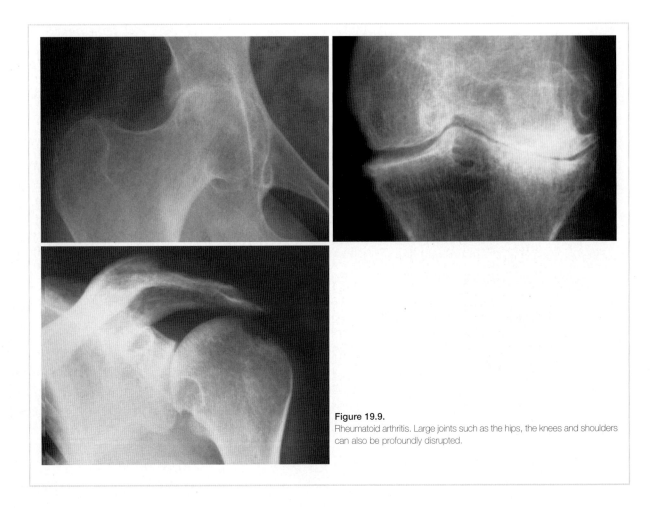

**Figure 19.9.**
Rheumatoid arthritis. Large joints such as the hips, the knees and shoulders can also be profoundly disrupted.

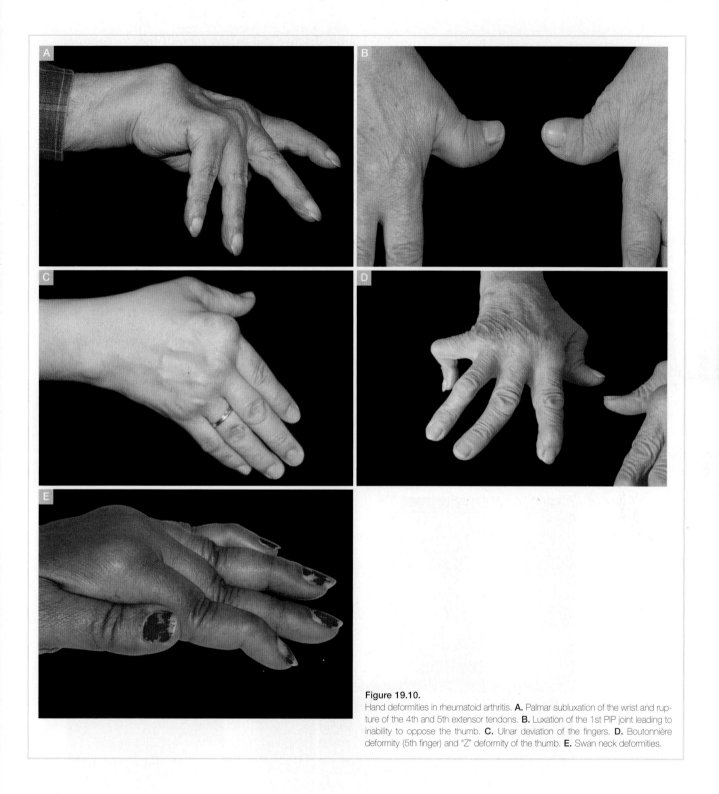

**Figure 19.10.**
Hand deformities in rheumatoid arthritis. **A.** Palmar subluxation of the wrist and rupture of the 4th and 5th extensor tendons. **B.** Luxation of the 1st PIP joint leading to inability to oppose the thumb. **C.** Ulnar deviation of the fingers. **D.** Boutonnière deformity (5th finger) and "Z" deformity of the thumb. **E.** Swan neck deformities.

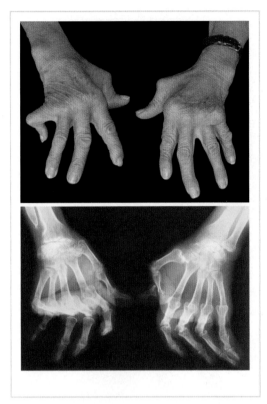

**Figure 19.11.** Rheumatoid arthritis. Joint deformity and disorganization can lead to profound functional disability.

Limited active and passive mobility is very common. Initially, it is due to articular swelling but, with time, it is caused by loss of cartilage, deformity and subluxation. These later lesions are irreversible (Figure 19.11.).

The feet are often deformed and painful, having a deep negative impact upon the patients' quality of life. Common deformities are calcaneovalgus foot (due to subluxation of the subtalar and talonavicular joints), secondary flatfoot caused by the collapse of the antero-posterior arch, anterior flatfoot with painful calluses under the MTPs and so-called "triangular foot" (Figure 19.12.). These deformities often cause conflict with footwear, frequently making corrective surgery necessary (see Chapter 14).

The cervical spine deserves special attention in rheumatoid patients. The joint between the arch of the atlas and the odontoid process of the axis is often affected. This can cause erosions in or even fracture of the odontoid process. The annular ligament that holds the odontoid process becomes lax or tears, resulting in

**Figure 19.12.**
Rheumatoid foot. **A.** Calcaneus varus. **B.** Flat foot (collapse of the transverse and the antero-posterior arches of the foot). **C.** Triangular forefoot. **D.** Collapse of the transverse arch of the forefoot leading to painful callosities.

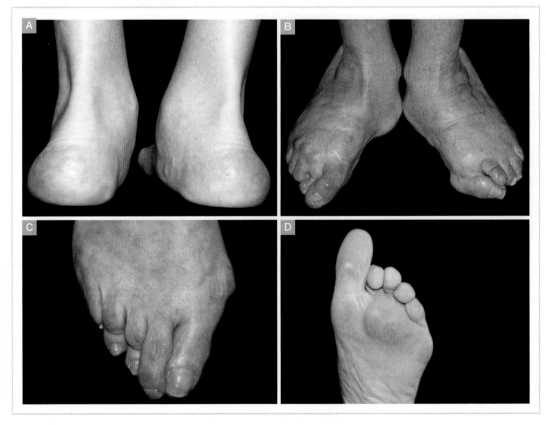

atlantoaxial subluxation, which may cause compressive myelopathy or even sudden death by compression of the cerebral trunk. This change occurs in about 50% of all patients with rheumatoid arthritis, although it is rarely severe enough to be life-threatening.

The symptoms associated with atlantoaxial subluxation (cervical cephalea, paresthesia of the limbs) appear very late and are not very reliable.

**Rheumatoid arthritis patients should be regularly checked for atlantoaxial subluxation.**

To do this, request lateral views of the upper cervical spine, in flexion and in extension. Note the distance between the anterior edge of the odontoid process and the posterior face of the arch of the atlas. There is anterior subluxation if it is greater than 3 mm (Figure 19.13.). Distances of more than 8 mm indicate an immediate risk of severe neurological lesion, making it wise to promote immediate immobilization with a rigid cervical collar and the consideration of surgery.

The other levels of the cervical spine may also be affected. There are sometimes multiple subluxations with profound disorganization of the cervical spine.

These late manifestations of rheumatoid arthritis can be completely prevented with sensible, timely treatment. Early diagnosis and referral to a specialist are, however, essential.

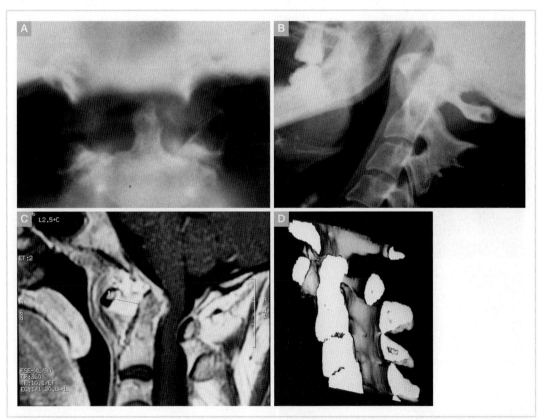

**Figure 19.13.** Rheumatoid arthritis. **A.** Erosion of the odontoid process of the axis (standard tomography). **B.** Anterior atlanto-axial subluxation. **C.** MRI – note the distance between the arch of the atlas and the dens, filled with inflamed tissue (under contrast). The spinal cord is compressed. **D.** 3D reconstruction of the same case.

## COMPLICATIONS AND EXTRA-ARTICULAR MANIFESTATIONS

### *Sicca syndrome (secondary Sjögren's syndrome)*

This consists of dryness of the mucosae due to inflammatory infiltration of the exocrine glands (see Chapter 25). It often accompanies rheumatoid arthritis. Clinically, it comprises dry eyes (xerophthalmia) and mouth (xerostomy). Lack of tears causes the patient's eyes to feel gritty ("as if I had sand in my eyes"), facilitates the occurrence of episcleritis, conjunctivitis and painful corneal ulcers, which may even perforate. Dryness of the mouth mainly causes discomfort and a stinging sensation. Patients have difficulty chewing and swallowing dry food and need to drink a lot of water.

### *Rheumatoid nodules*

These are hard, painless nodular lesions under the skin. The extension surface of the elbows and fingers are preferential locations. They sometimes appear in the viscera, such as the lungs (requiring differential diagnosis with neoplasm) or heart, causing conduction defects (Figure 19.14.). Their presence is associated with a more severe structural and functional prognosis.

### *Serositis*

The serous membranes of rheumatoid patients may be affected by inflammation leading to pain and effusion, especially in the pleura and pericardium. The situation is sometimes serious enough to warrant drainage.

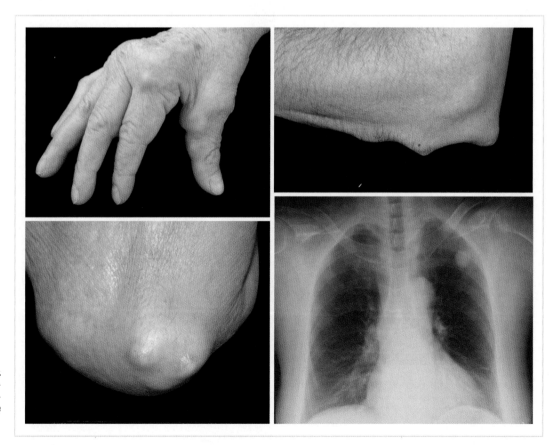

**Figure 19.14.** Rheumatoid nodules. Lung nodules may simulate cancer.

### Pulmonary fibrosis

This occurs in a considerable number of patients and can lead to significant respiratory impairment.

### Felty's syndrome

This consists in the association of rheumatoid arthritis with splenomegaly and leucopenia. The patient may have accentuated systemic signs, such as fever and weight loss. It requires timely, appropriate treatment by professionals with experience of this type of complication.

### Secondary amyloidosis

As with other chronic inflammatory diseases, prolonged, active rheumatoid arthritis can lead to the systemic deposition of amyloid protein, normally reflected by proteinuria (which can develop into a nephrotic syndrome and renal failure) and sensitive polyneuropathy. More rarely, the liver, heart, and other organs may also be affected. The sedimentation rate remains high even in the absence of any apparent inflammation. Definite diagnosis usually requires the demonstration of amyloid deposits, biopsies of the kidney, rectum or subcutaneous fat being the most productive for histological study.

### Rheumatoid vasculitis

Vasculitis is usually found only in patients with severe rheumatoid arthritis, who have serum rheumatoid factor. The inflammation tends to affect small vessels and is reflected by petechiae and necrotic ulceration of the lower extremities. It may also involve the kidneys. Although rare, it is one of the complications of the disease with worst prognosis and is associated with significant early to late mortality.

### Septic arthritis

Rheumatoid joints are particularly susceptible to infection. Early diagnosis is decisive. Suspect this possibility whenever a joint is highly inflamed in the absence of a general flare of the disease, i.e. an "out-of-phase" joint.[5]

## TREATMENT

The present paradigm in the treatment of rheumatoid arthritis can be summarized as follows:

> **The treatment of RA should begin as soon as possible, be as aggressive as necessary and as safe as possible.**

Our goal is to achieve remission of the disease, i.e. suppression of the signs of inflammation, as this is the best guarantee of comfort for the patient and of effective prevention of structural damage and long-term disability.

These objectives usually demand a variety of potentially highly toxic medications, which require careful monitoring of efficacy and safety and judicious adaptation of the treatment over time.

[5]To learn more about these and other systemic complications in rheumatoid arthritis, we suggest that you consult one of the many treatises on rheumatology.

### Educating patients and their families

An informed patient is the physician's best ally. It is essential that the patient understands, without drama, that rheumatoid arthritis can be treated very effectively, even though it is a chronic, incurable disease. The range, limitations, and potential toxicity of medications should be explained whenever this can be expected to influence the patient's compliance with the treatment and monitoring plan. The patient should know exactly which medications can be used "as necessary" to relieve pain and those that are under tight doctor control.

The patient should be advised to save his or her strength and to rest when necessary. Generally speaking, actively inflamed joints benefit from rest, as continuous movement tends to exacerbate the inflammatory process. On the other hand, once acute inflammation has subsided, it is important to perform strength and range-of-movement exercises to recover mobility and muscle power.

Most patients feel relief on applying cold packs to inflamed joints, while wet heat facilitates exercise in remission phases. Individual preferences vary, however, and should be respected.

The physician should pay considerable attention to the psychological and social dimensions of a disease of this kind, helping the patient to reduce the effects of the condition on his or her quality of life.

Medications used in the treatment rheumatoid arthritis can be classified into two main categories:

### Symptomatic medication

This aims at controlling pain and stiffness, making the patient more comfortable, but is not intended to prevent long-term structural damage.

**Anti-inflammatories** are extremely useful in these patients and are almost universally used. Bear in mind that rheumatoid arthritis in itself is a risk factor for gastropathy induced by these drugs, which therefore require special care in promoting the appropriate preventive measures. As pain and stiffness tend to be worse in the mornings, many patients achieve more benefit from taking a long-acting anti-inflammatory at night. The dose can be reinforced during the day, if necessary. The general guidelines for choosing and using anti-inflammatories are given in Chapter 30.

Simple analgesics are usually insufficient for controlling patients' pain.

**Glucocorticoids** are used as adjuvant therapy, especially during joint flares. They do a lot to relieve the symptoms and several studies suggest that they also prevent articular damage. However, given their long-term toxicity, these drugs should be used with care. In addition to other measures, prolonged treatment with glucocorticoids requires the prevention of osteoporosis (Chapter 30).

### Disease modifying agents

These agents are also called SAARDS – Slow Acting Anti-Rheumatic Drugs, or DMARDs – Disease Modifying Anti-Rheumatic Drugs. Symptomatic benefit from these agents can be marked (although delayed for several weeks), but they are aimed mainly at retarding or preventing the progressive destruction of the joints that dominates the long-term prognosis.

**DMARDs should be prescribed as soon as a definite diagnosis of rheumatoid arthritis is established.**

The most widely used at present is **methotrexate**, in weekly doses of 7.5–30 mg, orally. Its symptomatic and structural efficacy has been clearly established in clinical trials, although only a small number of patients achieve total remission. Toxicity is mainly hepatic and hematological and it therefore requires regular monitoring through blood tests. **Sulfasalazine** in doses of 2–3 gs a day is also effective in rheumatoid arthritis, although its ability to prevent structural damage is less reliable. Its toxicity is similar to methotrexate. **Hydroxychloroquine** is used today essentially as adjuvant treatment to methotrexate.

**Gold salts** and **D-penicillamine** were once used a lot to treat rheumatoid arthritis, but their high toxicity now limits their use to patients who are resistant to or intolerant of the alternatives.

Several biological therapies have been proved highly efficient in the control of inflammation and joint destruction in rheumatoid arthritis, changing the face of the disease. This is especially the case of TNF-α inhibitors, but several others are currently being investigated.

When maximum doses of isolated drugs do not achieve the desired effect or are not tolerated by the patient, current guidelines suggest moving to a combination of metrotretate with TNF-α inhibitor or other biological agents. These drugs have shown to significantly reduce disease activity and radiological progression in patients who do not respond sufficiently to methotrexate alone.

Ideally, treatment of rheumatoid patients is conducted within **multidisciplinary teams** involving rheumatologists, orthopedists and physiotherapists, with the support of allied health professionals like occupational therapists, podiatrists, psychologists and social service workers.

Good communication between primary and secondary care must be ensured, as GPs and nurses play an essential role in the regular monitoring of the patient.

### The role of the GP in rheumatoid arthritis

We have already stressed that early suspicion and referral is one of the most important contributions of the GP to his or her rheumatoid patient. The advantages of having rheumatoid arthritis treatment conducted by physicians with experience in this complex disease, from an early stage, has been repeatedly demonstrated.

The family doctor does not hand patients over to the specialist. S/he merely shares them as part of a system of joint responsibility, which naturally requires open, effective communication between those involved. The family doctor will continue to play an essential role in the success of treatment.

### Assessing disease activity and adapting treatment

The course of rheumatoid arthritis tends to fluctuate, with periods of remission or relative calm interspersed with inflammatory exacerbations. The inflammatory flares are associated with worsening pain, which tends, then, to persist over night and at rest. Morning stiffness lasts longer and the number of swollen and/or tender joints increases. Flares are accompanied by elevation of C-reactive protein levels and, later, of the erythrocyte sedimentation rate.

These exacerbations may follow changes in treatment or different kinds of trigger such as infection, surgery or even psychological stress. There is often no apparent trigger, however.

In coordination with the specialist in charge, the patient's GP can detect and treat aggravating factors and adapt the anti-inflammatory or corticosteroid treatment, once the patient's compliance with the established treatment plan has been guaranteed. If an "attack" persists, the patient's next visit to the specialist should be brought forward.

### *Monitoring for side effects and complications*

Rheumatoid patients are normally regularly monitored by their specialists. Several factors can, however, make the time between appointments quite long, while the patent's family doctor continues to provide support. Control of side effects and complications is essentially clinical. Nevertheless, because some side effects are initially asymptomatic, it is wise to perform some laboratory tests regularly, at intervals that vary according to the patient, his or her treatment and local conditions. Full blood count (anemia, leucopenia, thrombocytopenia), liver enzymes and albumin (liver toxicity), creatinine and urinalysis (kidney toxicity) and sedimentation rate or C-reactive protein (disease activity) are usually sufficient and appropriate whatever the treatment regime. There is no point in measuring rheumatoid factor repeatedly as the titer is not related to the activity of the disease.

The family doctor will communicate with the hospital physician if any significant alterations or other intercurrences arise that are beyond his or her field of action.

## ADDITIONAL PRACTICE
### CHRONIC ADDITIVE, SYMMETRICAL, PERIPHERAL POLYARTHRITIS

# CHRONIC, ASYMMETRICAL OLIGO- OR POLYARTHRITIS

20.

J.A.P. da Silva, A.D. Woolf, *Rheumatology in Practice*, DOI 10.1007/978-1-84882-581-9_20,
© Springer-Verlag London Limited 2010

# 20. CHRONIC, ASYMMETRICAL OLIGO- OR POLYARTHRITIS

When enquiry and clinical examination establish that the patient has chronic (lasting for more than 6 weeks) asymmetric oligo- or polyarthritis.[1] You identify a pattern that makes for the first step of diagnosis.

### *Second diagnostic step*

Psoriatic arthritis is at the top of the list of possible causes for this pattern of arthritis. This possibility will be considerably reinforced if other characteristic aspects of this condition are also present:

1. Cutaneous or ungual psoriasis – which, in most patients, is present before the arthritis sets in. A family history of psoriasis also point to this;

2. Axial involvement – reflected by inflammatory pain affecting the lumbosacral spine or, more rarely, other vertebral segments;

3. Asymmetric involvement of the small joints of the hands;

4. Inflammation of the distal interphalangeal joints;

5. Dactylitis – diffuse, accentuated inflammation of a digit, usually a toe;

**NB:** Differential diagnosis depends essentially on the distribution of the affected joints. In the face of chronic oligoarthritis which is predominantly proximal, several other possibilities have to be considered. This diagnostic context is dealt with in Chapter 21.

## PSORIATIC ARTHRITIS

As the name suggests, psoriatic arthritis appears in association with cutaneous psoriasis. Psoriasis is regarded as an immunogenetic disease, due to the chronic activation of T helper lymphocytes. The pathogenic mechanisms behind the articular involvement are still unclear. There is, however, a close histological and biological resemblance in the inflammatory synovial process to that described in rheumatoid arthritis. Psoriatic arthritis is also destructive and deforming. Although the prognosis varies considerably from one person to another, the disease can lead to severe, extensive articular destruction, and considerable disability. It has a marked tendency towards asymmetry and, in addition, involvement of the axial skeleton, distal interphalangeal joints and entheses are important for distinguishing it from rheumatoid arthritis.

Arthritis develops in 5–8% of patients with skin or nail psoriasis, resulting in a prevalence of about 0.1% in the general population. It is equally common in men and women, and its peak incidence is between the ages of 20 and 40, though it can appear at any age.

[1]When can we say "arthritis? See Table 17.1.

In about 85% of patients, psoriasis precedes the arthritis, thus facilitating the diagnosis. In 15%, however, they appear at the same time or the arthritis may precede psoriasis, making the diagnosis difficult.

Many reports suggest that psoriatic arthritis may be triggered by episodes of trauma or psychological stress, but this relationship is not clear. HIV infection can be accompanied by severe, explosive forms of psoriasis and psoriatic arthritis, with a poor prognosis for the joints.

## Psoriasis

An alert observer will find psoriatic lesions during the general clinical examination: typical hyperkeratotic, scaly, erythematosus lesions, in clearly delineated patches of variable size. If they are not obvious and there is a suspicion of psoriatic arthritis, the search should involve not only the usual places for these patches (scalp, elbows and knees), but also the whole body surface, including the ears, natal cleft and navel. On the palms and soles, psoriasis can look quite atypical to inexperienced eyes: the rash is known as palmoplantar pustulosis (Figure 20.1.).

Finger and toe nails are frequently affected, sometimes seriously – ungual dystrophy, and may require mycological examination to exclude a differential diagnosis of fungal infection. In other

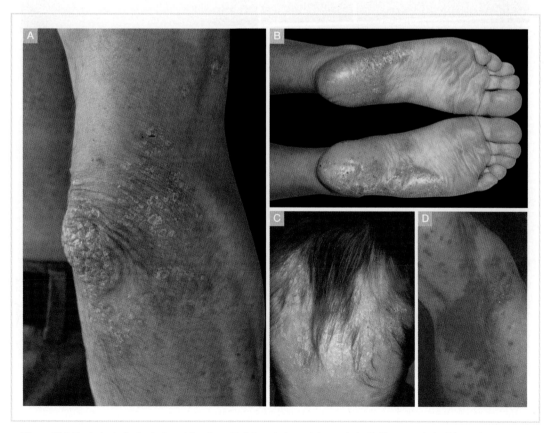

**Figure 20.1.** Psoriasis. **A.** Scaling lesions at the elbow. **B.** Palmo-plantar pustular psoriasis. **C.** Plaque psoriasis of the scalp. **D.** Inverse psoriasis (axilla).

cases, nail changes are more discreet, consisting of small pits (ungual pitting – Figure 20.2.). Look for them carefully. If you find more than 20 in the 10 fingernails, the diagnosis of psoriasis is confirmed. A pathognomonic aspect of psoriasis is distal onycholysis which looks like an "oil stain" under the nail.

The nails are more commonly involved in patients whose distal interphalangeal joints are affected. Other than this, there is no type of psoriasis particularly associated with arthritis. Even discreet skin lesions should suggest the diagnosis.

If in doubt, ask the opinion of a dermatologist.

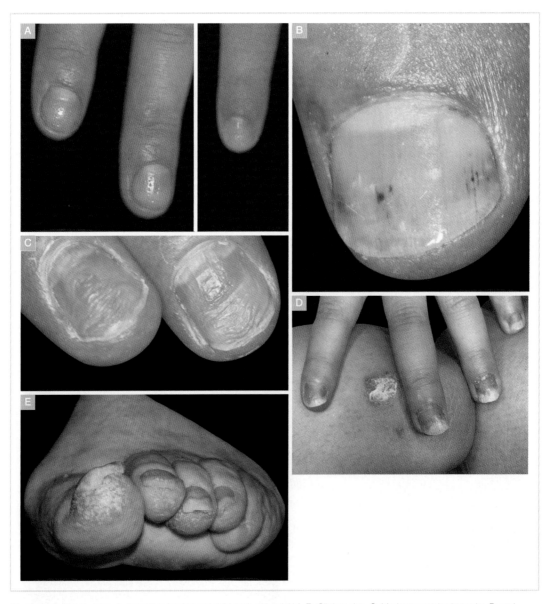

**Figure 20.2.** Nail psoriasis. **A.** Nail pitting (mother and child, both with arthritis). **B.** Oil drop sign. **C.** Moderate onychodystrophy. **D.** and **E.** Coarse onychodystrophy. (Courtesy: Prof. Américo Figueiredo and Dr. Manuel Salgado. Coimbra.).

### *Arthritis*

**There are five distinct patterns in psoriatic arthritis:**

1. Asymmetrical oligoarticular.

2. Rheumatoid-like.

3. Spondylitic.

4. Distal interphalangeal.

5. Mutilating.

Note that these forms are not mutually exclusive. Involvement of the axial skeleton can be associated with any other form.

### *TYPICAL CASES*
### 20.A ASYMMETRICAL OLIGOARTHRITIS

João António, a 32-year old patient, came to us with frank arthritis, which had begun insidiously 4 months before, affecting first the right index PIP, then the first left MTP and left ankle and the third toe on his left foot, which was diffusely swollen and red (Figure 20.3.). He denied any axial pain. The systematic enquiry was completely negative. He denied any personal or family history of psoriasis. He was taking an anti-inflammatory, with partial relief of pain.

The clinical examination confirmed arthritis in the spontaneously painful joints.

*How would you summarize the findings above?*[2]

*What do you think is the most probable diagnosis?*

*What would you do to find out more?*

Because of the distribution of the arthritis and the slight articular redness, we asked the patient's permission to give him a particularly thorough examination. We found discreet erythematous lesions in the natal cleft, which the patient had not mentioned because he had had them for a long time. His sedimentation rate was elevated (32 mm). X-rays of the affected joints were normal. A dermatologist confirmed psoriasis.

We diagnosed asymmetrical oligoarticular psoriatic arthritis and suggested treatment with anti-inflammatories and intra-articular injections of gluococorticoids. Four years later, the patient is well, with only occasional need for further glucocorticoid injections. No radiological changes have developed.

He may still need systemic immunosuppressants in the future.

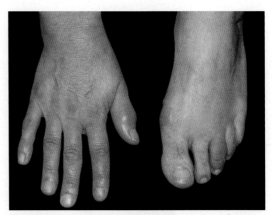

**Figure 20.3.** Clinical case "Asymmetrical oligoarthritis." Note the swelling and redness of the 3rd right PIP joint and the diffuse swelling of the 3rd left toe (dactilytis: "sausage digit").

[2] Asymmetrical oligoarthritis with involvement of the hands, no extra-articular manifestations.

## PSORIATIC ARTHRITIS – ASYMMETRICAL OLIGOARTICULAR FORM
### *MAIN POINTS*

This is the most common pattern of psoriatic arthritis (about 70% of cases).

It can affect practically all the joints, but has a particular tendency to involve the PIP, DIP, and MTP joints. The ankles, knees, wrists and elbows are also often affected (Figure 20.4.).

It may be accompanied by dactylitis (diffuse inflammation of an entire digit), which is particularly suggestive of the diagnosis.

Its course is unpredictable, with exacerbations and remissions. It may become polyarticular and be associated with involvement of the axial skeleton.

The prognosis varies, but it can be highly destructive and incapacitating.

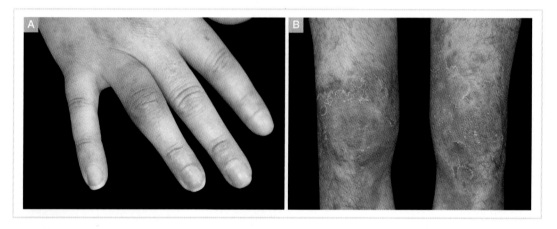

**Figure 20.4.**
Psoriatic arthritis: asymmetrical oligoarticular pattern. **A.** Note the swelling of the 4th right PIP joint and the suggestive blue tinge of the overlying skin. The left hand was not affected. **B.** Note the flexion deformity and swelling of the right knee, with psoriatic lesions in the vicinity.

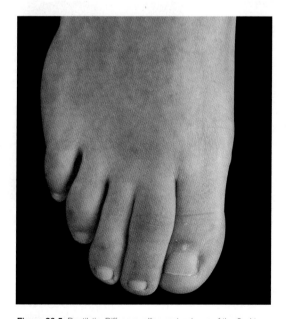

**Figure 20.5.** Dactilytis. Diffuse swelling and redness of the 2nd toe. The left foot was not affected.

Usually, joints affected by psoriatic arthritis show clear signs of inflammation with intense, fusiform swelling and a suggestive purplish discoloration of the skin.

Asymmetry in the hands is particularly significant if distal interphalangeal joints are affected. Dactylitis (Figure 20.5.), intense inflammation of the joints and tendinous sheaths of a digit, is rarely seen outside psoriatic arthritis. When the oligoarthritis affects only proximal joints, the differential diagnosis will have to be extended to other entities – see Chapter 21.

*TYPICAL CASES*

## 20.B. SYMMETRICAL POLYARTHRITIS

43-year old José Roberto was referred to our clinic with inflammatory polyarthralgia that had set in insidiously 5 years before and evolved additively ever since. On examination, we found symmetrical polyarthritis affecting the MCP, PIP and MTP joints, the right wrist and both knees. There was a clear ulnar deviation of the fingers of both hands. The DIPs had been spared (Figure 20.6.). He denied inflammatory axial pain.

His symptoms suggested rheumatoid arthritis… were it not for the psoriatic lesions spread over his body.

*Was it psoriatic arthritis or rheumatoid arthritis in a patient with psoriasis?*

*How could we find out?*

*What are the consequences of this distinction?*

His rheumatoid factor was negative. X-rays of his hands showed loss of joint space and subluxation of several MCPs, with no erosions or osteopenia. X-rays of his feet showed clear erosions in the fourth and fifth MTPs, with an enlargement at the base of the phalanx (Figure 20.7.). We assumed the diagnosis of rheumatoid-like psoriatic arthritis and began treatment with methotrexate. The patient later developed inflammation of distal interphalangeal joints.

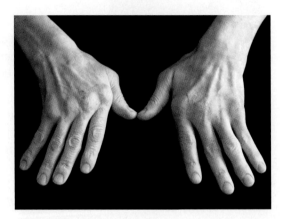

**Figure 20.6.** Clinical case "Symmetrical polyarthritis." The inflammatory process was well controlled by medication. Note the ulnar deviation of the fingers, muscle atrophy and scaling plaques in the dorsal aspect of the hands.

## PSORIATIC ARTHRITIS – rheumatoid-like form
*MAIN POINTS*

This is one of the most common forms of psoriatic arthritis.

It may be indistinguishable from seronegative rheumatoid arthritis.

The following factors suggest the diagnosis:

- psoriasis;
- persistently negative rheumatoid factor;
- involvement of DIP joints;
- some asymmetry;
- dactylitis;
- association of erosions and exostosis in x-rays; minimal periarticular osteopenia;
- tendency towards ankylosis of the joints.

Prognosis is generally more favorable than for rheumatoid arthritis, but still potentially incapacitating

Treatment follows the same lines as rheumatoid arthritis.

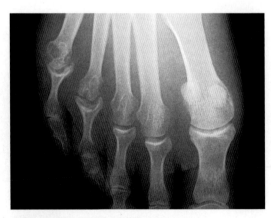

**Figure 20.7.** Clinical case "Symmetrical polyarthritis." Plain films of the feet show erosions of the 4th and 5th MTP joints, bilaterally, associated with an exostotic enlargement of the bases of the phalanxes. Osteopenia is quite mild taking into account the degree of joint destruction.

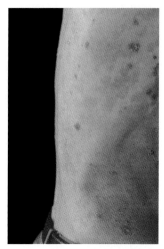

**Figure 20.8.** Clinical case "Nocturnal and diurnal thoraco-lumbar pain." Loss of lumbar lordosis and psoriactic lesions.

### TYPICAL CASES
### 20.C. NOCTURNAL AND DIURNAL THORACO-LUMBAR PAIN

Jorge Azevedo came to our clinic because of lumbar and thoracic pain that had begun about a year before. It was more intense on strenuous work days. Pain persisted at night and was accompanied by morning stiffness of variable duration (sometimes more than one hour). Movement in the morning relieved the pain a little.

*What are the most important points here?*

*Would the systematic enquiry be relevant?*

He denied any disturbances in bowel movements or problems in the eyes or mucous membranes. He had had diffuse psoriasis since the age of 27, like his father. He denied any other systemic manifestations.

Clinical examination showed loss of lumbar lordosis (Figure 20.8.) and pain in the right sacroiliac region on direct palpation and on mobilization of the sacroiliac joints (Figure 11.11.). Mobility was reduced in the lumbar spine (Schober 10→12.8 cm) and rotation of the thoracic spine elicited pain.

*How would you summarize these symptoms?*[3]

*What is your diagnosis?*

*On what have you based it?*

*What treatment would you suggest?*

A plain film showed asymmetrical sacroiliitis (Figure 20.9.).

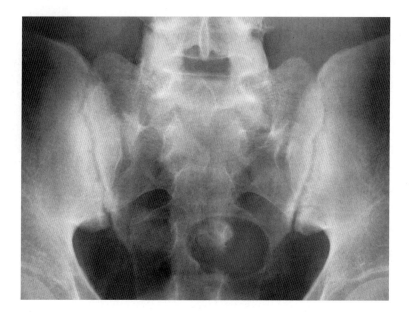

**Figure 20.9.**
Clinical case "Nocturnal and diurnal thoraco-lumbar pain." Pelvis antero-posterior radiograph. Notice the sclerosis surrounding the right sacroiliac joint and the blurring of the joint margins.

[3]Thoracic and lumbar pain and probable sacroiliitis, in a psoriatic patient.

We told the patient of our diagnosis of psoriatic spondylitis and began treatment with anti-inflammatories and regular exercises, with a good response. Over the next few years he also developed arthritis in some peripheral joints requiring local treatment and, finally, the introduction of sulfasalazin. This treatment improved the peripheral arthritis, but provided no additional relief of the axial pain.

---

**PSORIATIC ARTHRITIS – spondylitic form**
*MAIN POINTS*

Clinically, it can be indistinguishable from ankylosing spondylitis.

It is more common in carriers of the HLA-B27 antigen.

The radiological sacroiliitis is usually asymmetrical.

There may be irregular involvement of other segments of the spine, with the formation of coarse, asymmetrical exostoses.

It is often associated with arthritis of the limb joints (any of the four patterns mentioned), enthesopathy or ocular inflammation.

Treatment is based on anti-inflammatories and physiotherapy.

Classical DMARDs, like methotrexate and sulfasalazin, are useful for non-axial arthritis but ineffective on the spine.

Biological agents, as TNF-alpha inhibitors, are indicated in patients who remain highly symptomatic despite NSAIDs.

Injection of glucocorticoid in the sacroiliac joint often provides substantial, long-lasting relief of symptoms.

---

### Distal interphalangeal form

In a small percentage of patients there is predominant if not exclusive, sometimes symmetrical, rapidly deforming involvement of the distal interphalangeal joints of the hands. It is more common in males. This form is particularly associated with nail dystrophy and pitting (Figure 20.2.). Although it is deforming, the functional prognosis is usually good. Treatment is based on anti-inflammatories.

### Arthritis mutilans

This is a particularly aggressive form leading to rapid, massive destruction of the affected joints. It usually involves the MCPs and PIPs, leading to frank articular disorganization, with extensive loss of bone at the bone endings. This results in a phenomenon called telescoping, in which the affected segment can be mobilized towards the axis of the limb. Fortunately it is rare.

### Mixed patterns

Bear in mind that these forms are not mutually exclusive. In many cases, spondylitis is associated with peripheral involvement of varying patterns, the most common being asymmetrical oligoarticular. The association of inflammatory back pain with peripheral arthritis, makes psoriatic arthritis highly probable, especially if small joints are affected. Ankylosing spondylitis rarely involves the appendicular skeleton and the other types of spondyloarthropathy have a predilection for proximal joints.

### Evolution

Psoriatic arthritis has a fluctuating course, with partial remissions and sometimes dramatic flares. These have no relation in time with the evolution of the skin disease. A relatively slow onset in one or two joints is quite common, progressively extending to more joints. Joint destruction varies considerably from one patient to another, but joint erosion and subluxation are common. Some patients have a highly destructive and disabling arthritis with a special tendency to articular ankylosis.

As with other types of spondyloarthropathy, there is often inflammation of tendons and ligament insertions, especially in the Achilles tendon.

Psoriatic arthritis is not usually accompanied by extra-articular manifestations apart from psoriasis, but ocular inflammation and aortic insufficiency may occur. Severe, drawn-out cases without proper control may be complicated by secondary amyloidosis. Treatment requires regular monitoring for efficacy and safety.

### Differential diagnosis

The presence of psoriasis obviously plays a central role in differential diagnosis. The possibility that a patient with psoriasis may have some other type of arthritis should not be ruled out. However, if the pattern of articular involvement falls into one of the categories described above, the probability of psoriatic arthritis is very high. On the other hand, if the pattern is typical, a family history reinforces the diagnosis, even if the patient has no skin lesions. Problems arise if there is no psoriasis and the pattern is not typical.

Alternative possibilities vary according to the pattern of articular involvement.

An exclusively axial form must be differentiated from other causes of inflammatory lumbar or thoracic pain (Chapter 24). Note that the axial involvement of psoriatic arthritis tends to be asymmetrical and irregular, unlike the tendency towards symmetry and an ascending course in ankylosing spondylitis. The association of peripheral arthritis, especially if there is distal involvement, considerably reinforces the diagnostic possibility of psoriatic arthritis.

In cases of oligoarticular involvement the possibilities vary depending on whether the small joints of the hands are affected. Assymetrical involvement of the hands, leaves few alternative diagnoses: incipient rheumatoid arthritis? Gout? Sarcoidosis? An enquiry into the patient's personal history and associated manifestations is particularly important: a history of acute, recurring monoarthritis suggests gout, whereas erythema nodosum, respiratory difficulties and parotid enlargement favor sarcoidosis.

If the oligoarticular pattern is proximal (large joints), other types of seronegative spondyloarthropathy, including reactive arthritis, must be considered. The onset of reactive arthritis tends to be acute or subacute, however, and follows an infectious episode. It tends to clear up in less than 6 weeks and is almost always symmetrical when it affects the distal joints.

The distal interphalangeal form must be distinguished from nodal osteoarthritis. Note the typical bony nodes of osteoarthritis and the absence or scarcity of inflammatory signs. A rheumatoid-like pattern demands consideration of rheumatoid arthritis or another connective tissue disease.

### Diagnostic tests

What diagnostic tests are justified in this context of differential diagnosis?

### Laboratory

A full blood count may show anemia in chronic disease, but this is common to all types of chronic arthritis and does not assist in the differential. No other changes are expected. Erythrocyte sedimentation rate and C-reactive protein are usually mildly elevated, but may be normal in oligoarticular forms or in spondylitis. Rheumatoid factor may help in the differential diagnosis with rheumatoid arthritis. Note that it can be positive in up to 10% of patients with psoriatic arthritis, usually in low titre.

Liver and kidney tests will serve essentially to prepare and monitor treatment. Occasionally, raised liver function tests suggest liver involvement by sarcoidosis. If this possibility is considered, it worth requesting tests for angiotensin converting enzymes and serum calcium, chest x-ray and biopsies of the affected organs.

### Plain Films

As with rheumatoid arthritis, psoriatic arthritis should be diagnosed as early as possible, at a stage in which the only radiological changes are swelling of the soft tissue. In more advanced stages, more diagnostic changes may appear.

As a rule, an anteroposterior film of the pelvis gives a good view of the sacroiliac joints. Psoriatic sacroiliitis tends to be asymmetrical, unlike ankylosing spondylitis and spondylitis of inflammatory bowel disease (Figure 20.9.).

In more advanced stages, an x-ray of the affected segments of the spine can show large, horizontal exostoses of the vertebral bodies, looking like giant osteophytes, distributed asymmetrically. They affect separate segments of the spine. This aspect is very different from the fine, ascending, candle-flame calcifications found in ankylosing spondylitis (syndesmophytes).

When in doubt as to the existence of sacroiliitis or axial involvement, consider bone scintigraphy or, better still, CT or MRI of the sacroiliac joints.

Plain films of the hands and feet may be particularly informative, especially in the differential diagnosis with rheumatoid arthritis. Note the following aspects:

1. Distribution of the affected joints: asymmetry and (non-osteoarthritic) involvement of the distal interphalangeal joints suggests the diagnosis of psoriatic arthritis.

2. Psoriatic arthritis causes loss of joint space, just like rheumatoid arthritis and osteoarthritis. However, this occurs with minimal or absent periarticular osteopenia (unlike rheumatoid

arthritis), with erosions (unlike osteoarthritis) and the formation of exostoses looking like osteophytes (unlike rheumatoid arthritis). See Table 20.1. These distinguishing radiographic features are discussed in Chapter 10 and shown in Figure 10.41.

|  | Psoriatic arthritis | Rheumatoid arthritis | Nodal osteoarthritis |
|---|---|---|---|
| Wrists | ++ | ++ | – |
| MCP joints | + | +++ | – |
| PIP joints | + | +++ | +++ |
| DIP joints | + | – | +++ |
| Symmetry | – | +++ | + |
| Subchondral osteopenia | – | ++ | sclerosis |
| Erosion | ++ | ++ | rarely |
| Periarticular exostosis | + | – | ++ |

**Table 20.1.**
Radiological characteristics of common forms of hand arthritis.

X-rays of the other affected joints show varying degrees of destruction, depending on the location, duration and aggressiveness of the disease. Early, appropriate treatment can prevent this destruction to a great extent. Figure 20.10. shows x-ray images from patients with psoriatic arthritis.

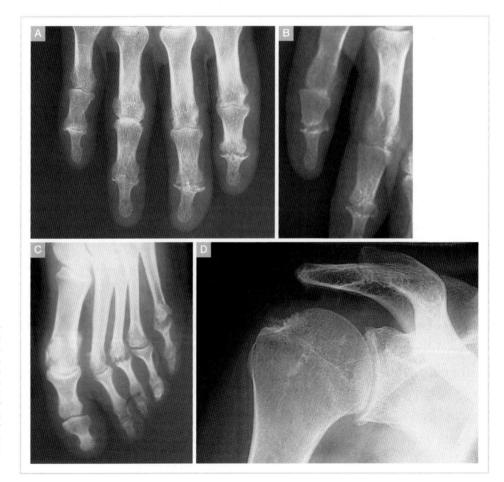

**Figure 20.10.**
Psoriatic arthritis – radiological features. **A.** and **B.** Hand involvement. Joint space loss and association of erosions with exostosis in DIP joints. **C.** Similar features in MCPs. **D.** Diffuse joint space loss in the shoulder joint. The irregularity of the upper pole of the greater tuberosity of the humerus suggests chronic local enthesitis.

### *Treatment*

In our opinion, the most appropriate advice for a GP strongly suspecting or with a firm diagnosis of psoriatic arthritis is to send the patient to a specialist as soon as possible, and to prescribe no treatment other than non-steroidal anti-inflammatories.

> **If you have good reason to suspect psoriatic arthritis,**
>
> **SEND THE PATIENT TO A SPECIALIST AS SOON AS POSSIBLE.**

The resources and treatment strategy used in psoriatic arthritis are generally very similar to those employed in rheumatoid arthritis.

In many patients with oligoarticular forms, treatment with anti-inflammatories and injections with glucocorticoids are enough for good symptomatic and structural control. The use of systemic corticosteroids should be avoided, except in particularly aggressive situations, due to the risk of exacerbation of skin psoriasis on withdrawal. Topical corticosteroids are used to treat psoriasis.

Intra-articular glucocorticoids are extremely useful and may even constitute the basic treatment in oligoarticular forms which show a good, long-lasting response to this treatment.

In polyarticular or resistant forms, it is necessary to use disease-modifying treatment. Methotrexate and sulfasalazyn are the most commonly used drugs. Cyclosporine A, like methotrexate, can improve both the arthritis and the psoriasis. Gold salts and TNF-α inhibitors are useful alternatives in cases that have not responded to other treatments. There may be a need for surgery, prosthesis or correction and the results are similar to those for rheumatoid arthritis.

It is better to treat axial pain with the judicious use of anti-inflammatories, accompanied by regular physical exercise and physiotherapy. Unfortunately, DMARDs are ineffective in the treatment of axial disease, with the exception of TNF inhibitors, which currently show promise of greater efficacy. Sacroiliitis with particularly severe symptoms can be treated with guided injections of corticosteroids with excellent results.

As a rule, patients with psoriatic arthritis who are referred to a rheumatology department will be followed up regularly. Their GPs still play an essential role, however, in monitoring the efficacy and safety of the treatment, as we mentioned when discussing rheumatoid arthritis.

## ADDITIONAL PRACTICE
### CHRONIC ASYMMETRICAL OLIGO- OR POLYARTHRITIS

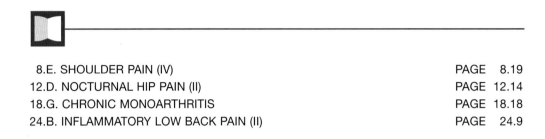

# CHRONIC PROXIMAL OLIGOARTHRITIS

21.

J.A.P. da Silva, A.D. Woolf, *Rheumatology in Practice*, DOI 10.1007/978-1-84882-581-9_21,
© Springer-Verlag London Limited 2010

# 21. CHRONIC PROXIMAL OLIGOARTHRITIS

t is not uncommon to see patients with clinically manifest, chronic, persistent arthritis involving a small number of large joints (2–4). Usually the joints of the lower extremities are affected: knees and ankle joints, followed in frequency by the elbows and wrists. The identification of these signs may be regarded as the first diagnostic step, and justifies a more detailed differential diagnosis strategy.

### Second diagnostic step

Table 21.1. shows the most important differential diagnoses.

**CHRONIC PROXIMAL OLIGOARTHRITIS**

*Most probable causes*

SERONEGATIVE SPONDYLOARTHROPATHY

- Reactive arthritis.
- Psoriatic arthritis (asymmetrical oligoarticular form).
- Arthritis of inflammatory bowel disease.

Unclassified oligoarthritis.

Behçet's disease.

Juvenile idiopathic arthritis.

Incipient rheumatoid arthritis.

Polymyalgia rheumatica.

**Table 21.1.**
The most probable causes of chronic proximal oligoarthritis.

---

**TYPICAL CASES**
**21.A. CHRONIC PROXIMAL OLIGOARTHRITIS**

Inês Pedrosa, aged 32, attended because of pain in both knees and the left ankle joint, which had started 6 months before. She was taking anti-inflammatories, which relieved the pain but did not reduce the swelling. She had no complaints in her lumbar spine, soles of her feet, or Achilles tendons.

The symptoms had begun insidiously in her left knee and had gradually progressed. She denied any gastrointestinal or urogenital infections in the preceding weeks. She was otherwise healthy and had no intestinal, cutaneous or mucosal manifestations of any kind. There was nothing significant in her personal or family history.

Our clinical examination confirmed the existence of synovitis in these joints with no appreciable effusion. Mobility of the lumbar spine was normal and an examination of the sacroiliac joints was unremarkable. We found no other abnormalities on a thorough general examination.

*What diagnoses do these symptoms suggest?*

*How would you justify them?*

*How would you investigate further?*

X-rays of the affected joints showed nothing abnormal. The x-ray of the sacroiliac joints was normal. The patient's sedimentation rate was 32 mm. IgM rheumatoid factor was positive at 1:40.

*What is your conclusion?*

*How important is the positive rheumatoid factor[1]?*

*How would you manage the patient?*

We diagnosed "unclassified oligoarthritis" and proposed treatment based on anti-inflammatories and corticosteroid injections in the inflamed joints, followed by exercises. We informed the patient that an exact diagnosis was not possible at that stage but that it did not preclude effective treatment. The disease might evolve over time enabling a more concrete diagnosis later and suggesting necessary changes to the treatment.

Differential diagnosis naturally requires special attention to criteria that will enable us to distinguish between the different conditions.

### Age at onset and gender

Juvenile idiopathic arthritis appears before the age of 16. It affects boys and girls equally. This is disease falls into a category of its own and is dealt with in Chapter 28.

Seronegative spondyloarthropathies have a clear predilection for young, male patients with the exception of psoriatic arthritis, which usually appears a little later and affects men and women equally.

### Form of onset

Acute onset strongly suggests reactive arthritis. As a rule, these conditions settle down in a matter of weeks. In some cases, however, they can become chronic. Generally, the alternative diagnoses have a subacute or chronic onset and persist.

### Recent infection

A history of nasopharyngeal, gastrointestinal or genitourinary infection in the 2 or 3 weeks preceding the onset of the arthritis strongly suggests reactive arthritis. An infection may, however, have gone unnoticed, especially when the patient attends after many months or even years of evolution. Our enquiry must always look into this.

---

[1]Does a positive rheumatoid factor mean a diagnosis of rheumatoid arthritis? No, because the clinical examination was not compatible and the x-rays did not support this theory either. See Tables 19.2. and 19.3. Although rarely, the onset of rheumatoid arthritis can be like this, but it can only be confirmed by the appearance of typical characteristics.

### *Associated inflammatory back pain or enthesopathy*

Its presence, even if unsure, reinforces the possibility of seronegative spondyloarthropathy and the appropriate tests should be requested.

### *Associated manifestations*

A history of chronic, recurrent diarrhea, especially if bloody or associated with fever, suggests inflammatory bowel disease which may be complicated by arthritis. The joint disease activity will tend to follow the flares and remissions of the intestinal disease. An endoscopy may be justified because treatment is different from that of the other conditions.

We should look carefully for a personal or family history of psoriasis or other skin lesions. Cutaneous or mucosal manifestations suggesting reactive arthritis (Chapter 23) are absent in the chronic phase of the disease. Their presence in the onset phase of arthritis can reinforce the possibility of this diagnosis.

Any associated oral and/or genital ulceration should be investigated, as it is suggestive of Behçet's disease.

Occasionally, rheumatoid arthritis may start in proximal joints and remain limited to this pattern for a few months, before adopting its characteristic distribution.

### **Diagnostic tests**

The diagnostic tests required will depend on the clinical examination. Skin lesions of an uncertain nature may require dermatological evaluation and possibly a biopsy. A full blood count and acute-phase reactants may show the changes expected in a chronic inflammatory disease. Investigation of infectious agents that may be the cause of reactive arthritis is unproductive in the chronic phase, unless we suspect urethral infection by *Chlamydia*. With this exception, the treatment will not be affected by the exact etiological diagnosis, which makes it relatively unimportant. Elevated rheumatoid factor suggests rheumatoid arthritis, after other causes for this serological marker have been ruled out. In children, it is essential to test for antinuclear antibodies and examine the eyes.

Whenever possible, we should take synovial fluid and conduct a cellular and bacteriological analysis and test for crystals. In most cases, we will find fluid with unspecified inflammatory characteristics. In some patients there will be a predominance of lymphocytes, which is associated with a good structural prognosis. As a rule, a synovial biopsy is unproductive, but it should be done, including a bacteriological culture, if the x-rays show destruction. Although rare, several joints may be involved in infectious arthritis, particularly by fungus or mycobacterium.

All patients should undergo an x-ray of the sacroiliac joints as sacroiliitis, which may not elicit symptoms, is typical of spondyloarthropathy. X-rays of the affected joints may provide clues. Erosions of the sacroiliac joint are exceptional in reactive arthritis or arthritis associated with inflammatory bowel disease, though they are relatively common in psoriatic and rheumatoid arthritis.

If these elements allow a precise diagnosis, the treatment will be dictated by the condition.

Suspected temporal arteritis requires a biopsy of the artery and rapid initiation of the appropriate treatment while awaiting the histology report.

### *Treatment*

If the symptoms suggest polymyalgia rheumatica, we should first check for signs of temporal arteritis.

**Patients with suspected temporal arteritis should be referred urgently to a specialist.**

If there are no such symptoms and the patient has no peripheral arthritis, we suggest moderate dose corticotherapy (no more than 15 mg of prednisolone a day). Patients with polymyalgia usually feel considerable benefit in a few days, and sometimes the symptoms clear up completely. This response reinforces the diagnosis. Although it does not completely rule out seronegative rheumatoid arthritis, it is a good choice of treatment for this condition too. If the improvement is not so dramatic, we should seek expert advice.

Treatment should be continued chronically, accompanied by measures to prevent osteoporosis and monitoring for other side effects. The dose is progressively reduced to between 5 and 10 mg/day after 4–8 weeks. The natural history of the condition dictates that treatment will last for about 2 years. The risk of recurrence is high if it is discontinued earlier. Most patients can stop the treatment without recurrence by 4 or 5 years.

If the condition reappears after reducing the doses, consideration should be given to sending the patient to a specialist for further investigation and the possible addition of immunosuppressants as steroid-sparing agents.

# ACUTE OLIGO- OR POLYARTHRITIS

FEBRILE ARTHRITIS
ARTHRITIS WITH
MUCOCUTANEOUS
MANIFESTATIONS

23.

J.A.P. da Silva, A.D. Woolf, *Rheumatology in Practice*, DOI 10.1007/978-1-84882-581-9_23,
© Springer-Verlag London Limited 2010

# 23. ACUTE OLIGO- OR POLYARTHRITIS
## FEBRILE ARTHRITIS
## ARTHRITIS WITH MUCOCUTANEOUS MANIFESTATIONS

This syndrome involves the rapid onset (days or weeks) of oligo- or polyarticular synovitis. It is often, but not invariably, associated with concomitant cutaneous and/or mucosal manifestations, with or without fever. In many cases, symptoms appear two to three weeks after an infection of variable severity. Young people predominate.

### TYPICAL CASES
### 23.A. ARTHRITIS AND CONJUNCTIVITIS

We had known Manuel Roseiro, a 36-year old medical sales rep, for some time. He came to see us because he was not feeling well. He described intense pain and demonstrated marked swelling in both wrists and the left knee, which had begun suddenly three days before. He evidently also had conjunctivitis (Figure 23.1.). He denied any fever or rash.

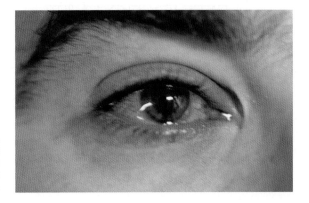

**Figure 23.1.**
Clinical case "Arthritis and conjunctivitis." Bilateral conjunctivitis in a patient with acute arthritis.

*How would you interpret these data?*

*Would you like to have any additional information? What?*

In answer to our questioning, he denied any high-risk sexual behavior, drug abuse or recent contact with blood products. He did describe a short bout of diarrhea that had affected several members of the family during a recent trip. The diarrhea had resolved spontaneously in all of them in 2 or 3 days, seemingly without sequelae…

*Summarize the problems.*[1]

*What is your diagnosis?*

*What would you do next?*

We concluded that the most likely diagnosis was postdysenteric reactive arthritis. We began treatment with anti-inflammatories. The laboratory tests showed an increase in acute phase reactants, moderate leucocytosis and slightly elevated transaminases. The stool culture was negative.

The symptoms resolved gradually over 2–3 weeks.

[1]Conjunctivitis and acute oligoarthritis in a young man, following dysentery.

### Second diagnostic step

Table 23.1. shows the most important possibilities to be considered after defining this context.

In this context, the systematic enquiry should be incisive when asking about infections in the 2 weeks preceding the onset of the articular symptoms, focusing particularly on intestinal, pharyngeal and sexually transmitted infections. The absence of any prior infection suggests possibilities other than reactive arthritis. Mucocutaneous manifestations such as erythema, palmoplantar pustulosis, balanitis, urethritis, conjunctivitis, oral or genital ulceration, pseudo-folliculitis and others should be carefully investigated. The presence of fever with arthritis is particularly common in Still's disease. The pattern of distribution in the joints can vary. A proximal oligoarticular pattern is the most common, but some conditions, like post-viral arthritis may be polyarticular, symmetrical and distal.

Gouty arthritis may be mistaken for acute oligo- or polyarthritis. We will, however, always find a history of typical recurring monoarthritis. Although an uncommon presentation, the onset of rheumatoid arthritis or lupus may be acute or subacute with predominant symptoms of fever, weight loss or lymphadenopathy.

| **ACUTE OLIGO- OR POLYARTHRITIS** **FEBRILE ARTHRITIS** **ARTHRITIS WITH MUCOCUTANEOUS MANIFESTATIONS** *Most probable causes* |
|---|
| REACTIVE ARTHRITIS: |
| • Postdysenteric; |
| • Post-sexually transmitted disease; |
| • Post-streptococcal. |
| Viral arthritis. |
| Still's disease (systemic juvenile idiopathic arthritis, adult Still's disease). |
| Gonococcal arthritis. |
| Behçet's disease. |
| Polyarticular gout. |
| Rheumatoid arthritis. |
| Systemic lupus erythematosus. |

**Table 23.1.** Most common causes of acute oligo- or polyarthritis.

## REACTIVE ARTHRITIS

### Concept and pathogenesis

Reactive arthritis consists of inflammation of the synovium triggered by an infection at a site distant from the joint. If the organism is located and proliferates in the joint, the diagnosis is not reactive but septic arthritis, in which case a bacteriological culture of the synovial fluid should be positive.

The mechanisms underlying articular involvement in reactive arthritis are complex and the fine detail still the subject of debate. For practical purposes, however, we can consider that it is due to antigenic similarities between constituents of the infectious agent and the affected articular and extra-articular tissue. As a result, antibodies and lymphocytes sent to fight an aggressor have a cross-reaction with self antigens, causing inflammation at a joint.

This cross-reaction is not common to everyone. Only a small percentage of people affected by any given infection develop reactive arthritis. It depends on antigenic similarity and the

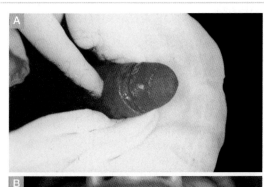

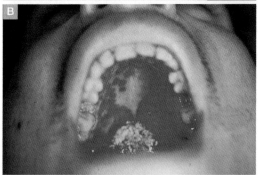

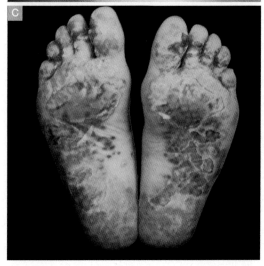

**Figure 23.2.** Clinical case "Acute polyarthritis (II)." Muco-cutaneous lesions started 1 week before the onset of arthritis affecting: **A.** The penis (circinate balanitits), **B.** The hard palate and **C.** the soles (keratoderma blenorrhagicum).

nature of the "self" HLA antigens involved in the presentation of the antigen to T lymphocytes. The HLA B27 antigen is particularly favorable to this type of reaction and is very often found in patients with reactive arthritis.

## TYPICAL CASES
## 23.B. ACUTE POLYARTHRITIS (II)

Vítor Cardoso, a 24-year old hotel employee, was admitted to the ER with asymmetrical polyarthritis that had started 3 weeks before, with additive involvement of the wrists, right knee, and several joints in the hands and left foot. He was confined to bed by the intense pain.

The clinical examination confirmed severe inflammation of these joints with local heat and redness. He also had mucocutaneous lesions that had appeared a week before the arthritis, affecting the glans of the penis (Figure 23.2A.), hard palate (Figure 23.2B.) and soles of his feet (Figure 23.2C.), and erythematous papules on his buttocks and thigh. He also said that he had had bilateral red eye, which had resolved in the meantime.

*How would you summarize these symptoms?*[2]

*What possible diagnoses would you suggest?*

*What aspects of his history still needed to be looked into?*

He denied any recent infection but had an unprotected casual sexual encounter about 4 weeks before. After insistent questioning he admitted having a purulent urethral discharge for about 2 weeks.

The full blood count showed marked leukocytosis. His sedimentation rate was high at 77 mm/h. Of the bacteriological and serological tests, only the serology for Chlamydia trachomatis was highly positive. A culture of the urethral discharge confirmed the presence of this bacterium.

The diagnosis of reactive arthritis after a sexually transmitted disease was confirmed.

The patient was treated with tetracycline, anti-inflammatories and a 4-week course of oral corticosteroids.

His symptoms cleared up without any sequelae.

[2]Acute-onset polyarthritis with mucocutaneous manifestations, in a young man.

## REACTIVE ARTHRITIS
### MAIN POINTS

This is a sterile inflammation of the joint, triggered by a distant infection.

The arthritis appears 2 or 3 weeks after the infection.

It normally involves large joints and can be migratory.

Its onset is typically acute and it can be accompanied by enthesopathy, tendonitis and dactylitis.

It can also be accompanied by systemic manifestations such as fever and anorexia or, rarely, visceral involvement like carditis or nephritis.

Mucocutaneous manifestations are common, as are urethritis, anterior uveitis or conjunctivitis.

It particularly affects young adults. Susceptibility is increased in those expressing the HLA B27 antigen.

There is usually leukocytosis and the sedimentation rate is very high.

The most common causal infections are located in the digestive tract, genitourinary system and pharynx. They may occur in the absence of obvious infection.

Severity varies from simple joint pain to incapacitating polyarthritis.

Recovery is usually spontaneous.

## The most common agents

Almost all infections can cause reactive arthritis in a genetically predisposed host. It is, however, most often associated with the infections shown in Table 23.2.

| Type of infection | Infectious agent |
|---|---|
| Urogenital | Chlamydia trachomatis |
| | Ureaplasma urealyticum |
| Digestive tract | Yersinia enterocolitica |
| | Yersinia pseudotuberculosis |
| | Salmonella sp. |
| | Shigella sp. |
| | Campylobacter |
| Respiratory tract | Streptococcus |
| | Chlamydia pneumonie |

Table 23.2.
Infections most commonly associated with reactive arthritis.

We occasionally come across cases of reactive arthritis caused by one of a variety of other agents, including invasive parasites like Strongyloides stercoralis.

## Symptoms

### Arthritis

In most cases, the onset of the arthritis is rapid, taking only a few days, in the 2 or 3 weeks following the infection. It is predominantly oligoarticular, and asymmetrical, preferentially involving the knees, ankles joints, elbows and wrists. It may occasionally by migratory. Post-viral arthritis tends to be more generalized, sometimes taking on a pattern of acute, symmetrical, polyarthritis.

Occasionally, reactive arthritis involves the sacroiliac joints, which is one reason why it is included in the large group of seronegative spondyloarthropathies.

The affected joints present accentuated local heat and may be red, which is rarely seen in other conditions (Figure 23.3.).

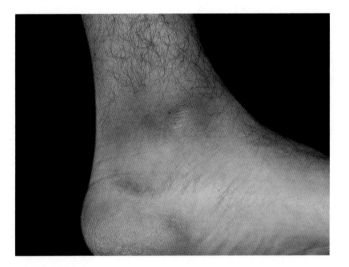

**Figure 23.3.**
Redness of the affected joints is common in reactive arthritis.

In almost all cases the patient is a young adult. This is due not only to the fact that this age group is the most exposed to some of these infections (STDs for example), but also because arthritis tends to appear immediately after the first exposure to the infectious agent.

These two aspects, rapid-onset arthritis in a young adult, should immediately make us think of this syndrome.

The prognosis is, as a rule, highly favorable.

Almost all cases of reactive arthritis resolve spontaneously in a few weeks or months, without any sequelae.

Only a small percentage will become chronic, with destructive peripheral arthritis or persistent spondylitis. If the arthritis persists for more than six weeks, this is termed chronic arthritis.

### Extra-articular manifestations

These often, but not always, accompany Reactive arthritis is often, but not always, accompanied by a variety of manifestations, which may suggest the agent responsible. Figures 23.2A.–C. show some of these. Conjunctivitis (Figure 23.1.) is common, but iridocyclitis (anterior uveitis) is particularly worrying, as it can lead to permanent damage (Figure 23.4.).

The association of arthritis, urethritis and conjunctivitis is known as Reiter's syndrome or partial Reiter's if only two of the features are present. Many authors use this name today as a synonym of reactive arthritis.

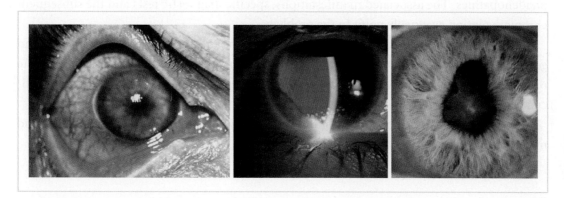

**Figure 23.4.**
Anterior uveitis.
(Courtesy: Prof.
Rui Proença).

### Rheumatic fever

Rheumatic fever is a form of reactive arthritis, triggered after an oropharyngeal infection by group A β-hemolytic streptococci.

For several decades before the introduction of antibiotics, this particular form of reactive arthritis was the subject of special attention because it was very common, and was the principal cause of cardiac valvopathy in adults. The disease is now very rare in the developed world and its diagnosis requires a definite demonstration of the established criteria (see Chapter 28).

Post-streptococcal reactive arthritis, however, is still quite common. It is much more benign than rheumatic fever as there is no visceral involvement.

### Differential diagnosis

Differential diagnosis of reactive arthritis is necessary particularly when there is no appreciable history of recent infection. In this case, we have to consider other causes of acute or subacute arthritis accompanied by fever or mucocutaneous manifestations.

Still's disease predominates in children, but can also affect adults. It deserves special consideration if the symptoms are predominantly systemic with fever and an evanescent rash. The fever persists during the arthritis and its profile is characteristic, with daily peaks accompanied by exacerbation of the erythema. Lymphadenopathy and involvement of the liver and spleen are common. The symptoms last for more than 6 weeks. Note that, as a rule in reactive arthritis, the fever of the triggering infection has already subsided when the articular symptoms appear.

We should suspect gonococcal arthritis (i.e. a septic arthritis) in all sexually active adults with oligo- or polyarthritis and fever. The arthritis is generally migratory and accompanied by manifest tenosynovitis. There are often erythematous papules, pustules or vesicles on the skin of the trunk and limbs. There are important systemic manifestations suggesting sepsis in its initial stages, followed by the onset of septic arthritis, which usually affects the knee, ankle joints, elbow and/or wrist. A bacteriological examination of synovial fluid from an affected joint shows *Neisseria gonorrhea*.

Occasionally, both rheumatoid arthritis and lupus can present with rapid-onset polyarthritis accompanied by systemic manifestations such as fever, weight loss and even lymphadenopathies. The associated manifestations, specific diagnostic tests and the subsequent chronic evolution eventually point to the problem.

Behçet's disease is a type of vasculitis and its symptoms are dominated by recurrent oral and genital ulceration. It may usually present with a proximal oligoarticular arthritis of subacute onset. The patient may, however, have fever and cutaneous manifestations, like pseudo-folliculitis which, together with the ulcers, suggest this rheumatic syndrome (see Chapter 25).

Reactive arthritis confined to one joint is rare and requires differentiating from septic and microcrystalline arthritis.

### Diagnostic tests

In this context, tests serve two purposes:

### 1. Confirming the prior infection and its nature

The studies requested will depend on the symptoms and the results of our routine examinations. They may include bacteriological tests of feces, and exudate from the pharynx, rectum, cervix or urethra, for example. In patients with urogenital involvement it is important to conduct serological tests and cultures of the urethral exudate for *Neisseria gonorrhea* or *Chlamydia*.

Several serological testes are available for many of the infections potentially involved. Note that evidence of a recent infection requires the presence of IgM antibodies, preferably with elevation of levels in subsequent tests. HIV-infected patients may develop Reiter's syndrome and it may be necessary to test for retroviruses.

It is important to point out that these tests will be negative in a large number of patients with symptoms suggesting reactive arthritis, either because the infection is due to other agents, or because it has already been controlled with antibiotics. This is not usually a problem clinically because treatment is not dependent on accurate diagnosis of the triggering infection.

> **Once reactive arthritis has started, specific antibiotic treatment does not change the course of the articular inflammation, except in the case of Chlamydia.**

The only exception seems to be reactive arthritis from *Chlamydea trachomatis* and it therefore merits more detailed investigation with serology and tests of cervicourethral exudate.

It may also warrant a full blood count, liver and kidney tests or a chest x-ray, for example, to look for indirect signs of the type of infection. Inflammatory intestinal disease favors the occurrence of reactive arthritis, as it increases intestinal permeability to bacterial antigens. The presence of suggestive signs or symptoms may justify a colonoscopy.

### 2. Aiding differential diagnosis

A full blood count and sedimentation rate or reactive C protein are usually conducted and show the changes described. They also help to monitor the activity of the disease. Other tests can be postponed until after 6 weeks, unless the symptoms strongly suggest some other diagnosis from the start. Depending on the case, they may include rheumatoid factor, antinuclear antibodies and ferritin (lupus, Still's disease), a dermatological examination, etc. If we suspect septic arthritis, a bacteriological test of the synovial fluid is essential. It will be sterile with high polynuclear counts in the case of reactive arthritis.

### Treatment

When the symptoms suggest reactive arthritis, we suggest the following approach in terms of primary care.

---

**REACTIVE ARTHRITIS**

*MANAGEMENT IN PRIMARY CARE*

Guaranteeing that the causal infection has been properly treated (in the patient and his/her sexual partner, where appropriate).

Reassuring the patient – it will all clear up soon with no long-term sequelae.

Monitoring extra-articular involvement.

Treatment with non-steroidal anti-inflammatories and partial rest.

Managing extra-articular manifestations.

Referring the patient to a specialist if the arthritis lasts for more than 6 weeks, reappears when treatment is discontinued or if there is visceral involvement.

---

Treatment of the rare forms that develop into chronicity is along the same lines as those described for rheumatoid arthritis, preferably by specialists.

## VIRAL ARTHRITIS

*TYPICAL CASES*
### 23.C. ACUTE POLYARTHRITIS (III)

Óscar Rodrigues, a 34-year old surgeon, came to us with generalized pain that had set in suddenly over the previous 2 days. On examination, we found synovitis of practically all the joints including the MCPs, PIPs and MTPs which were swollen, hot, slightly red and extremely sensitive to touch and mobilization. The patient denied any kind of recent infection. Our general examination did not find any cutaneous or mucosal abnormalities and there was only slight sensitivity to palpation of the right hypochondrium.

*Give a brief description of the symptoms.*[3]

*Consider the possible diagnoses and tests.*

The tests showed a sedimentation rate of over 100 mm/h, lymphocytosis and discreetly elevated transaminases. We prescribed a non-steroidal anti-inflammatory, which greatly improved the pain and stiffness. The serological tests were positive for HepBsAg and HepBeAg, confirming acute hepatitis B, with associated arthritis. In the following weeks the patient developed severe cholestatic hepatitis. The arthritis disappeared spontaneously in about two weeks with no articular sequelae.

*TYPICAL CASES*
### 23.D. ACUTE OLIGOARTHRITIS

Jorge Monteiro, a 37-year old computer operator, came to us with pain and swelling, which had started in the left ankle joint and extended to the right knee and wrist over the following 2 weeks. The patient described recurrent diarrhea in the previous months, but none recently. He said that he had had a fever 2 months before, with no precise diagnosis, but it had responded to antibiotics.

On examination, we confirmed arthritis in the above locations and also found generalized lymphadenopathy. Track marks on his right forearm confirmed that he was a drug user.

*How would you define this condition?*[4]

*What diagnoses would you consider and why?*

*What investigation would you opt for?*

The laboratory tests confirmed HIV infection.

The polyarthritis responded to anti-inflammatories and the patient began treatment for the viral infection, with good results.

[3] Acute, symmetrical, predominantly peripheral polyarthritis in a young man.

[4] Acute oligoarthritis in a young male drug addict, associated with diarrhea, fever and lymphadenopathies.

## VIRAL ARTHRITIS
### MAIN POINTS

It presents as acute, sometimes febrile, oligo- or polyarthritis.

It may take on a pattern of symmetrical, peripheral polyarthritis, simulating rheumatoid arthritis.

It is often accompanied by erythema and other manifestations typical of the underlying viral disease.

As a rule it resolves spontaneously in 1–3 weeks with no sequelae.

Parvovirus B19 arthritis may become chronic, with symptoms similar to rheumatoid arthritis.

The treatment is for the underlying disease, together with anti-inflammatories.

There is a great variety of viruses that may cause arthritis, either by direct synovial infection or by cross-immunological reaction.

There basically five types of virus associated with arthritis in the industrialized world:

- Hepatitis B virus;

- Hepatitis C virus;

- Human Immunodeficiency Virus (HIV);

- Parvovirus B19;

- Rubella virus.

In underdeveloped countries there are many more.

Although they are generally benign and self-limiting it is important to recognize these types of arthritis, not only to control the associated manifestations, but also to avoid other inappropriate diagnoses and treatments. The onset of the arthritis is usually acute, with or without fever, and is accompanied by other manifestations of viral infection: erythema, lymphadenopathy, opportunistic infections, jaundice, etc. The predominant articular pattern is symmetrical, peripheral polyarthritis not dissimilar to rheumatoid arthritis. It is usually self-limiting, resolving spontaneously in 10–14 days.

HIV infection is associated with a variety of rheumatic manifestations, including septic arthritis, Reiter's syndrome, psoriatic arthritis, undifferentiated spondyloarthropathy, aseptic necrosis, Sjögren's syndrome and viral or toxic polymyopathy. These conditions often become chronic, unlike the self-limiting course of the other viral rheumatic conditions.

About 10% of patients with arthritis associated with Parvovirus B19 have chronic non-erosive polyarthritis. It is associated with an infection in the upper respiratory tract and typical facial erythema ("slapped-cheek disease").

Arthritis associated with hepatitis virus B and C infection generally appears in the pre-jaundice phase of the disease and is associated with an increased risk of later complications, such as necrotizing vasculitis (hepatitis B) and cryoglobulinemia (hepatitis C).

In our enquiry, it is important to cover the epidemiological and clinical aspects of the different infections (Table 23.3.).

The treatment is essentially symptomatic.

| | HIV | Parvovirus B19 | Hepatitis B & C | Rubella |
|---|---|---|---|---|
| Accompanying manifestations | Psoriaform rash<br>Fever<br>Lymphadenopathy<br>Infections | Sore throat<br>Fever<br>Cough, diarrhea<br>Generalized rash<br>Intense facial redness | Nausea, vomiting<br>Elevated liver enzymes<br>Jaundice (later) | Erythema<br>Fever<br>Coriza<br>Lymphadenopathy |
| Risk factors | Sexual promiscuity<br>Drug abuse | Season (spring and winter)<br>Respiratory transmission | Sexual promiscuity<br>Exposure to blood products | Contact with patients<br>Season (spring and winter) |
| Tests | ELISA, Western Blot | Anti-parvovirus B19 IgM antibodies | AgHBs and HBe, IgM anti HBc or anti HCV | IgM antibodies, anti-rubella |

**Table 23.3.**
Distinguishing characteristics of viral arthritis.

## STILL'S DISEASE

*TYPICAL CASES*
### 23.E. FEBRILE ARTHRITIS

João Rodrigo, a 19-year old student, was brought to our department with oligoarthritis involving both knees and his right wrist, which had set in progressively over the previous 4 weeks. His temperature was high with daily peaks of over 39°C, accompanied by chills and a mild skin eruption on his torso. The patient complained of aggravated precordial pain when he bent forward. He had lost about 4 kg. He described an identical episode when he was 12, which had resolved after hospitalization and prolonged treatment with anti-inflammatories and corticosteroids, which he had stopped when he was 14. He had been asymptomatic since then.

Our physical examination confirmed arthritis and identified splenomegaly and axillary and cervical lymphadenopathy. His temperature profile is shown in Figure 23.5.

*Make a list of the problems.*[5]

*How do they fit in with the possible diagnoses?*

*What tests would you request?*

[5]Febrile, recurring oligoarthritis accompanied by chest pain, skin eruptions, splenomegaly, adenomegaly and weight loss.

His sedimentation rate was 72 mm in the 1st hour. The full blood count showed 17 G/l leukocytosis, with 82% neutrophils. Transaminases were elevated and ferritin was 1,240 mg/dl.

Rheumatoid factor and antinuclear antibodies were negative. The blood cultures were negative, as was serology for bacteria and viruses, including HIV. The echocardiography showed mild pericardial effusion, with no valvular changes.

In view of these data, we considered it highly likely that this was a recurrence of Still's disease and began treatment with anti-inflammatories and corticosteroids. They produced a frank improvement in the arthritis and temperature (Figure 23.5.). The symptoms and signs recurred whenever we reduced the dose of prednisolone to less than 20 mg/day. The patient is currently well and being treated with methotrexate as a steroid-sparing agent and 10 mg/day prednisolone.

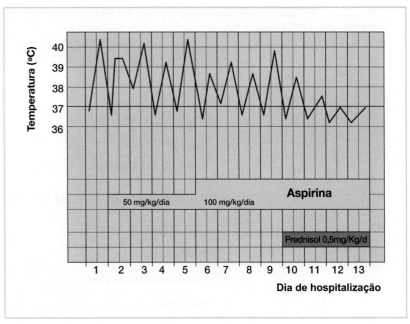

Figure 23.5. Clinical case "Febrile arthritis." Temperature profile.

Still's disease is a systemic disease of unknown cause that includes manifestations of arthritis of variable severity. It usually affects children (systemic juvenile idiopathic arthritis), but also appear in adults (so-called Adult Still's disease).

The arthritis is usually oligoarticular, and predominates in the large joints of the lower limbs. If not properly treated, it may become chronic, with variable destructive effects.

It is almost always accompanied by fever with a characteristic pattern: daily peak (>39°C) then returning to normal. Most patients present a discreet macular, evanescent, pinkish rash on the trunk, which is exacerbated during febrile episodes (Figure 23.6.). There is often lymphadenopathy and hepato-splenomegaly. Patients show anorexia and a marked deterioration in their general condition.

During the course of the disease there may be hepatic, pericardial or pleural involvement.

The lab tests show elevated sedimentation rate and accentuated neutrophilia with anemia. Rheumatoid factor and antinuclear antibodies are usually negative, facilitating differential diagnosis with rheumatoid arthritis and lupus. A very high concentration of ferritin is common and is suggestive of the diagnosis.

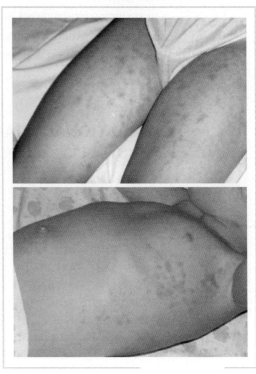

Figure 23.6. Typical rash of Still's disease. A nonpruritic maculo-papular rash which typically appears during peaks in temperature and subsides with defervescence. (Courtesy: Dr. Manuel Salgado. Coimbra.)

Table 23.4. shows the criteria for diagnosing Still's disease.

| *All the following:* |
| --- |
| Fever ≥ 39°C; |
| Joint pain or arthritis; |
| Rheumatoid factor < 1:80; |
| Antinuclear antibodies < 1:100. |
| *Associated with at least two of the following:* |
| Leukocytosis (> 15 G/l); |
| Typical rash; |
| Pleurisy or pericarditis; |
| Hepatomegaly, splenomegaly or polyadenopathy. |

**Table 23.4.**
Criteria for diagnosing
Still's disease.[6]

Differential diagnosis involves considering a variety of conditions, such as rheumatoid arthritis, lupus, vasculitis, bacterial endocarditis, tuberculosis, leukemia, lymphoma, reactive arthritis, chronic viral infection, TB etc.

### Treatment

On suspicion or diagnosis of Still's disease in a child or adult, we should send the patient to a specialist immediately with symptomatic treatment only.

The management is based on anti-inflammatories and corticosteroids, though, in severe cases, it may require aggressive immunosuppressant treatment.

## ADDITIONAL PRACTICE
### ACUTE OLIGO- OR POLYARTHRITIS

[6]Cush JJ et al. Adult-onset Still's disease: clinical course and outcome. Arthritis Rheum 1987; 30: 186–194

# INFLAMMATORY LOW BACK PAIN

24.

J.A.P. da Silva, A.D. Woolf, *Rheumatology in Practice*, DOI 10.1007/978-1-84882-581-9_24,
© Springer-Verlag London Limited 2010

# 24. INFLAMMATORY LOW BACK PAIN

In patients with lumbar pain, we must investigate the rhythm of the pain and other associated aspects that may be alarm signals of a specific or even sinister underlying pathology (Chapter 11).

It is essential to establish the rhythm of the pain.

Inflammatory lumbar pain, i.e. pain that persists or worsens at night and early morning, is relieved by movement and is accompanied by morning stiffness, requires special attention. It may or may not be accompanied by peripheral synovitis.

In any case, inflammatory low back pain identifies one of our "first-step diagnoses."

---

### TYPICAL CASES
### 24.A. INFLAMMATORY LOW BACK PAIN (I)

Jorge Humberto, a 22-year old student, complained of lumbar pain that had been getting steadily worse for the last 3 years. The pain was worse in the morning when it was accompanied by stiffness, which improved over time, more quickly if he did some exercises. It worsened again if he sat for any length of time. The pain sometimes woke him at night and he felt he had to get up and move about. At the start, the pain was only localized to the buttocks and lower lumbar region, but recently it had begun to affect the upper lumbar and thoracic spines.

He denied any involvement of other joints and any systemic manifestations, including gut and mucocutaneous abnormalities. His mother had had similar complaints since she was young.

---

*Consider the most important aspects of this case.*

*How would you define the problem?[1]*

*How would you assess the patient? (See below)*

## Second diagnostic step

The main diagnoses possible for these symptoms are shown in Table 24.1.

---

### INFLAMMATORY LOW BACK PAIN

#### Most probable causes

SERONEGATIVE SPONDYLOARTHROPATHIES.

- Ankylosing spondylitis;
- Psoriatic arthritis (spondylitic form);
- Reiter's syndrome;
- Spondylitis of inflammatory bowel disease;

Behçet's disease.

Infectious or aseptic discitis.

Neoplastic lesion.

**Table 24.1.**
Main causes of inflammatory lumbar pain.

---

[1]Chronic inflammatory low back pain in a young man with no systemic manifestations. Note the family history.

In view of these possible diagnoses, our enquiry must be well focused in order to identify associated articular and systemic manifestations, such as mucocutaneous, gut, ocular and general manifestations that will help distinguish between these conditions. The clinical examination should include a very careful investigation of the spine looking for the signs of sacroiliitis.

---

*TYPICAL CASES*

**24.A. INFLAMMATORY LOW BACK PAIN (I) – Continued**

On clinical examination, we found some limitation of mobility of the lumbar spine (Schober 10 → 13 cm), where palpation was diffusely painful along the mid-line. Mobilization and direct palpation of the sacroiliac joints triggered bilateral pain.

*What diagnoses can you think of?*

*What would you do to find out more?*

An x-ray of the pelvis showed bilateral blurring and erosions of the sacroiliac joints. The lumbar spine showed no changes except perhaps some squaring of the vertebral bodies.

We told Jorge that he had ankylosing spondylitis and explained the nature of the condition. We advised him to follow a regular exercise plan and prescribed a long-acting anti-inflammatory to take at night.

# SERONEGATIVE SPONDYLOARTHROPATHIES

*Concept*

This name covers a variety of arthropathies, which have some characteristics in common (see main points, below).

They all mostly affect young patients, with the exception of psoriatic arthritis, which can start later. The others usually begin in the late teens and twenties. Spondyloarthropathies are two to three times more common in men than in women.

**SERONEGATIVE SPONDYLOARTHROPATHIES**
*MAIN POINTS*

A chronic, systemic inflammatory disease with a predilection for the sacroiliac and vertebral joints ("spondyloarthropathies").

Central clinical symptoms: inflammatory lumbosacral pain.

Limited mobility of the spine.

Variable involvement of joints in the limbs, depending of the type of disease.

Enthesopathy – inflammation of the tendon and ligament insertions.

Often associated with ocular (anterior uveitis), cutaneous (psoriasis, keratoderma blenorrhagica, etc.), mucosal and intestinal (inflammatory bowel disease) manifestations,

Typical radiological aspects: sacroiliitis is the most specific manifestation.

Genetic predisposition linked to HLA-B27.

Absence of rheumatoid factor ("seronegative").

Symptoms respond well to non-steroidal anti-inflammatories.

> **This generic name includes the following diseases:**
>
> - Ankylosing spondylitis;
> - Spondylitis of inflammatory intestinal disease;
> - Psoriatic arthritis;
> - Reiter's syndrome;
> - Reactive arthritis.
>
> *and, for those cases which do not fit into the above, a condition designated as*
>
> - Undifferentiated spondyloarthropathy.

Spondylitis of inflammatory bowel disease is clinically and radiologically indistinguishable from ankylosing spondylitis. In fact, they are very probably different aspects of the same disease, as if the bowel is investigated thoroughly it is s often found to have varying degrees of intestinal wall inflammation, even in the absence of clinical manifestations. Spondylitis evolves independently of the intestinal disease.

Ankylosing spondylitis is the most common and most typical of the seronegative spondyloarthropathies.

---

### ANKYLOSING SPONDYLITIS
### *MAIN POINTS*

Chronic inflammatory disease with a strong predilection for the axial skeleton.

Its onset is usually in the teens or twenties.

It is equally common in both sexes but is more severe in men.

Symptoms are dominated by inflammatory lumbosacral pain.

Sacroiliitis is universal, with typical progressive, ascending involvement of the spine.

Chronic and persistent, evolving progressively to ankylosis.

Enthesopathy and anterior uveitis are often associated.

Occasional involvement of peripheral joints.

Genetic and family predisposition linked to HLA B27.

---

### *Clinical and radiological signs of seronegative spondyloarthropathies*
### *Sacroiliitis*

Clinical and/or radiological sacroiliitis is the paradigm of these types of arthritis. The main complaint related to sacroiliitis is inflammatory lumbosacral pain, radiating to the buttocks. The clinical examination confirms sacroiliac inflammation, with pain on palpation and mobilization of these joints (Chapter 11).

Radiologically, sacroiliitis is easiest to view on an anteroposterior radiograph of the pelvis, with specific angles for these joints (Figure 24.1.). The x-ray images may remain normal for a long time. The first changes are the enlargement of the joint space, followed by sclerosis and blurring of the articular borders, especially in the lower third (Figure 24.1A.). There may be peri-articular erosions (Figure 24.1A. and B.). The blurring of the joint becomes more pronounced (Figure 24.1C.). In the final stages, complete bone ankylosis sets in ("phantom" joints – Figure 24.1D.).

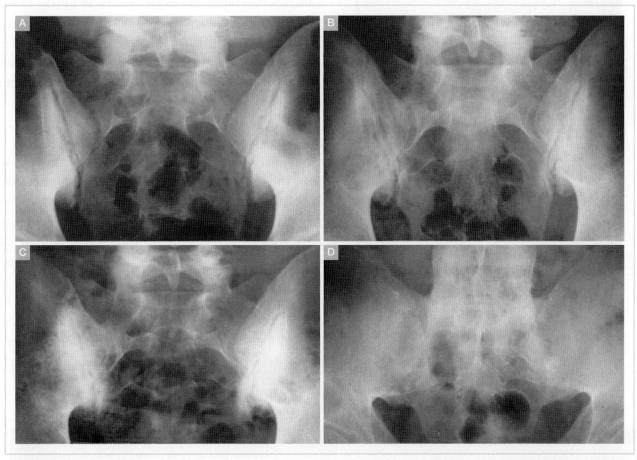

**Figure 24.1.** Progression of radiological features of sacroiliitis. (Vd. explanation in the text.) Radiographs **A.** to **C.** were taken at four yearly intervals from a single patient with ankylosing spondylitis.

In ankylosing spondylitis and spondylitis of inflammatory intestinal disease, sacroiliitis is normally bilateral and symmetrical. In psoriatic arthritis and Reiter's syndrome it is often asymmetrical (Figure 24.2.).

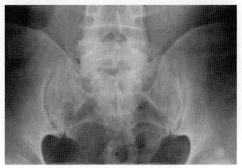

**Figure 24.2.** Assymetrical sacroiliitis suggests psoriatic arthritis or Reiter's syndrome.

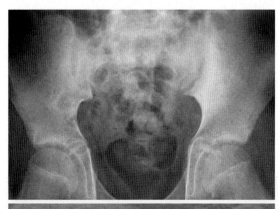
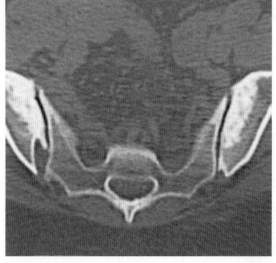

**Figure 24.3.** Osteitis condensans ilii. This radiological aspect is relatively common in young people and may be mistaken for sacroiliitis. *Notice that sclerosis does not affect the sacrum and the joint margins are not affected.* A CT or MRI scan may be needed to clarify the diagnosis. (Courtesy: Dr. Manuel Salgado.)

In its initial stages, radiological sacroiliitis may be confused with *osteitis condensans ilii*, a particularly common condition in childhood and adolescence, in which there is sclerosis on the iliac (but not the sacral) side of the joint (Figure 24.3.).

Any doubts about the existence of sacroiliitis may warrant a CT scan or MRI of these joints, as they are much more sensitive and specific for this diagnosis (Figure 24.4.). Scintigraphy shows an increase in uptake of the radioisotope, but often leaves doubts as to whether the inflammation is bilateral.

NB: the absence of radiological sacroiliitis does not rule out the diagnosis if the clinical symptoms are typical (see Table 24.3.)

### Spondylitis

Inflammatory involvement of the spine is common in these conditions and its onset may be ascending from the lumbosacral spine (which is typical of ankylosing spondylitis) or it may affect separate segments, as in psoriatic arthritis or reactive arthritis (Reiter's syndrome). It is reflected by local pain which is also inflammatory, limited mobility and possible impairment of breathing.

In time, these lesions tend to cause frank limitation of mobility of the spine, which may even be completely immobilized (assessed by Schobber's test). In advanced forms, we often find loss of the lumbar spine and thoracic

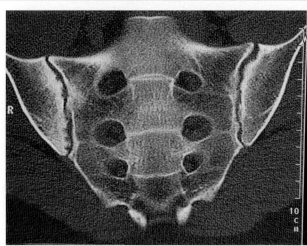
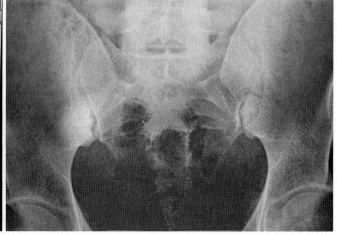

**Figure 24.4.** CT scan showing sacroiliitis in a patient with recent onset inflammatory low back pain and dubious plain film. Bone sclerosis affects both sides of the joints and there are prominent erosions.

kyphosis, with anterior projection of the head and neck and markedly limited mobility (Figure 24.5.). Thoracic expansion may be limited by the involvement of the costovertebral joints. Curiously, the pain diminishes or even disappears after ankylosis sets in.

Radiologically, ankylosing spondylitis is characterized by the appearance of small calcifications of the intervertebral ligaments

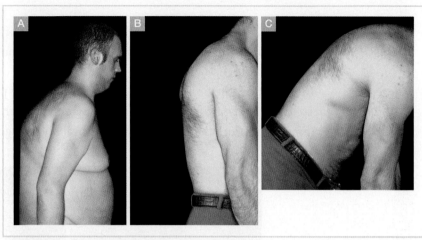

Figure 24.5. Ankylosing spondylitis. Patient with low back pain for 10 years, without any treatment or postural care. A. Limited extension of the dorsal and cervical spine. B. and C. Straightening and rigidity of the lumbar spine when the patient is asked to flex the trunk.

growing vertically from one vertebral body towards the adjacent body, which look like candle flames – syndesmophytes (Figure 24.6.). Quite early on, the anterior border of the vertebral bodies may lose its normal concave shape, due to the combination of erosion and bone apposition

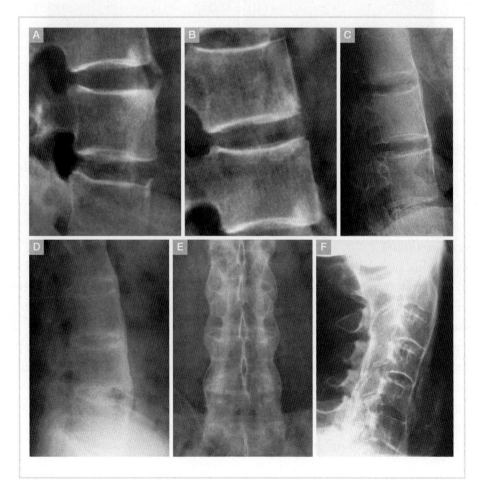

Figure 24.6. Ankylosing spondylitis. A. Syndesmophytes. B. Vertebral body squaring – flattening of the anterior aspect of the vertebral body. C. Calcification of the anterior vertebral ligament. D. Calcification of ligaments and annulus fibrosus of intervertebral disks. E. "Bamboo spine." F. Ankylosis of the cervical spine.

("squaring"). The progressive calcification of intervertebral ligaments results in the so-called "bamboo spine" which can extend along the whole spinal column. Involvement of the thoracic joints limits chest expansion.

In psoriatic arthritis and Reiter's syndrome there are no fine syndesmophytes, but rather coarse exostoses that are similar to osteophytes (but without loss of disk space) and project asymmetrically from the border of the vertebral body (Figure 24.7.).

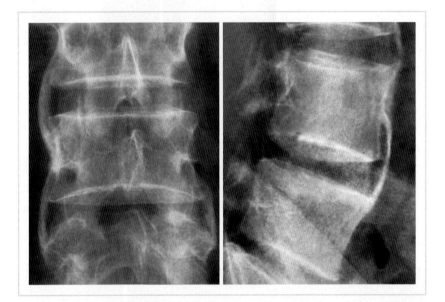

**Figure 24.7.**
Coarse assymetrical syndesmophytes – suggesting psoriatic arthritis or Reiter's syndrome. (Courtesy: Dr. Pratas Peres.)

### Enthesopathy

This is a common but not universal manifestation of these diseases. It is usually reflected by Achilles tendonitis and pain in the sole of the foot, generally associated with plantar fasciitis or inflammation of the ligaments in the tarsal joints.

### Peripheral arthritis

Adult ankylosing spondylitis primarily affects the spine. Involvement of peripheral joints is relatively uncommon and if it occurs, it is the large joints which are usually affected. However, when the disease appears in children or adolescents, involvement of the limb girdle joints is common (shoulders and hip), and may develop into ankylosis.

Psoriatic arthritis and Reiter's syndrome often involve appendicular arthritis. The patterns associated with psoriatic arthritis were described in Chapter 23. Reiter's arthritis is usually acute, asymmetrical oligoarthritis, with a preference for the large joints of the lower limbs.

Inflammatory intestinal disease may be associated with appendicular arthritis in a pattern similar to that of Reiter's syndrome. Unlike spondylitis however, its course is related to and mirrors the relapses and remissions of the bowel disease.

---

**TYPICAL CASES**

**24.B. INFLAMMATORY LOW BACK PAIN (II)**

Manuel Rodrigues, a 37-year old business manager, complained of pain in his right buttock and the base of his spine, which bothered him particularly at night and sometimes on certain movements. Long car journeys were particularly uncomfortable. He had noticed slight stiffness of the spine, but felt that the pain got better rather than worse when he moved.

It had all begun 7 years before with pain and swelling in the knees and left ankle joint, associated with conjunctivitis and rash. The problem had been attributed to venereal disease. The pain resolved, with the exception of the lumbar discomfort, which had gotten worse.

The clinical examination showed pain on palpation and mobilization of the right sacroiliac joint, with no other alterations.

---

*Summarize the clinical case.*[2]

*What do you think is the most probable diagnosis?*

An x-ray of the pelvis showed advanced sacroiliitis on the right side, with erosions and sclerosis. The left sacroiliac joint appeared normal. There were no visible changes in the spine.

We diagnosed spondylitis as a sequela of Reiter's syndrome. The causal infection had resolved long ago. We suggested that the patient underwent an image-guided injection in the right sacroiliac joint, which yielded excellent results. The procedure was repeated 2 years later when the symptoms recurred.

## Systemic manifestations

These are frequent and important for an accurate diagnosis of the type of seronegative spondyloarthropathy.

Psoriasis points to psoriatic spondylitis. Intestinal manifestations, like bloody diarrhea and pain, suggest inflammatory intestinal disease. Reiter's syndrome is frequently accompanied by mucocutaneous manifestations such as erythema, keratoderma blenorrhagica, mouth ulcers, conjunctivitis and urethritis (Chapter 23).

Ankylosing spondylitis may be associated with anterior uveitis and conjunctivitis. Occasionally, the patient complains of episodes of discreet, generally non-bloody diarrhea. Ankylosing spondylitis may also be associated with aortic valve insufficiency, which is rarely clinically significant. In severe forms without proper treatment, there may be moderate respiratory impairment due to limitation of thoracic expansion, sometimes complicated by apical pulmonary fibrosis. The kidneys are rarely affected by glomerulonephritis, but secondary amyloidosis is an important cause of death in severe, drawn-out forms.

---

[2]Chronic oligoarthritis with inflammatory back pain associated with mucocutaneous manifestations.

| | Ankylosing spondylitis | Spondylitis of inflammatory intestinal disease | Psoriatic spondylitis | Reiter's syndrome |
|---|---|---|---|---|
| Sacroiliitis | Symmetrical | Symmetrical | Asymmetrical | Asymmetrical (Inconstant) |
| Spondylitis | Ascending Syndesmophytes Symmetrical Bamboo spine | Ascending Syndesmophytes Symmetrical Bamboo spine | Intermittent Exostoses Asymmetrical | Intermittent Exostoses Asymmetrical |
| Peripheral arthritis | Rare (children) Proximal | Oligoarthritis Proximal (Inconstant) | Oligoarticular Polyarticular Distal interphalangeal joints | Oligoarticular Asymmetrical |
| Systemic manifestations | Aortic insufficiency Acute anterior uveitis | Inflammatory intestinal disease | Psoriasis | Urethritis Conjunctivitis Keratodermia Erythema |

**Table 24.2.** Characteristics distinguishing between spondyloarthropathies.

## Undifferentiated spondyloarthropathy

Many patients have enough typical manifestations of spondyloarthropathy to meet the diagnosis criteria, though they do not have the additional manifestations that enable us to establish the specific subtype. For example, a young patient with dactylitis, Achilles tendonitis and inflammatory lumbar pain shows no radiological changes.

In these circumstances and for practical purposes, the patient is classified as suffering from undifferentiated spondyloarthropathy. This is the second most common form of seronegative spondyloarthropathies! In time, many cases evolve into typical ankylosing spondylitis. The treatment strategy is practically the same.

| One of the following: |
|---|
| Inflammatory lumbar pain |
| or |
| Asymmetrical arthritis or arthritis of the lower extremities |

| Associated with one or more of the following |
|---|
| Family history of ankylosing spondylitis, psoriasis, uveitis, reactive arthritis or inflammatory intestinal disease. |
| Psoriasis. |
| Inflammatory bowel disease. |
| Urethritis, cervicitis or acute diarrhea in the month preceding the arthritis. |
| Pain in the buttocks, may alternate sides. |
| Enthesopathy (Achilles tendonitis or inflammation of the plantar fascias or tendons). |
| Definite radiological sacroiliitis. |

**Table 24.3.** The European Spondyloarthropathy Study Group criteria for classifying seronegative spondyloarthropathy.[3]

## Diagnostic criteria

With this information, we can assess whether our patient meets the classification criteria for these diseases (Table 24.3.).

Note that the presence of radiological changes is not essential to the diagnosis.

[3]Dougados M, et al. The European Spondyloarthropathy Study Group preliminary criteria for the classification of spondyloarthropathy. Arthritis Rheum 1991; 34: 1218–1227.

# 25. SYSTEMIC SYNDROMES CONNECTIVE TISSUE DISEASES. VASCULITIS. RAYNAUD'S PHENOMENON.

## *Concept*

Under the heading of connective tissue diseases (CTDs), we include a very broad spectrum of conditions that are all systemic and are all of immunological and inflammatory origin (although of unknown etiology). Their systemic nature (several organs and tissues are affected) derives from the ubiquitous distribution of connective tissue and vessels, which are the site of the pathological changes found.

---

**WE GROUP THE FOLLOWING CONDITIONS UNDER THE HEADING OF DIFFUSE CONNECTIVE TISSUE DISEASES:**

Rheumatoid arthritis;

Systemic lupus erythematosus;

Progressive systemic sclerosis;

Polymyositis/dermatomyositis;

Overlap syndromes;

Sjögren's syndrome;

Vasculitis.

---

Rheumatoid arthritis has been dealt with in its own chapter, as arthritis predominates in its clinical presentation, while systemic manifestations are rarer and usually less prominent/conspicuous. As a result, differential diagnosis is different from that described here.

Still's disease (in adults or children), which was addressed in Chapter 23, should be included in this context of differential diagnosis, as it comprises the association of arthritis and exuberant systemic manifestations.

This chapter deals with the remaining conditions, in which there is often arthritis, though systemic symptoms often predominate and may involve practically all the body's systems and organs.

The pathogenesis of the different CTDs varies considerably from one disease to another. For reasons of clinical pragmatism, these aspects will only be touched on superficially.

## WHEN TO SUSPECT CONNECTIVE TISSUE DISEASE

The typical CTD patient is a woman aged between 20 and 40, although these conditions can appear in all ages and both sexes. The different types of vasculitis form a highly heterogeneous group of conditions with different preferences in terms of age and gender.

The clinical pattern may be quite discreet at the beginning, requiring a high degree of suspicion and consideration of all the signs and symptoms originating in different systems. We should bear in mind that these diseases vary substantially, depending on the type, and also from one patient to another. The same disease may present in many different ways. One patient may have constitutional and mucocutaneous manifestations, while another may have the renal pathology as dominant.

# SYSTEMIC SYNDROMES
## CONNECTIVE TISSUE DISEASES
## VASCULITIS
## RAYNAUD'S PHENOMENON

**25.**

J.A.P. da Silva, A.D. Woolf, *Rheumatology in Practice*, DOI 10.1007/978-1-84882-581-9_25,
© Springer-Verlag London Limited 2010

More recently, some studies have demonstrated highly favorable results with TNF-α inhibitors, which seem to be capable of significantly affecting the symptoms and long-term functional and structural progression. Their current cost has limited their use to particularly severe forms that are resistant to ordinary treatment.

### WHEN SHOULD THE PATIENT BE REFERRED TO A SPECIALIST?

Patients with uveitis should be seen by an ophthalmologist.

Patients with suspected inflammatory intestinal disease may benefit from being examined by a rheumatologist or gastroenterologist.

Patients with peripheral arthritis, incapacitating axial pain or neurological manifestations, in spite of the appropriate treatment, should see a rheumatologist.

All patients should be seen and instructed by a physiotherapist, at least once.

## ADDITIONAL PRACTICE
### INFLAMMATORY LOW BACK PAIN

### Treatment

The occurrence of peripheral arthritis is inconstant and its treatment is dealt with in other chapters. Here, we will focus our attention on the treatment of axial involvement, taking ankylosing spondylitis as an example. The same principles will be applied to the other cases.

### Educating the patient

This is a chronic disease that will affect the patient for the rest of his or her life. It is therefore important to explain to the patient the nature of his or her affection, its probable evolution and treatment and what s/he should do to minimize its repercussions.

We should first reassure the patient. Even with highly ankylosing forms, patients can maintain good general functional capacity with no significant changes in life expectancy. The spine may become limited, but they will be able to lead a normal life, with some adjustments. In women, the course of ankylosing spondylitis is usually very favorable, with no significant ankylosis.

It is important to help the patient find a way to be patient with and tolerant of the pain and limitations, in order to prevent the psychological problems that only increase the suffering.

**Posture** The spine will tend towards ankylosis. If this happens, it is important for it to be in the best possible position. If we do not educate the patient, s/he will tend towards loss of the lumbar spine lordosis with thoracic and cervical kyphosis (Figure 24.5.). Patients should be encouraged to adopt a correct posture, especially in bed, and to use a firm mattress and low pillow.

**Exercise and physical therapy** This is one of the basic pillars of the treatment. The patient should be instructed to do exercises two or three times a day. The movements will focus on flexibility of the lumbar, thoracic and cervical spine, and on breathing exercises to expand the thorax. These exercises help to relieve the pain and retard the ankylosing evolution of the disease.

It is very important for the patient to have early access to a physiotherapy center to receive treatment and, more especially, instruction.

Almost all countries have associations of spondylitis patients, to whom they provide an extremely useful service. Encourage your patient to join.

### Medication

Pharmaceutical treatment of the mild forms is aimed mainly at relieving the pain and stiffness. Anti-inflammatories are the basis of the therapy and should be properly suited to the rhythm of the pain and the patient's tolerance. As a rule, it is a good idea to use long-acting anti-inflammatories taken at night to prevent nocturnal and morning pain. The patient will find his or her own rhythm.

In some cases, the sacroiliac pain can be incapacitating and resistant to anti-inflammatories. An intra-articular corticosteroid injection guided by ultrasound or CT can usually achieve long-term relief of the symptoms. Oral corticosteroids are of no proven benefit.

Some patients experience a significant improvement with prolonged use of salazopyrin (2–3 g/day) Patients with recurring diarrhea benefit from this regimen, even when the existence of inflammatory intestinal disease has not been demonstrated.

# DIAGNOSTIC TESTS

## Lab tests

When the spondyloarthropathy is limited to the spine, acute phase reactants can be quite discrete, reflected by mild to moderate elevation of the sedimentation rate and reactive C protein. Rheumatoid factor is positive in less than 10% of patients and is low. There is no association with antinuclear antibodies.

Determining the HLA-B27 antigen is not essential in primary health care, unless the diagnosis is exceptionally difficult. It is only a marker of risk. It is present in about 50% of patients with psoriatic spondylitis, 60–85% of cases of Reiter's and more than 90% of people with ankylosing spondylitis. The prevalence of this antigen in the general population varies from 5 to 10% in most of the world, rising to 50% in the Haida Indians for example. Only about 10% of HLA-B27 carriers develop spondyloarthropathy, although the risk is about six times greater than that of the rest of the population. Identifying it thus increases the probability of spondyloarthropathy in a doubtful case, but, alone, it never establishes or rules out the diagnosis.

Note that the presence of HLA-B27 is associated with an increased risk of uveitis, regardless of whether or not there is spondyloarthropathy.

## Differential diagnosis

When dealing with inflammatory low back pain with no associated peripheral arthropathy, there are two diagnoses that we must always rule out, because they are serious and treatable:

**Spondylodiscitis** – attach importance to the association of fever, weight loss, and clearly localized pain on palpation of the lumbar spine or unilateral sacroiliitis, as well as the absence of other signs of spondyloarthropathy. Onset in middle-aged and elderly patients practically excludes spondyloarthropathy, which almost always appears in young people. Acute phase reactants are quite high, there is leukocytosis and the radiographic findings are highly distinctive (see Chapter 11).

**Lumbar metastases** can cause continuous daytime and nocturnal pain, which may suggest an inflammatory rhythm. Note the absence of morning stiffness or of improvement with movement. Attach importance to systemic complaints compatible with neoplasm and the absence of other characteristics of spondyloarthropathy. Age is, once again, important.

Behçet's disease is a form of vasculitis that can occasionally affect the sacroiliac joints and lumbar spine resulting in inflammatory lumbar pain. In our systematic enquiry we almost always find associated recurring oral and/or genital aphthosis. Skin lesions may appear but are different (Chapter 25).

If the patient is seen for the first time in the advanced stages of the disease, with established ankylosis, diffuse idiopathic skeletal hyperostosis (DISH) should be considered (Chapter 11).

In practice, consider the possibility of CTD whenever a patient has one or more of the manifestations described below, either simultaneously or successively.

---

*TYPICAL CASES*
### 25.A. ARTHRALGIA, FEVER AND FATIGUE

Isabel Marques, a 32-year old shop assistant, was sent to us by her doctor with apparently unconnected manifestations. The predominant problem was joint pain, especially in the morning and affecting the small joints of the hands in particular. The pain was relieved by anti-inflammatories. These symptoms had appeared about 4 months previously. She complained of extreme fatigue and recurring episodes of fever (37.5–38°C), without an obvious cause. She denied any muscular, digestive, respiratory, neurological or cutaneous problems.

---

*What would you do if you were her doctor?*

*What other information would you find useful?*

Given the persistent nature of her complaints, her doctor had recently requested tests for rheumatoid factor and antinuclear antibodies. Both were positive. Her sedimentation rate varied from 20 to 35 mm in the first hour. In view of these results, he requested an urgent appointment with us.

In our systematic enquiry, we detected the existence of Raynaud's phenomenon since the age of 15. Her personal history included hospitalization for pleuritic type chest pain with no precise diagnosis being made.

The clinical examination revealed pain on palpation of the MCPs and PIPs in both hands, with doubtful swelling. There were no other changes.

*How would you summarize this clinical pattern?[1]*

*What possible diagnoses would you consider?*

Lab tests showed leucopenia, proteinuria (0.7 g in 24 h), positive antinuclear antibodies with a homogeneous pattern (1:320) with anti-dsDNA, anti-ssDNA, anti-Sm, anti-and e anti-La antibodies. The x-ray of the hands was normal.

Our patient had systemic lupus erythematosus. We were happy that we were able to intervene before any irreversible lesions developed.

## MANIFESTATIONS SUGGESTING CTD

### 1. Constitutional

The CTDs are often accompanied by a discrete increase in body temperature, which tends to be worse during episodes of marked disease activity. The onset of the disease is often characterized by substantial weight loss. Both fever and weight loss are common manifestations in the CTDs, but can be particularly marked in systemic vasculitis.

---

[1]Systemic symptoms in a young woman with polyarthralgia, Raynaud's, recurring hyperthermia and probable pleurisy.

The patients often complain of tiredness, easy fatigability and headaches, which can be incapacitating.

In some cases we find lymphadenopathy suggesting lymphoma.

## 2. Joints
### Polyarthritis

This is a very common manifestation. In almost all patients its pattern is similar to that of rheumatoid arthritis: chronic, symmetrical, additive and peripheral, with an insidious onset. As a rule, the inflammatory signs in the joints are subtle when compared to the degree of pain and morning stiffness.

## 3. Skin
### Photosensitivity

This is an inflammatory erythematous reaction triggered by exposure to ultraviolet rays (sunlight, fluorescent lighting, or computers). As is to be expected, it predominates in the exposed areas – face, chest, hands and forearms although other areas may also be affected. Do not mistake first-degree sunburn, which is common in pale-skinned people, for photosensitivity. There must be an inflammatory skin reaction.

In many cases, we find an erythematous eruption in all the exposed areas. Butterfly-wing exanthema, which is highly typical of lupus, is also photosensitive. Infiltrated, discoid, scarring-type lesions are also common in systemic lupus (lesions in discoid or chronic lupus Figure 25.1.).

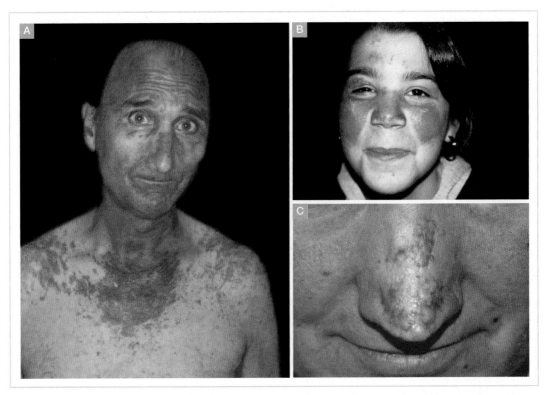

**Figure 25.1.**
Fotosensitivity. **A.** Facial erythema of sun exposed areas (courtesy: Prof. Américo Figueiredo). **B.** Butterfly rash (highly suggestive of systemic lupus erythematosus). **C.** Chronic or discoid lupus.

### Cutaneous sclerosis

It generally begins in the fingertips and face, extending progressively, sometimes to the entire skin surface. It is reflected by thickening of the skin, which becomes taut and tight, making it difficult to pinch (Figure 25.2.). It acquires a waxy shine. The condition normally appears as part of progressive systemic sclerosis.

### Rash

The rash may have a variety of appearances. A slightly scaly erythematose eruption on the backs of the phalanges is common in systemic lupus erythematosus. Gottron's papules are small, reddish lesions on the knuckles. They suggest dermatomyositis.

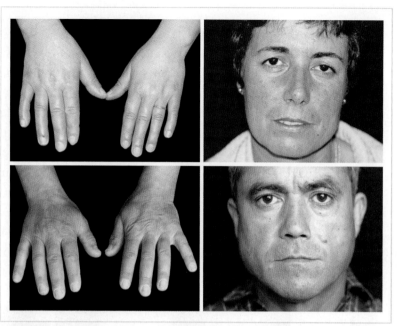

**Figure 25.2.** Cutaneous sclerosis. Thickening of the skin and subcutaneous tissue with loss of skin wrinkles and a waxy, shiny look. The skin is tight and adherent to deeper structures.

Heliotrope rash over the eyelids is a characteristic purplish discoloratioin which is highly suggestive of dermatomyositis (Figure 25.3.).

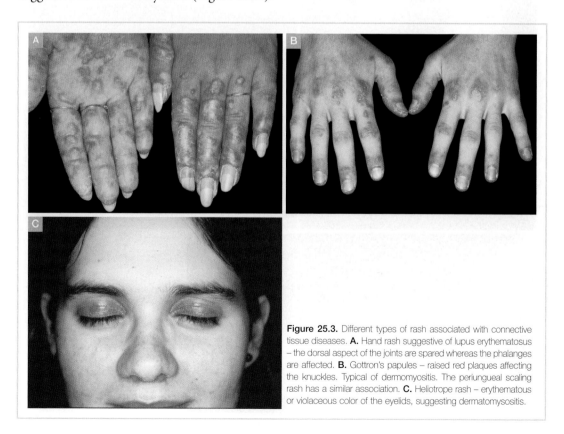

**Figure 25.3.** Different types of rash associated with connective tissue diseases. **A.** Hand rash suggestive of lupus erythematosus – the dorsal aspect of the joints are spared whereas the phalanges are affected. **B.** Gottron's papules – raised red plaques affecting the knuckles. Typical of dermomyositis. The periungueal scaling rash has a similar association. **C.** Heliotrope rash – erythematous or violaceous color of the eyelids, suggesting dermatomysositis.

## *Vasculitic lesions*

These are due to ischemia of areas of skin of varying size resulting from the inflammatory obliteration of the vessels. One such manifestation is palpable purpura (Figure 25.4A.). On running your hand over these purple lesions, they are felt to be raised, which distinguishes them from ordinary thrombocytopenic purpura. It is differentiated from inflammatory erythema, however, as the lesions do not "blanche" or disappear when pressed.

Livedo reticularis looks like a network of pale purple mottling, generally on the limbs and of more sinister implication if found on the trunk (Figure 25.4B.).

Small brownish plaques are visible in some patients with CTD, reflecting cutaneous infarctions (Figure 25.4C.).

Bloody vesicles and pustules or necrotic ulceration are more serious, however. They usually appear on the lower limbs (Figure 25.4D.). The condition can develop into gangrene of the digits or large areas of skin (Figure 25.4E.).

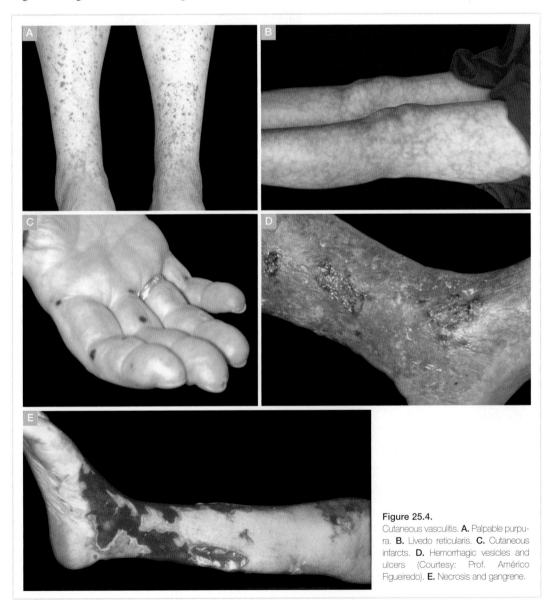

**Figure 25.4.**
Cutaneous vasculitis. **A.** Palpable purpura. **B.** Livedo reticularis. **C.** Cutaneous infarcts. **D.** Hemorrhagic vesicles and ulcers (Courtesy: Prof. Américo Figueiredo). **E.** Necrosis and gangrene.

### Raynaud's phenomenon

This consists in episodic vasomotor ischemia, clinically translated into a three-phase alteration in the color of the hands or other extremities (e.g. feet or ears), caused by exposure to cold or emotional stress. It usually begins with accentuated pallor followed by cyanosis then redness, and is often accompanied by pain or paresthesia (Figure 25.5.). Even without these three phases, pallor should be considered synonymous with Raynaud's. Cyanosis of the extremities (acrocyanosis) is suggestive but less specific.

Raynaud's phenomenon associated with the CTDs is usually bilateral, which is not the case when it is triggered by local mechanical causes.

Repeated episodes, sometimes accompanied by vasculitis, can cause important trophic changes, with loss of substance in the pads of the fingers, or even gangrene.

NB: Strictly speaking, Raynaud's phenomenon is a vascular and not a cutaneous process.

### Telangiectasia

Fine facial telangiectasia is common in progressive systemic sclerosis (Figure 25.6.).

### Hair loss

We should regard this as important if it exceeds the normal hair loss that occurs in autumn and spring. In many patients, there is unquestionable, usually diffuse, alopecia (Figure 25.7.).

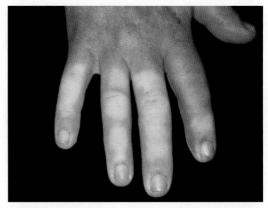

**Figure 25.5.** Raynaud's phenomenon. This color change of the extremities is due to vasomotor dysregulation and may occur with all forms of connective tissue diseases.

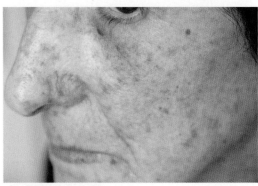

**Figure 25.6.** Facial telangiectasia. Especially common in the limited form of systemic sclerosis. Notice associated cutaneous sclerosis.

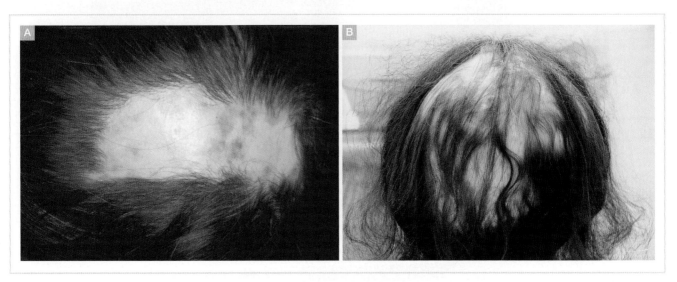

**Figure 25.7.** Alopecia. Severe hair loss may develop in different connective tissue diseases but is more frequent in systemic lupus. **A.** Scarring discoid lupus causing alopecia (Courtesy: Prof. Américo Figueiredo) **B.** Diffuse alopecia in a patient with systemic lupus.

## DIFFUSE CONNECTIVE TISSUE DISEASES

### *Most common clinical signs*

Polyarthritis or polyarthralgia

Raynaud's phenomenon

Photosensitivity

Oral and/or genital ulcers

Cutaneous sclerosis

Serositis

Dry cough or dyspnea

Sicca syndrome

Proximal muscular weakness

Unexplained fever

Accentuated fatigue

Predominance in young women

## *4. Mucosae*
### *Mouth and genital ulcers*

More than four episodes of aphthae a year is considered significant. Ulcers associated with CTDs can be particularly deep and painful. The association with genital ulcers (not just itch) should also be sought.

The mouth is also often affected by superficial, painless ulcers that tend to affect the hard palate (Figure 25.8.).

### *Xerostomia and xerophthalmia*

These terms mean dryness of the mouth and eyes, respectively. The patient may describe the former as a burning sensation in the eyes, with frequent irritation, as if there was sand in his or her eyes. Dryness of the mouth can cause soreness in the mouth and pharynx, and difficulty in speaking for any length of time or in chewing and swallowing dry food. Together, these symptoms are described as the sicca syndrome. They may reflect primary Sjögren's syndrome or it may be "secondary" to another CTD.

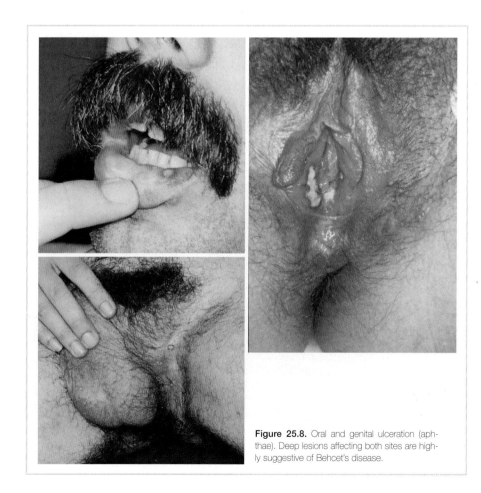

**Figure 25.8.** Oral and genital ulceration (aphthae). Deep lesions affecting both sites are highly suggestive of Behcet's disease.

### 5. Eyes

In CTDs, the eyes are often affected by sicca syndrome and the resulting risk of infection as well as episcleritis and painful ulceration of the cornea. Some forms of vasculitis can, however, have dramatic effects on the eyes as a result of optical ischemia (especially Wegener's granulomatosis and temporal arteritis) or posterior uveitis lesions, which can develop almost unnoticed into blindness (Behçet's disease).

### 6. Serosae

Pleurisy and aseptic pericarditis are common in CTDs, reflected only by typical pain, with or without effusion, which may be visualized by plain film (Figure 25.9.) and echocardiography.

### 7. Lungs

The most common pulmonary involvement in CTDs is progressive pulmonary fibrosis, resulting in dyspnea and possibly respiratory impairment. This condition is particularly common in systemic sclerosis and some forms of myositis. More rarely, acute, sterile pneumonitis or pulmonary nodules may appear on chest radiography. Dyspnea is the most common symptom and can be associated with any of these alterations. Pulmonary hypertension, which is linked to systemic sclerosis, can also cause dyspnea and is difficult to detect as the chest x-ray may be normal.

### 8. Blood vessels

In addition to vasculitic lesions and Raynaud's phenomenon, any episodes of arterial or venous thrombosis should be sought. Intermittent claudication of the jaw or upper limbs may also be manifestations of vasculitis.

### 9. Pregnancy

Take into account any history of repeated miscarriages of unknown cause. It may be a manifestation of the antiphospholipid antibody syndrome, often associated with CTD.

### 10. Central nervous system

Convulsions and psychosis can be manifestations of systemic lupus erythematosus or, more rarely, of other CTDs. Polyneuropathy and mononeuritis multiplex may appear as a result of metabolic and vascular disturbances.

### 11. Muscles

Diffuse muscular pain is frequent and usually non-specific. Pay special attention to signs of proximal weakness – difficulty in brushing hair, walking up stairs or getting up from a chair. Such manifestations warrant assessment of serum muscle enzyme levels. Elevated levels suggest myositis.

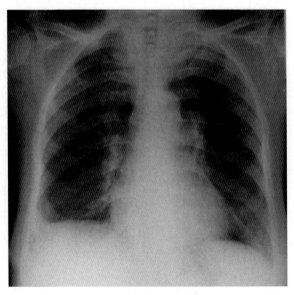

**Figure 25.9.** Pleural effusion (*right side*) in a patient with rheumatoid arthritis.

### 12. GI track

Dysphagia is one of the symptoms of progressive systemic sclerosis and severe forms of myositis. Diarrhea may also occur, sometimes with malabsorption. Vasculitis of abdominal vessels may present with intermittent episodes of acute abdominal pain or gastric hemorrhage and is difficult to diagnose unless there is a high index of suspicion.

### 13. Blood

Hemolytic anemia, leucopenia or thrombocytopenia without obvious cause should suggest this possibility in the appropriate clinical context.

### 14. Kidney

Hypertension, elevated serum creatinine, proteinuria and casts in the urine are some of the manifestations of renal involvement common in lupus and other CTDs, and they are usually insidious in onset and may go unnoticed. Massive proteinuria can be complicated by nephritic syndrome with generalized oedema.

> **Do not wait for your patient to present all or even a large number of these manifestations. Any association is significant. When in doubt, it is better to ask for too many tests and be sure than to postpone the diagnosis of these diseases.**

## SECOND DIAGNOSTIC STEP

The aspects described above should raise the suspicion of a diffuse connective tissue disease (first diagnostic step). Often, we will already suspect what type of condition we are dealing with, given the relative specificity of some of the manifestations.

When faced with a justified clinical suspicion, we think it is perfectly appropriate for a GP to request only basic tests (see below) and refer the patient to a specialist without delay.

In fact, given the rarity and potential severity of these conditions, detailed assessment and treatment of connective tissue diseases should be left to specialists. For this reason, we will only describe the basic aspects of the different CTDs.

### Subtypes of connective tissue disease

Consideration of the predominant clinical manifestations and the changes in basic lab tests, on the whole, makes it relatively easy to reach a conclusion, not only as to the existence of CTD, but also as to the type of disease in question (Table 25.1.).

### Overlap syndromes

It is common for patients to present an association of manifestations typical of different CTDs. In fact, in this type of disease, it is important to bear in mind the concept of the clinical spectrum. Some patients will be suffering from pure lupus or myositis, while others will show varying

| | Systemic lupus erythematosus | Progressive systemic sclerosis | Dermatomyositis polymyositis | Mixed connective tissue disease | Vasculitis |
|---|---|---|---|---|---|
| Constitutional symptoms | ++ | – | + | + | +++ |
| Arthritis | +++ | + | + | +++ | + |
| Diffuse swelling of the hands | Rare | ++ | Rare | ++ | – |
| Photosensitivity | +++ | + | +++ | + | – |
| Cutaneous sclerosis | – | +++ | – | + | – |
| Erythema | ++ | – | ++ | + | – |
| Vasculitic lesions | + | + | Rare | Rare | +++ |
| Raynaud's | + | +++ | + | ++ | + |
| Hair loss | ++ | ++ | Rare | Rare | Rare |
| Xerophthalmia | ++ | ++ | + | ++ | – |
| Serositis | ++ | – | – | ++ | – |
| Arterial and venous thrombosis* | + | Rare | Rare | Rare | +++ |
| Miscarriages* | + | Rare | Rare | Rare | Rare |
| CNS | + | Rare | Rare | Rare | + |
| Muscular | – | + | +++ | ++ | + |
| Digestive | – | ++ | + | ++ | – |
| Hematological | +++ | – | – | ++ | – |
| Renal | +++ | ++** | Rare | + | ++ |
| Pulmonary | + | ++ | + | ++ | ++*** |

**Table 25.1.** Manifestations associated with the different connective tissue diseases. The number of crosses reflects the weight of the manifestation as an argument in favor of a diagnosis.
*In anti-phospholipid antibody syndrome
**Hypertensive crisis, drop in creatinine clearance
***Cavitary nodules – Wegener's granulomatosis.

degrees of one pattern or another. SLE/progressive systemic sclerosis, SLE/dermato-polymyositis and PSS/dermato-polymyositis overlaps are common.

Mixed connective tissue disease is an independent condition, with its own clinical and immunological characteristics.

## LAB TESTS

From our description it is obvious that a patient with suspected CTD should undergo the following tests: full blood count, sedimentation rate, reactive-C protein, albumin, serum creatinine and urine summary. If the last of these tests indicates proteinuria, it should be followed by a 24 hour urine collection so that creatinine clearance can be calculated and 24 hour protein excretion estimated.

In all cases, an immunofluorescence test for antinuclear antibodies (ANAs) should be requested. It is considered positive, whenever the level is above 1:80. Lower levels are non-specific and are common in healthy elderly people.

A significant level of ANAs reinforces the diagnosis, although it can be found in varying percentages of patients, depending on the disease in question. Note that ANAs are not exclusive to CTDs. They can also be found in chronic hepatitis, primary biliary cirrhosis, idiopathic thrombocytopenic purpura, type I diabetes (about 25% of patients!), with administration of several drugs, etc. They are present in 8% of the healthy population and this percentage increases with age (25% at the age of 65!). ANAs may also be induced by a wide variety of medical products, with or without symptoms suggesting drug-induced lupus. On the other hand, a considerable percentage of CTD sufferers do not test positive for ANAs.

The pattern of immunofluorescence gives some indication of the most probable type of CTD (Figure 25.10.).

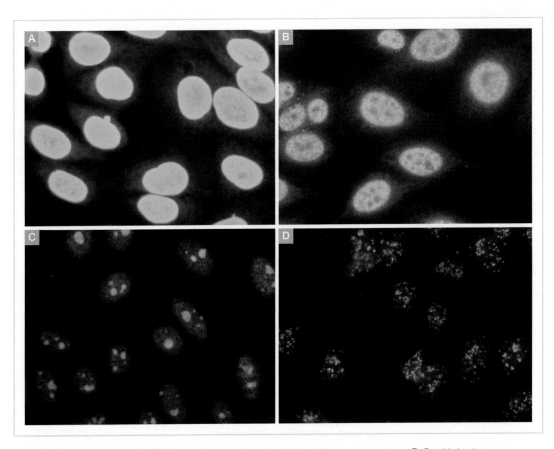

**Figure 25.10.** Antinuclear antibodies. Immunofluorescence on Hep2 cells. **A.** Homogeneous pattern. **B.** Speckled pattern. **C.** Antinucleolar pattern. **D.** Anti-centromere pattern. (Courtesy: Dr. Helena Azevedo. Coimbra.)

## CONNECTIVE TISSUE DISEASES
### *Primary health care guidelines*

When combined with suggestive symptoms, a significant level of ANAs warrants sending the patient to a specialist without wasting any more time on other tests which are better dealt with by a physician with experience in CTDs.

Avoid prescribing treatment other than non-steroidal anti-inflammatories.

There may be a very wide variety of additional tests to ascertain the exact nature of the disease and the organs affected, choose the treatment and assess prognosis. Suspected muscular involvement warrants a serum muscle enzyme estimation (creatinophosphokinase and/or aldolase) and an electromyogram and possibly imaging (MRI is sensitive). If we suspect pleural effusion or respiratory impairment, a chest x-ray may be helpful. The same goes for an ECG and echocardiography for pericarditis and pulmonary hypertension. Dysphagia may warrant endoscopy and esophageal manometry. The complexities of a case may justify a whole variety of tests, which do not fall within the scope of our text.

If the immunofluorescence test is positive, and only then, it may be worthwhile for the specialist to conduct a more accurate antibody tests aimed at specific nuclear antigens. This may be very helpful in making a precise diagnosis and establishing the prognosis (Table 25.2.).

| | Systemic lupus erythematosus | Progressive systemic sclerosis | Dermatomyositis Polymyositis | Mixed connective tissue disease | Sjögren's syndrome |
|---|---|---|---|---|---|
| ANAs (%) | 95 | 90 | 60–80 | 95–100 | 80 |
| Pattern | Nuclear Peripheral Homogeneous | Anti-centromere Anti-nucleolar | | Speckled | |
| ds-DNA | 50 | < 5 | < 5 | < 5 | < 5 |
| ss-DNA | 60–70 | 10–20 | 10–20 | 10–20 | 10–20 |
| Sm | 30–40 | < 5 | < 5 | < 5 | < 5 |
| Histones | 70 | < 5 | < 5 | < 5 | < 5 |
| SSA (anti-Ro) | 30–40 | < 5 | 10 | < 5 | 60–70 |
| SSB (anti-La) | 15 | < 5 | < 5 | < 5 | 45–60 |
| RNP | 35–45 | 20 | 15 | 95–100 | < 5 |
| Jo-1 | < 5 | < 5 | 30 | < 5 | Rare |
| Scl 70 | < 5 | 20–30* (15**) | < 5 | < 5 | < 5 |
| Centromere | < 5 | 5* (50–90**) | < 5 | < 5 | < 5 |

**Table 25.2.** Approximate percentages of patients with positive antinuclear antibodies and specificities predominant in some CTDs.
*In the generalized form of PSS
**In the limited form – CREST.

Note that lupus typically presents antibodies against a variety of antigens, while the specificity of autoantibodies for other CTDs is more selective.

# SYSTEMIC LUPUS ERYTHEMATOSUS

This may be regarded as the paradigm of the diffuse connective tissue diseases. It is the most common and can affect practically all the body's organs and systems.

Its prevalence varies from 10 to 40 per 100,000 population. It affects nine times more women than men. The most common age is from 20 to 40, but its can affect all age groups. It is most common and severe in black and Asian women.

It is the autoimmune disease *par excellence*, and its pathogenesis is dominated by the development of auto-antibodies against a variety of omnipresent antigens. Some cause direct cytotoxicity (inducing cytopenia, for example), while others lead to lesions in the organs by deposition of immunocomplexes (e.g. glomerulonephritis). Underlying these features is a multi-factorial genetic predisposition.

---

*TYPICAL CASES*

**25.B. ARTHRITIS AND SKIN CONDITIONS**

Ana Esteves complained to her family doctor of extreme fatigue that had developed over the previous 3 months, for which she could find no explanation except perhaps stress. She was 37 years old. She described pain in the left anterior chest wall, which she attributed to anxiety though it was worse when she breathed in. She mentioned pain in the hands, especially in the morning. She had fevers of 37.8°C in the evening. Her doctor had found nothing abnormal on physical examination except for discrete malar erythema. He had asked for routine tests, which showed slight anemia and a total leukocyte count of 3.2 G/l (17% lymphocytes). Her platelet count was normal. The sedimentation rate was elevated at 37 mm, but reactive-C protein was normal. There were no changes detected in the urine.

---

*Summarize this information.*[2]

*How would you interpret it?*

*What would you do?*

Suspecting systemic lupus erythematosus, her doctor asked our department to see her and we confirmed the diagnosis. She tested positive for antinuclear antibodies with a homogeneous pattern (1: 320), with positive anti-dsDNA, ss-DNA and Sm. We began treatment with low doses of corticosteroids and hydroxychloroquine. Two years later, her doctor noted significant proteinuria (>0.5 g/day). A renal biopsy revealed diffuse membranoproliferative glomerulonephritis. We began treatment with monthly pulses of cyclophosphamide, associated with high doses of corticosteroids.

[2]Systemic syndrome in a young woman with inflammatory polyarthralgia, fatigue, pleuritic pain, fever, leucopenia, lymphopenia and unexplained anemia.

## SYSTEMIC LUPUS ERYTHEMATOSUS
### MAIN POINTS

It is the most common diffuse connective tissue disease.

It affects women more than men with peak incidence between age 20 and 40. It can appear at any age, however.

It can affect multiple organs and systems.

Constitutional signs, peripheral arthritis and skin and mucosal manifestations are predominant symptoms.

Serositis (pleura, pericardium) and hematological changes (anemia, leucopenia, thrombocytopenia) are common.

Involvement of the kidneys or CNS signifies a bad prognosis.

Almost universal presence of antinuclear antibodies detected by immunofluorescence, with specificity for a variety of nuclear antigens.

Mortality, which is high in the absence of appropriate treatment, is quite low with early, appropriate treatment.

The most common manifestations on presentation are **constitutional symptoms** (fever, tiredness), arthritis, **cutaneous and mucosal changes** (Figures 25.1., 25.3. and 25.11.), **serositis**, **Raynaud's phenomenon** (Figure 25.5.) and **hematological alterations** (hemolytic anemia, leucopenia, thrombocytopenia). The persistent tiredness is often marked and incapacitating.

As a rule, the **arthritis** in lupus is peripheral, symmetrical and sometimes migratory. Inflammatory signs are usually minimal. It does not normally cause erosions or deformities, though some patients develop ligamental laxity leading to deformity of the hands, with reducible subluxations (Jaccoud's arthropathy).

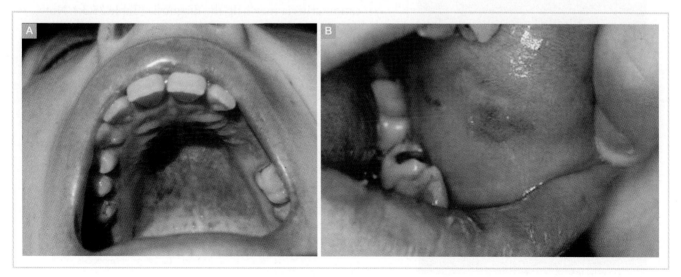

**Figure 25.11.** Mucous lesions in systemic lupus erythematosus. **A.** Palate erosions. **B.** Oral ulcers.

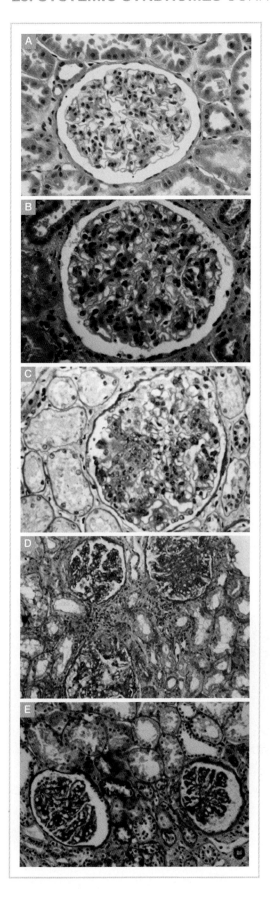

There is **kidney involvement** in about 50% of all patients, and it is present from the start in about half of these cases. It usually consists of glomerulonephritis of a variety of histological types, mainly due to deposition of immunocomplexes (Figure 25.12.). The first revealing abnormalities are casts in the urine and proteinuria, which may progress to nephrotic syndrome Elevated creatinine and high blood pressure reflect more severe renal disease. Without aggressive immunosuppressant therapy, the condition can progress to end stage renal failure requiring renal replacement therapy or renal transplantation.

A possible complication is vasculitis of varying severity, often reflected by periungueal micro-infarctions.

The **central nervous system** is often affected but, fortunately, in most patients this involves headaches and slight cognitive alterations. More rarely, however, there may be convulsions or psychotic alterations that may be very difficult to treat.

SLE is usually a relapsing and remitting condition. It is important to note that attacks are often heralded by the same symptoms and abnormal lab test results that marked the inaugural episode. Fever is a common problem in lupus patients and can make differential diagnosis between increased disease activity and infection particularly difficult, requiring detailed examination and investigation and careful treatment.

The American College of Rheumatology SLE classification criteria may help the diagnosis (Table 25.3.). Note, however, that they are only guidelines and not absolutely required for diagnosis.

**Figure 25.12.**
Histological features of lupus nephritis. **A.** Normal glomeruli. **B.** Mesangial nephritis (Class II: mild mesangial proliferation with normal capillary walls). **C.** Focal glomerulonephritis (Class III: mesangial and endothelial proliferation; focal necrosis; some glomeruli are not affected). **D.** Diffuse glomerulonephritis (Class IV: proliferative and necrotizing lesions; all glomeruli are affected). **E.** Diffuse membranous glomerulonephritis (Class V: diffuse thickening of the basal membrane). (Courtesy: Dr. Jorge Pratas. Coimbra.)

| Criterion | Description |
|---|---|
| Malar rash | Fixed, smooth or raised erythema over the malar eminences, usually sparing the naso-labial cleft. |
| Discoid rash | Raised, scaly erythematous patches. Atrophic scarring common in old lesions. |
| Photosensitivity | Rashas a result of an uncommon reaction to sunlight described by the patient or observed by the doctor. |
| Oral ulcers | Usually painless oral or nasopharyngeal ulcers observed by the doctor. |
| Arthritis | Non-erosive arthritis involving two or more peripheral joints, characterized by pain on pressure, swelling or effusion. |
| Serositis | a) **Pleuritis** – convincing history of pleuritic pain or pleural rub found by the doctor or pleural effusion<br>Or<br>b) **Pericarditis** – documented by EKG, pericardial rub or evidence of pericardial effusion. |
| Renal disorder | a) **Persistent proteinuria** – over 0.5 g in 24 hours or higher than +++ if not quantified<br>Or<br>b) **Urinary casts** – granular, tubular or mixed urinary casts of erythrocytes and hemoglobin. |
| Neurologic disorder | a) **Convulsions**<br>Or<br>b) **Psychosis** – if there are no drug-related causes or known causal metabolic changes, e.g. uremia, ketoacidosis or electrolytic disturbances. |
| Hematologic disorder | a) **Hemolytic anemia** with reticulocytosis<br>Or |
| Immunologic disorder | b) **Leucopenia** – less than 4,000/mm$^3$ on two or more occasions<br>Or<br>c) **Lymphopenia** – less than 1,500/ mm$^3$ on two or more occasions<br>Or<br>d) **Thrombocytopenia** – less than 100,000/mm$^3$ in the absence of drug-related causes |
| Antinuclear antibody | a) **Anti-dsDNA**, native anti-DNA antibody (ds-double strand) at abnormal levels<br>Or<br>b) **Anti-Sm** – antibody against the Sm nuclear antigen<br>Or<br>c) **Antiphospholipid antibodies**<br>1. Abnormal levels of type IgG or IgM anticardiolipin antibodies<br>2. Positive test for lupus anticoagulant, with standard methodology<br>3. False positive tests for syphilis for at least 6 months confirmed by Treponema pallidum immobilization tests or fluorescent antibody absorption test. |
| | An abnormal titer of antinuclear antibody by immunofluorescence or an equivalent assay at any point in time in the absence of drugs. |

*The case will be classified as systemic lupus erythematosus if four or more criteria are present simultaneously or sequentially.*

**Table 25.3.** The American College of Rheumatology criteria for classifying systemic lupus erythematosus, established in 1982 and updated in 1997.[3]

[3]Tan EM, Cohen AS, Fries JF, et al. The 1982 revised criteria for the classification of systemic lupus erythematosus. Arthritis Rheum 1982; 25: 1271–1277.

Hochberg M. Updating the American College of Rheumatology revised criteria for the classification of systemic lupus erythematosus. Arthritis Rheum 1997; 40: 1725–1734.

Ambulatory monitoring of these patients, with the support of their GP, should pay special attention to:

- Infection – lupus patients are highly susceptible to intercurrent infections. Fever, especially with high peaks, requires very careful assessment.

- Elevated creatinine or hypertension reflect the development or exacerbation of a renal lesion.

- Control of blood pressure and serum lipids – coronary disease is currently one of the main causes of death in these patients.

- Limiting the side effects of treatment, particularly corticosteroids.

- Thrombosis and thrombophlebitis can cause pulmonary thromboembolism and often reflect associated antiphospholipid syndrome.

- Pregnancy in patients with lupus requires careful monitoring right from the start, or even prior to conception to ensure the safety of mother and fetus.

- Persistent hip or knee pain may reflect aseptic necrosis.

- Chest pain or dyspnea may be the result of pleurisy, pericarditis or lupus pneumonitis, which requires timely treatment.

- Early detection of exacerbations of the disease, which frequently include the same manifestations that marked the initial episode.

Thanks to the new strict monitoring strategies for these patients, with timely, aggressive treatment of the complications, it has been possible to change radically the vital and functional prognosis of lupus. Today, average 10 year survival from diagnosis is over 90%. The main causes of death are superinfection and coronary disease.

Treatment is based on the careful (symptomatic) use of anti-inflammatories, corticosteroids and steroid-sparing immunosuppressive agents in carefully titrated doses depending on the activity, extent and severity of the disease. Anti-malarial drugs are also widely used. Patients with lupus should avoid exposure to sunlight and use ultraviolet A and B sun block on a regular basis. The treatment has to be constantly adapted to progression and tolerance, with appropriate action in case of intercurrences or complications.

For all these reasons, lupus patients should be monitored from the start by experienced specialists, with access to a multidisciplinary team, in close collaboration with their GP.

# PROGRESSIVE SYSTEMIC SCLEROSIS

This is an enigmatic disease where pathogenesis is concerned. Its pathological process is dominated by excessive deposition of collagen, resulting in sclerosis of the skin and other connective tissues. The thickening of the vascular walls and associated phenomena of vasculitis with consequent tissue ischemia plays an important role in the progression of the disease.

It is, fortunately, a rare disease affecting women more than men (3:1), with its peak incidence between the ages of 40 and 60.

> *TYPICAL CASES*
>
> **25.C. RAYNAUD'S AND EDEMA OF THE HANDS**
>
> Odete Janito, 43-year old housewife, was sent to us with pain, stiffness and diffuse, persistent swelling in both hands, which had begun insidiously about 18 months before. When asked, she described recurring episodes of hand pallor and pain triggered by exposure to cold since she was 26.
>
> On inspection of her hands there was obvious diffuse edema, not focussed on the joints as well as discrete distal cyanosis. The skin was stretched and puffy, with loss of the normal skin folds. The pads of her fingers had small depressions with focal loss of substance (Figure 25.13.).

*How would you summarize this information?*[4]

*Would you go back to the systematic enquiry? What questions would you ask?*

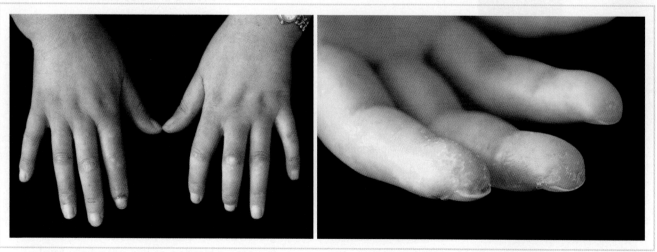

**Figure 25.13.** Clinical case "Raynaud's and edema of the hands." Notice the diffuse edema, not limited to the joints, and the thickening of the skin. Focal scarring lesions at the fingertips, resulting from digital infarcts.

[4]Diffuse edema and thickening of the skin in the hands, associated with Raynaud's phenomenon.

During the systematic enquiry, the patient described difficulty in swallowing solid food, dryness of the mouth and sore eyes. She said that she tired easily and experienced dyspnea with moderate exercise.

In our physical examination there was loss of facial folds and tapering of the nose, which we confirmed by comparing her appearance with that in an old photo. She presented discrete malar telangiectasia. The skin of her trunk was also thickened and difficult to fold (Figure 25.14.).

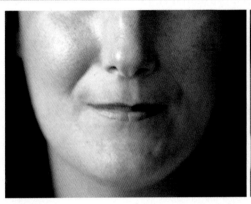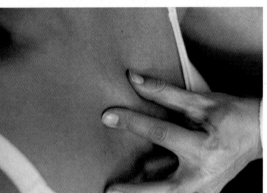

**Figure 25.14.** Clinical case "Raynaud's and edema of the hands." Tight waxy skin affecting the face. With time the nose tends to become pinched even beak-like, and the lips thinner. Thickened skin on the chest wall, establishing "diffuse" disease.

*What diagnosis does this information suggest?*

*How would you investigate this patient further?*

Full blood count and routine tests were normal, with only a slightly elevated sedimentation rate. Rheumatoid factor was negative and thyroid hormone levels were normal. Antinuclear antibodies were positive at 1: 640, with a speckled pattern. Further investigation revealed anti-centromere antibodies. X-rays of the chest, hands and feet showed no alterations, apart from swelling of the soft tissue.

There was regular stenosis of the two distal thirds of the esophagus, and associated hypomotility confirmed by esophageal manometry (Figure 25.15.). Nailfold capillaroscopy showed substantial capillary irregularities.

Two months later the patient was hospitalized urgently with digital ischemia and a risk of gangrene in several fingers. She required treatment with prostacyclin infusions. In the third year of follow-up she presented with severe arterial hypertension and rapidly progressive renal failure. Fortunately, thanks to the early detection of this potentially fatal complication, it was possible to administer timely, effective treatment with an angiotensin converting enzyme inhibitor.

**Figure 25.15.** Clinical case "Raynaud's and edema of the hands." Diffuse stenosis of the esophagus. Hypomotility of the medium and lower segments demonstrated by esophageal manometry.

Initial presentation is dominated by intense Raynaud's phenomenon, found in 90% of patients which, as a rule, precedes the other manifestations of the disease by several years.

Cutaneous sclerosis often begins in the digits and face. At the beginning there is almost always an edematous phase, characterized by firm, diffuse non-articular swelling of the skin of the hands, with accentuated stiffness (Figure 25.13.). This phase resolves progressively leaving thickened, hard skin, adherent to deep tissues with loss of normal skin flexibility and a waxy appearance. The stretched, thickened tissue appears to limit joint mobility. In the face, the skin fold creases lessen or disappear completely and the mouth may appear puckered, with limited opening. There are often telangiectasia in the localized form of the disease (Figure 25.16.).

In some patients this scleroderma is limited to the face and to the fingers and toes (sclerodactaly) or to the extremities below the wrists and ankles. In others the alteration is more extensive and can involve the entire limb and body.

It is not unusual for the Raynaud's phenomenon to get worse leading to severe trophic alterations of the fingers and toes, sometimes with acute ischemia and gangrene or progressive loss

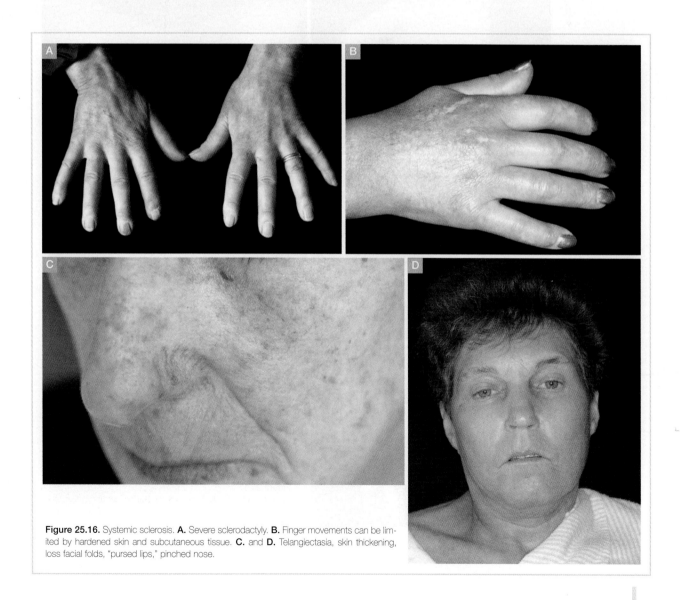

**Figure 25.16.** Systemic sclerosis. **A.** Severe sclerodactyly. **B.** Finger movements can be limited by hardened skin and subcutaneous tissue. **C.** and **D.** Telangiectasia, skin thickening, loss facial folds, "pursed lips," pinched nose.

of digit leading to tapering of the fingers (Figure 25.17.). In x-rays, in severe forms, there may be re-absorption of the distal phalanges (acro-osteolysis) and calcified deposits in the pads of the digits (calcinosis).

The most common visceral manifestation in PSS is dryness of the mucosae (secondary Sjögren's syndrome) and loss of the striated muscle of the esophagus causing dysmotility leading to dysphagia and gastro-esophageal reflux (Figure 25.15.). In advanced phases, patients may present esophageal stenosis secondary to esophagitis and recurring diarrhea due to dysmotility and ascending bacterial colonization.

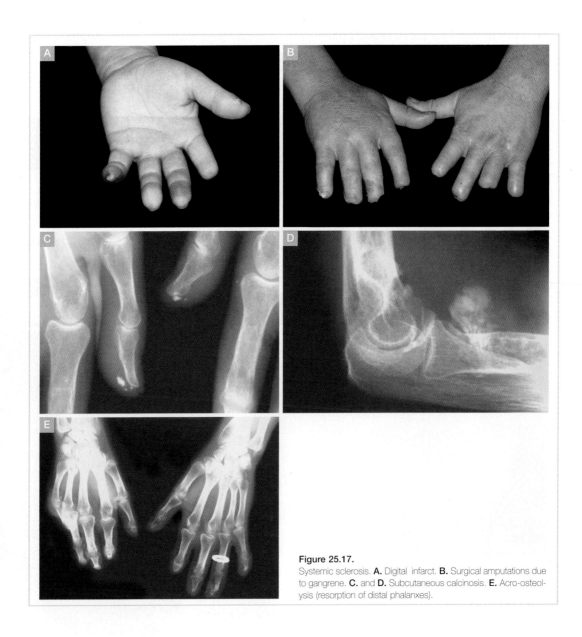

**Figure 25.17.**
Systemic sclerosis. **A.** Digital infarct. **B.** Surgical amputations due to gangrene. **C.** and **D.** Subcutaneous calcinosis. **E.** Acro-osteolysis (resorption of distal phalanxes).

The lungs may be affected by interstitial fibrosis and pulmonary arterial hypertension, with a secondary effect on the heart. Exercise dyspnea and unproductive cough often herald pulmonary involvement. The kidneys are especially affected by vascular sclerosis, which, initially, may cause alterations in renal function. Renal involvement can culminate in a severe hypertensive crisis with rapidly progressing kidney failure (sclerodermal renal crisis), which may be fatal even with timely appropriate intervention.

On the basis of the physical examination and immunological profile, progressive systemic sclerosis is divided into two subtypes:

### Generalized form

The scleroderma involves not only the fingers and face but also the proximal parts of the limbs and torso. Pulmonary fibrosis and involvement of the digestive tract are the dominant systemic manifestations. Sclerodermal renal crisis is the complication most feared. Generalized scleroderma is associated with anti-Scl 70 antibodies, found in 30% of patients.

### Limited form

Previously known by the acronym CREST syndrome, derived from: calcinosis, Raynaud's, sclerodactaly, esophageal dysmotility and telangiectasia. In this form, the scleroderma is usually limited to the digits or distal upper and lower limbs. It is common for patients to present esophageal involvement and pulmonary hypertension develops in around 25% of the cases. Pulmonary fibrosis is less common than in the generalized form. Telangiectasia presents as fine vascular spider-like shapes on the face (Figure 25.16C.). Raynaud's phenomenon is particularly marked. Limited systemic sclerosis associated with the anti-centromere antibody, found in about 80% of LSS patients.

---

**PROGRESSIVE SYSTEMIC SCLEROSIS**
*MAIN POINTS*

A systemic connective tissue disease with cutaneous, vascular and visceral involvement.

Predominates in females, with peak incidence between ages 40 and 60.

Common clinical manifestations include:

- Raynaud's phenomenon;
- Edema, thickening and retraction of the skin;
- Arthralgia;
- Telangiectasia;
- Pulmonary fibrosis, and arterial and pulmonary hypertension;
- Dysphagia;
- Sicca syndrome;
- Arterial hypertension and renal failure.

Antinuclear antibodies present.

---

## TREATMENT

Patients with suspected PSS should be referred to a rheumatologist. Treatment is often unsatisfactory and is largely symptomatic, based on the predominant manifestations. Its aim, first and foremost, is to prevent and relieve ischemia and fibrosis. Angiotensin converting enzyme inhibitors are the drugs of choice for treating the scleroderma renal crisis and have radically changed its prognosis.

### *Polimyositis/Dermatomyositis*

This is an inflammatory process of unknown etiology affecting predominantly the muscles, though it can also involve the skin and internal organs. The coexistence of cutaneous manifestations characterizes dermatomyositis. Incidence is from 2 to 10 new cases per million per year.

It affects more women than men (2–3:1). The distribution of age of onset is bi-modal, with one peak in childhood and another around the age of 40. Some forms appear as a paraneoplastic syndrome, predominating around the age of 60.

The clinical manifestations are dominated by proximal, symmetrical loss of muscle strength, which sets in progressively. Patients have difficulty in going up and down stairs or getting up from a low seat, though, once standing, they are able to walk on tiptoe. It becomes difficult for patients to raise their arms for any length of time when brushing their hair, for example, though manual dexterity is not affected. The neurological examination confirms the lack of strength and should exclude sensory neurological deficit.

If left to take its course, the condition can progress to other muscle groups and cause difficulty in swallowing and breathing, with respiratory failure that may be fatal. There may be spontaneous myalgia or palpation tenderness but it is variable.

Arthralgia or even arthritis is common and tends to adopt a similar pattern to rheumatoid arthritis. There is often fever.

Some patients, especially anti-Jo-1 antibody carriers, develop interstitial pulmonary fibrosis, which can lead to respiratory failure. Cardiac involvement most often consists of abnormal rhythm, though there may be myocarditis presenting with signs of cardiac insufficiency.

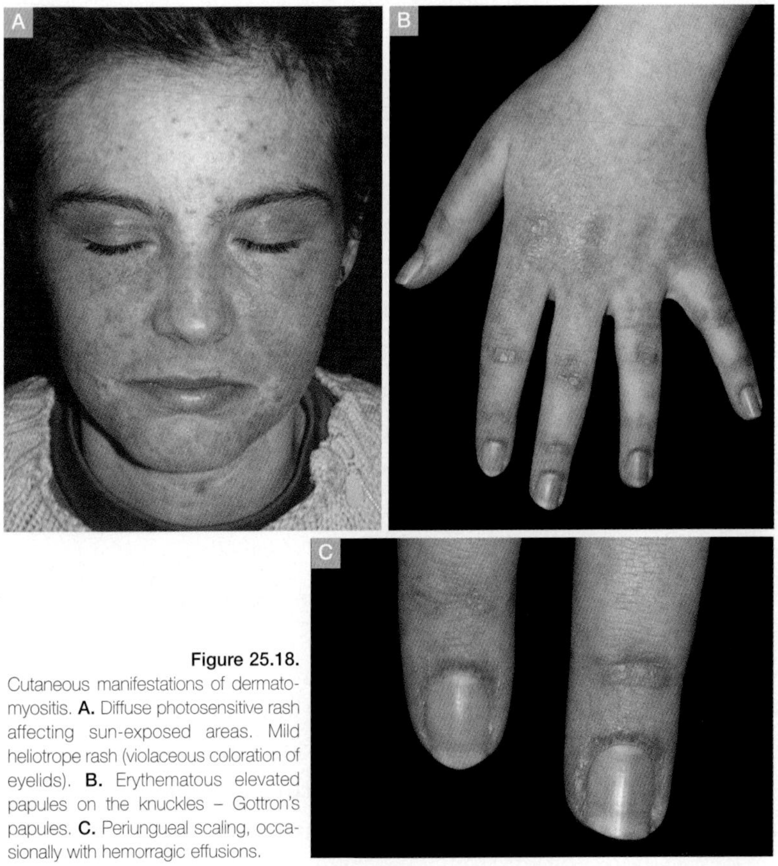

Cutaneous manifestations are present in dermatomyositis and consist of photosensitivity, with diffuse erythema in areas exposed to sunlight and characteristic red pearly patches over the knuckles (Gottron's papules). The heliotrope rash, a purplish discoloration of the eyelids, is less common but highly characteristic of the condition (Figure 25.18.). When it occurs in children, dermatomyositis is often complicated by subcutaneous calcifications, which may be extensive.

**Figure 25.18.**
Cutaneous manifestations of dermatomyositis. **A.** Diffuse photosensitive rash affecting sun-exposed areas. Mild heliotrope rash (violaceous coloration of eyelids). **B.** Erythematous elevated papules on the knuckles – Gottron's papules. **C.** Periungueal scaling, occasionally with hemorragic effusions.

*TYPICAL CASES*

## 25.D. RASH AND LACK OF MUSCLE STRENGTH

José Almeida, a 62-year old farmer, was admitted by the ER in a serious condition: congestive heart failure, uncontrolled diabetes, arterial hypertension, aspiration pneumonia, Cushingoid facies and generalized lack of strength, which had been keeping him bedridden.

It had all started 2 years before with progressive loss of strength, which he had first noticed when going upstairs and which had progressively prevented him from getting up alone or combing his hair. He described several episodes of fever with no apparent cause. He had been treated with antibiotics and later with corticosteroids, to little effect. The condition had been complicated by the onset of arrhythmia, arterial hypertension and diabetes, which required multiple, poorly tolerated therapy. In recent weeks he had noticed increasing difficulty in breathing and he often choked. Finally, he had developed a cough with abundant sputum.

The patient's face and hands were covered with erythema with some scarring (Figure 25.19.).

*Make a short list of this patient's clinical problems.*

*What possible diagnoses would you look into and how?*

The patient's muscle enzymes were very high, in association with anemia and marked elevation in his sedimentation rate. An electromyogram confirmed the existence of polyphasic complexes typical of myopathy. We conducted a muscle biopsy and immediately began immunosuppressant treatment with methotrexate associated with corticosteroids, insulin and general support. The patient required assisted ventilation for several weeks. The biopsy revealed inflammatory infiltration associated with muscle fiber necrosis. He did recover, however, over time. The diabetes and arterial hypertension settled with a reduction in the dose of corticosteroids. He regained normal cardiac function and, in time, his ability to walk and take care of himself, was only slightly limited.

Elevated muscle enzymes are almost universal in these patients, while antinuclear antibodies are found in most. Some have antibodies against the Jo1 nuclear antigen, which is associated with greater prevalence of pulmonary fibrosis.

The association of dermatomyositis with neoplasm suggested by some studies is not universally accepted. Some authors suggest, however, that patients should undergo immediate studies for neoplasm, especially if the disease appears after the age of 55 or if there are systemic symptoms reinforcing the possibility of a malignancy.

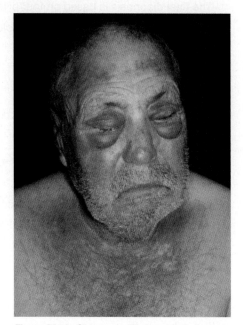

**Figure 25.19.** Clinical case "Rash and lack of muscle strength."

## INFLAMMATORY MYOPATHY
### *MAIN POINTS*

It is characterized by acute or chronic inflammation of the muscles.

Proximal lack of muscle strength in the limbs is the cardinal symptom. Myalgia is inconsistent.

Skin lesions such as photosensitive erythema, Gottron's papules and heliotrope rash characterize dermatomyositis.

There may be arthritis, erythema, or pulmonary and cardiac involvement.

Elevated muscle enzymes are almost invariable.

Antinuclear antibodies are found in most patients (approximately 70%).

An electromyogram, muscle biopsy and MRI confirm the diagnosis.

Differential diagnosis includes a multiplicity of causes of muscle weakness. The proximal distribution of weakness, if well characterized, is highly suggestive of a muscular condition, while ruling out polyneuropathy.

Look into the patient's regular medication. Corticosteroids, lipid-lowering agents, zidovudine, colchicine and anti-tuberculous drugs are part of the long list that can induce myopathy. Note any fever. It may be a form of septic myositis (abscess). Rule out the possibility of myopathy of endocrinal cause: hypothyroidism, Addison's disease, hypo- or hyperparathyroidism, hypocalcemia, etc. In the elderly, it is worth considering polymyalgia rheumatica. Differential diagnosis with neurological diseases, such as muscular dystrophy and myasthenia gravis, may be very difficult and requires a multidisciplinary approach.

The **final diagnosis** is based on four pillars:

- Symmetrical lack of proximal muscle strength, confirmed by the doctor, with no apparent cause;
- Elevated muscle enzymes;
- Electromyogram (characteristic polyphasic complexes);
- Muscle biopsy.

## PRIMARY CARE

Reduced proximal muscle strength, associated with persistently elevated muscle enzymes and the absence of any potentially responsible drugs, justifies referring the patient to a specialist without delay.

The treatment of polymyositis/dermatomyositis may be difficult and drawn out. It involves corticosteroids and immunosuppressants, such as methotrexate and azathioprine. The potentially fatal complications require urgent, aggressive measures which are usually only available in specialist centers.

## MIXED CONNECTIVE TISSUE DISEASE

This is characterized by the association of aspects typical of two or more connective tissue diseases and the isolated presence of anti-ribonucleoprotein antibodies (anti-U1 RNP).

---

**THE FOLLOWING CLINICAL MANIFESTATIONS PREDOMINATE:**

- Polyarthritis, which is peripheral and symmetrical but often associated with diffuse, extensive edema of the hands. It can vary from a discreet form like the arthritis of lupus to erosive forms similar to rheumatoid arthritis;
- Raynaud's phenomenon is found in about 85% of patients;
- Myositis;
- Interstitial pulmonary fibrosis;
- Sclerodactylia, telangiectasia, photosensitivity;
- Esophageal dysmotility in more than 50% of patients;
- Sjögren's syndrome in about half the patients.

---

The diagnosis is based on these overlapping clinical characteristics and on the demonstration of antinuclear antibodies by immunofluorescence with U1 RNP specificity.

## OVERLAP SYNDROMES

It is not uncommon to find patients whose clinical manifestations and lab tests show associations of elements characteristic of more than one CTD. There may, for example, be an association of malar rash and glomerulonephritis with myositis (SLE/PM overlap syndrome), or sclerodactaly, Raynaud's and myositis (PSS/PM overlap syndrome). These patients do not present the typical immunological pattern of diffuse connective tissue disease (anti-RNP),? which is a separate condition, and tend rather to associate antibodies typical of the overlapping conditions.

The treatment depends on the existing manifestations.

## UNDIFFERENTIATED CONNECTIVE TISSUE DISEASE

It is not uncommon to find patients with mild clinical manifestations compatible with CTD and positive antinuclear antibodies without the alterations as a whole enabling us to make a definite diagnosis.

The most common complaints are migratory arthralgia, Raynaud's phenomenon and discreet photosensitivity. When the clinical manifestations and lab tests do not allow us to make a definite diagnosis of any specific type of CTD, the patient should be classified as having undifferentiated connective tissue disease and should be kept under clinical monitoring and symptomatic treatment. Many cases will eventually evolve into a typical pattern.

## SJÖGREN'S SYNDROME

The principal manifestation of Sjögren's syndrome is dry syndrome: dryness of the eyes (xerophthalmia) and mouth (xerostomia). This manifestation is due to inflammatory infiltration of the exocrine glands.

The clinical pattern consists of sore eyes with recurring episodes of red eye. Lack of lubrication of the cornea can be complicated by painful ulceration (identifiable using the Rose Bengal test and an examination with a slit lamp) and, more rarely, perforation (dry keratoconjuntivitis). Tear production can be quantified by Schirmer's test. This test uses small strips of calibrated filter paper the end of which is inserted under the lower lid for 5 minutes (Figure 25.20.). If less than 5 mm of the paper is moistened, this is a classification criterion for this disease. Eye dryness may be helped by regular use of artificial tears to lubricate the cornea and prevent ulceration.

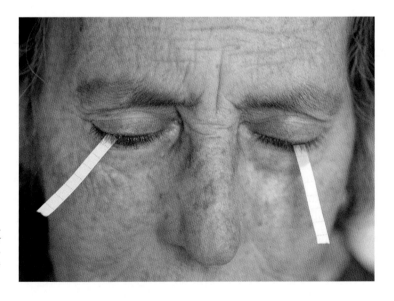

**Figure 25.20.**
Schirmer's test. Quantifies tear production through the moisturizing of filter paper fit under the inferior eyelid for 5 minutes.

It is important to exclude other causes of eye dryness: antidepressants, parasympathomimetics, diabetes or even a congenital lack of lachrymal glands.

Oropharyngeal dryness is reflected mainly by discomfort and soreness in the mouth, with difficulty chewing dry foods. It is associated with a high prevalence of dental caries and periodontitis. The parotids may develop calculi in the excretory ducts with obstruction that leads to sometimes painful recurring hypertrophy with the risk of superinfection. The involvement of the salivary glands can be demonstrated on scintigraphy or sialography (Figure 25.21.).

The infiltration of other exocrine glands may be reflected by dyspareunia and biliary (cholestasis) or pancreatic (acute or chronic pancreatitis) obstruction.

In most cases, Sjögren's syndrome is associated with other connective tissue diseases, like rheumatoid arthritis, lupus and progressive systemic sclerosis (**secondary Sjögren's syndrome**). This association does not change the basic treatment of the disease, apart from the need for the regular use of artificial tears, and ophthalmologic examination and relief of dryness of the mouth.

In other patients, the syndrome is isolated with no accompanying manifestations that enable us to diagnose another CTD (**primary Sjögren's syndrome**). Its course is indolent and progressive. It affects nine times more women than men.

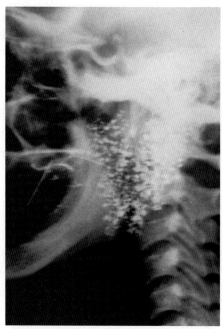

**Figure 25.21.** Sialography in a patient with Sjögren's syndrome. Hypertrophy and dilatation of the parotid gland ducts, 24 hours after contrast was applied.

### *Primary Sjögren's syndrome*

In primary Sjögren's syndrome it is not unusual to find **discreet non-erosive synovitis**. **Raynaud's phenomenon** is common without telangiectasia or cutaneous sclerosis. Accentuated, chronic **hypergammaglobulinemia** may be reflected by **orthostatic purpura**, i.e., aggravated by standing for a long time (Waldenstrom's purpura). It may also involve the lungs (dry cough, interstitial fibrosis), stomach (atrophic gastritis), kidneys (renal tubular acidosis and kidney stones), liver (cholestasis with inflammation of the bile ducts or primary biliary cirrhosis), or blood vessels (vasculitis – 5% of patients).

Lab tests usually show greatly elevated sedimentation rate and polyclonal hypergammaglobulinemia. In the absence of any associated disease, reactive-C protein may be normal (the high sedimentation rate is due to gammopathy). Rheumatoid factor and antinuclear antibodies are almost always found, with a **high prevalence of anti-SSA and anti-SSB**. The presence of these autoantibodies in the context of other CTDs is

---

## SJÖGREN'S SYNDROME
### *MAIN POINTS*

Dryness of the mucosae is the main manifestation.

It may appear in association with other CTDs (secondary Sjögren's syndrome) or in isolation (primary Sjögren's syndrome).

#### *Primary Sjögren's syndrome:*

- Polyarthritis;
- Raynaud's phenomenon;
- Orthostatic purpura;
- Interstitial fibrosis;
- Renal tubular acidosis;
- Cholestasis;
- Elevated sedimentation rate;
- Polyclonal hypergammaglobulinemia;
- Rheumatoid factor (almost constant);
- Antinuclear antibodies;
- Anti-Ro (SSA) and anti-La (SSB);
- Watch out for lymphoma transformation.

also associated with sicca syndrome. In order to reach a final diagnosis it may be necessary to perform a biopsy of the minor salivary glands (labial biopsy), to demonstrate a lymphocytic infiltrate.

In practical terms, a diagnosis of primary Sjögren's syndrome should lead to a similar strategy as that proposed for lupus: regular clinical and laboratory follow-up, with treatment depending on the significant manifestations. There is one additional concern. Patients with this syndrome have a 40 fold greater risk of developing lymphoma. The signs suggesting this include fever, night sweats, adenopathy or hepatomegaly, monoclonal gammopathy and reduction in IgM levels.

### *Treatment*

The treatment of Sjögren's syndrome is symptomatic. The aim is to keep the mucosae moist and prevent complications.

The patient should be told to apply false tears regularly and often, as this is essential in preventing keratoconjuntivitis sicca. A lubricating gel with more long-lasting action can also be used. The patient should be warned of the drying effect of heat, air conditioning and dry wind and advised to wear protective glasses and use a humidifier at home. Contact lenses are not recommended. It is advisable to have regular eye check-ups. Patients should avoid smoking and drugs with anticholinergic effects.

It is important to tell patients to have heightened oral hygiene, brushing their teeth after each meal and paying regular visits to the dentist. The symptoms of xerostomia are very hard to relieve and many patients learn to carry water with them all the time. Sugar-free chewing gum can be useful. Dyspareunia can be relieved by using vaginal creams.

Medications do not play much of a role in this syndrome. Anti-inflammatories may be necessary to treat the arthritis. Corticosteroids and immunosuppressants should be reserved for significant extra-glandular involvement.

## VASCULITIS

The different forms of vasculitis constitute potentially fatal systemic syndromes caused by inflammation of the walls and periphery of arteries and/or veins, and arterioles and/or venules with resulting tissue ischemia.

Most patients with vasculitis present one of two types of clinical pattern:
1. Lesions of cutaneous vasculitis (Figure 25.4.) – typical of small-vessel vasculitis and vasculitis associated with connective tissue diseases;
2. Predominant constitutional symptoms: fever, anorexia and weight loss in a clinical context suggesting a neoplastic or infectious disease. There is often polyarthritis. These are the most common manifestations of severe necrotizing vasculitis.

The secret of the diagnosis in these cases is to systematically look for symptoms or signs of the skin, muscle, nervous system or vital organ impairment pointing to local ischemia: arterial and venous thromboses, arterial hypertension, bloody nose discharge, sight loss, mononeuropathy, pulmonary infiltration, etc.

There is a wide variety of vasculitic syndromes, grouped according to the size of the vessels affected and by the dominant clinical pattern. They are generally rare diseases, and so we have only presented a summary of the most common forms – Table 25.4.

| Vasculitic syndrome | Preferential age | Sex (M:F) | Predominant clinical characteristics |
| --- | --- | --- | --- |
| Polyarteritis Nodosa | 40–60 | 2:1 | Fever, weight loss, livedo reticularis, mono- or polyneuropathy, arterial hypertension. |
| Wegener's granulomatosis | 30–50 | 1:1 | Sinusitis, mouth ulcers, otitis, hemoptysis, pulmonary nodules, nephritis. |
| Churg-Strauss's granulomatosis | 40–60 | 2:1 | Severe asthma, atopic eczema, mono- or polyneuropathy, pulmonary infiltration, eosinophilia. |
| Leukocytoclastic vasculitis | 30–50 | 1:1 | Often associated with other CTDs and drugs, palpable purpura, maculopapular erythema, skin ulceration. |
| Henoch-Schonlein purpura | 5–20 | 1:1 | Palpable purpura, maculopapular erythema, skin ulceration (usually in lower limbs and buttocks), abdominal pain, bloody diarrhea, nephritis with deposition of IgA. |
| Giant cell arteritis | 60–75 | 1:3 | Temporal pain, masticatory claudication, stiffness of the scapular and pelvic girdles, double vision, sudden sight loss. |
| Behçet's disease | 20–35 | 1:1 | Mouth and genital ulcers, pseudo-folliculitis of the skin, uveitis (sight loss), thrombophlebitis, arthritis. |
| Urticarial vasculitis | | | Palpable purpura, urticarial lesions with residual scarring, skin nodules and ulcers. |

**Table 25.4.** The most common vasculitic syndromes: age group, sex and main clinical manifestations.

They are accompanied by intense acute phase reaction and often neutrophilia or eosinophilia. A final diagnosis requires a biopsy of the affected tissue. An angiogram can be very useful in identifying lesions of the viscera. Syndromes with renal and pulmonary involvement are often associated with an anti-neutrophil cytoplasmic antibody (ANCA).

Vasculitis can rapidly lead to irreversible or even fatal organic lesions. It requires early, aggressive treatment with corticosteroids and immunosuppressants, especially cyclophosphamide.

**If you suspect vasculitis, refer the patient to a specialist as soon as possible.**

# RAYNAUD'S PHENOMENON

Clinically, Raynaud's phenomenon is characterized by a sudden change in the skin color of the extremities (mainly fingers, toes and ears).

It typically involves three successive phases: pallor, cyanosis and redness (Figure 25.22.). Only a small percentage of these patients present the three phases. Pallor is considered the most specific manifestation of Raynaud's. Cyanosis alone, as a reaction to cold (acrocyanosis), is much less specific and can be found in a variety of benign conditions, such as lupus pernio ("chilblains").

Crises are brought on by exposure to cold and emotional stress. It is caused by a vasospastic phenomenon of complex pathogenesis affecting microcirculation, i.e. arterioles, capillaries, arterio-venous shunts and venules.

It is an extremely common condition in clinical practice and affects about 10% of the population. This percentage can go up to 25% in cold climates (much more common in women than in men).

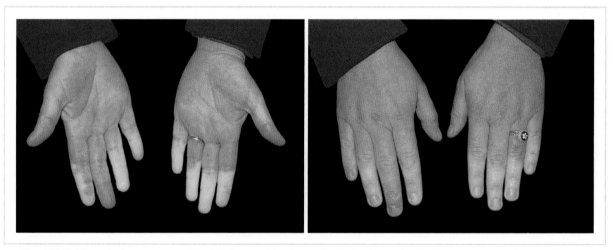

**Figure 25.22.** Raynaud's phenomenon translates clinically as a sudden change of coloration affecting the skin of extremities (fingers, toes, ears). Typically, pallor (figure) is followed by cyanosis and redness (reactive hyperemia). (Courtesy: Dr. Manuel Salgado. Coimbra.)

---

*TYPICAL CASES*

**25.E. RAYNAUD'S AND GENERALIZED PAIN**

Elizabete Macedo, a 43-year old PE teacher, was sent to us because of intense pain in almost all joints and changes in the color of her hands suggesting Raynaud's phenomenon. According to her GP, all the tests had been negative, including sedimentation rate and antinuclear antibodies. He still suspected systemic lupus erythematosus, however.

*Comment on this suspected diagnosis.*

*What additional information would you like to have?*

Our enquiry confirmed typical, three-phase Raynaud's phenomenon, particularly exuberant in winter, which had started at the age of 25. She had also noticed that it was exacerbated by stress but there had never been any significant trophic alteration of the hands. The pain was migratory and diffuse, having developed for about 13 years, with no deformities. She described occasional transitory edema in her hands. Our systematic enquiry ruled out any significant general symptoms, except for tiredness. She denied any cutaneous or mucosal changes or respiratory, ocular or other manifestations. She was taking oral contraceptives and smoked about 15 cigarettes a day.

*Think about your diagnosis and subsequent investigation again.*

The clinical examination was completely normal. We found no skin lesions or signs of arthritis, but 13 of the 18 typical points of fibromyalgia were extremely tender.

In fact, the different tests performed up to then were normal, including sedimentation rate, reactive-C protein and antinuclear antibodies. The thyroid function tests that we then requested were normal.

*What is your diagnosis?*

*How would you treat the patient?*

We explained to the patient carefully that her pain was due to fibromyalgia and gave her appropriate advice. The Raynaud's phenomenon could be primary but was very probably related to the contraceptives and smoking, which we strongly advised her to give up. The patient opted for an intra uterine device and stopped smoking. Four months later, the pain still persisted with a slight improvement but there had been no more episodes of Raynaud's in spite of outdoor activities in the middle of autumn.

Raynaud's phenomenon can be of varying severity, ranging from a mild or moderate form with no general repercussions to a severe form with ulceration and ischemic gangrene of the extremities, occasionally requiring amputation (Figure 25.17.). In particularly severe cases, vasospasm can also occur in the internal organs, causing primary pulmonary hypertension, Prinzmetal's angina or even myocardial infarction

The importance of Raynaud's phenomenon can therefore go far beyond a mere alteration in visible color and be life threatening.

### Etiology and significance

For didactic purposes, we can consider two main types of Raynaud's phenomenon, from the etiological point of view: primary and secondary.

In primary or idiopathic Raynaud's phenomenon, (also called "Raynaud's disease"), as the name suggests, it is not possible to find an underlying cause in spite of exhaustive investigation.

### Drug-related

Oral contraceptives
b-blockers
Anti-histamines
Ergotamine derivatives

### Toxic

Smoking
Caffeine
Heavy metals
Polyvinyl chloride

### Traumatic

Vibration, percussion
Local trauma (e.g. using crutches)

### Regional neurological or vascular compromise

Thoracic outlet syndrome
Carpal tunnel syndrome
Embolism
Thrombosis
Accelerated atherosclerosis

### Diffuse connective tissue diseases

Systemic sclerosis
Systemic lupus erythematosus
Polymyositis/dermatomyositis
Rheumatoid arthritis
Sjögren's syndrome
Vasculitis
Overlap syndromes
Cryoglobulinemia

### Miscellaneous

Hidden neoplasm
Arterial hypertension
Hematological diseases (e.g. cryoglobulinemia, Waldenström's macroglobulinemia)
Cardiovascular diseases (e.g. angina, intermittent claudication, heart failure)

**Table 25.5.** The most common causes of Raynaud's phenomenon.

It accounts for 85% of the total number of outpatient cases. This high percentage cannot justify less care in excluding underlying causes. Given the potential severity of linked conditions some authorities recommend clinical follow-up for at least 2 years even if systematic investigation for associated causes remains negative.

Table 25.5. shows the conditions most commonly associated with Raynaud's phenomenon.

Diffuse connective tissue diseases should always be considered. It is, however, important to bear in mind that these are relatively rare diseases and therefore account for a very small percentage of cases of Raynaud's phenomenon found in family medicine. Additional manifestations compatible with these diseases, especially in young females, should reinforce our suspicions and suggest appropriate tests.

## Diagnostic strategy

Unilateral Raynaud's phenomenon is generally associated with regional compression such as thoracic outlet syndrome, proximal arterial thrombosis or the use of vibratory machinery. Other cases are usually bilateral.

Our clinical enquiry should be thorough in a systematic search for risk factors, including medications that are "above suspicion" and symptoms suggesting an associated disease. A general clinical examination is naturally necessary, with special attention to the proximal sections of the limbs, if the phenomenon is unilateral.

Tests and scans should be requested on the basis of clinical findings suggesting one condition or another. Because of their sensitivity in detecting a variety of causes, a full blood count, simple biochemistry and protein electrophoretic strip, sedimentation rate, rheumatoid factor, antinuclear antibodies, urine summary and a chest x-ray are usually performed. An electromyogram, ultrasound with Doppler and even an arteriogram may be worth considering if we suspect neurological or vascular compromise.

If these tests and scans are negative, the need for additional investigation will depend on the severity of the manifestations and, possibly, on their response to general treatment. In most cases, Raynaud's phenomenon is discreet and well-tolerated. In these circumstances, it is enough to maintain regular clinical monitoring to check for warning signs, with no need for further investigation.

In the case of more severe manifestations or an association of symptoms suggesting an unknown cause, more precise studies may be warranted, usually under the care of a specialist.

An important investigation is capillaroscopy. It involves viewing the morphology of the capillaries of the ungual bed through a microscope. Megacapillaries, irregular diameter or other anomalies are highly suggestive of an underlying systemic disease (Figure 25.23.).

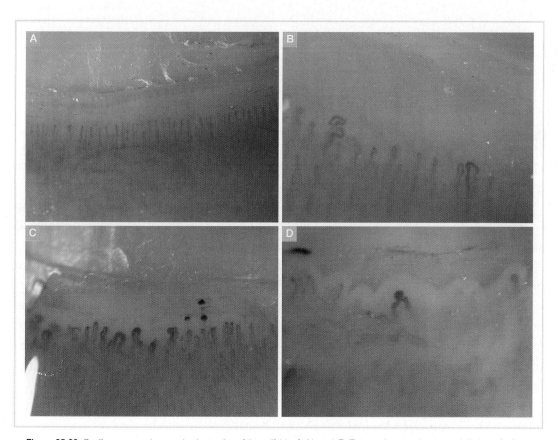

**Figure 25.23.** Capillaroscopy: microscopic observation of the nailfolds. **A.** Normal. **B.** Tortuous loops and segmental dilations. **C.** Giant capillaries, disorganization of capillary architecture and hemorrhage. **D.** Loss of capillaries ecapillary neoformation.

Figure 25.24. shows a diagram of our proposed diagnostic approach.

## Treatment

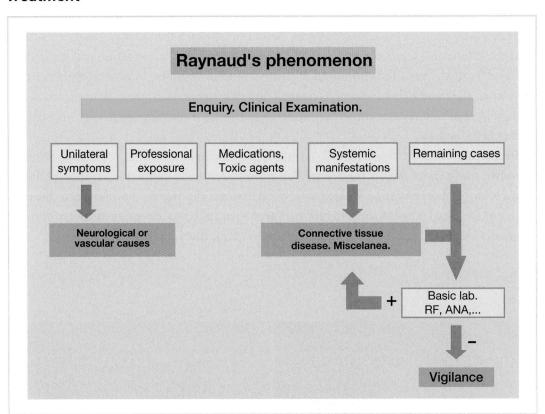

**Figure 25.24.**
Diagnostic strategy
for Raynaud's phe-
nomenon.

Treatment of Raynaud's phenomenon depends on the frequency and severity of the episodes.

The removal or treatment of the etiology identified is naturally of primordial importance whenever possible. This recommendation includes environmental and drug factors.

In all cases, it is essential to tell the patient to avoid exposure to cold and to "wrap up" in warm clothes, socks, gloves, and scarf and heat their homes if necessary. They should also avoid alcohol and coffee, and giving up smoking should be considered compulsory.

Treatment with medications should be reserved for patients whose attacks are more frequent or severe or who have ischemic lesions.

The medications used most are calcium channel antagonists, especially nifedipine. The recommended doses are 10–20 mg 3 times a day, though long-acting formulations can be used to improve compliance. Angiotensin converting enzyme inhibitors can be tried as an alternative. In many cases, treatment can be discontinued in spring and summer, depending on the temperature and response to treatment.

If there are significant trophic lesions, sweet almond oil or other moisturizing products can be applied. Nitroglycerin ointment (0.25%) or patches can also be used regionally under strict clinical supervision. Local infections warrant prescribing antibiotics. Referral to a specialist is fully justified in these cases.

Other medications should be reserved for use by specialists, not only because they require experience but also because they are only justified in severe, resistant conditions, usually associated with severe underlying diseases. These include serotonin receptor antagonists, sympatholytics, alpha-adrenergic antagonists and intravenous prostacyclin. Surgical treatment may be necessary in severe cases, with gangrene: digital sympathectomy, microsurgical revascularization or even amputation.

## ANTIPHOSPHOLIPID ANTIBODY SYNDROME

This condition has only recently been described and is characterized by the production of autoantibodies against phospholipids, resulting in prothrombotic diathesis with a variety of manifestations.

This syndrome should be suspected whenever one or more of the manifestations shown in Table 25.6. are present.

Repeated miscarriages with no apparent cause

Recurring arterial or venous thromboses

Livedo reticularis

CVAs in young people

Transitory coronary ischemia

Unexplained thrombocytopenia

**Table 25.6.** Common manifestations in antiphospholipid antibody syndrome.

More rarely, the syndrome is associated with cardiac valve vegetations and cardiac vasculopathy.

It may appear as an independent syndrome – so-called primary APS or in association with a variety of connective tissue diseases, particularly lupus.

Abnormal lab tests suggesting this condition include a false positive VDRL and isolated prolongation of the activated partial thromboplastin time and dilute Russell's viper venom test.

To make the diagnosis it is necessary to quantify antiphospholipid antibodies, such as anti-cardiolipin (IgG more significant than IgM), anti-$\beta$2 glycoprotein and lupus anticoagulant. Clinical and laboratory investigation for possible connective tissue disease is naturally warranted.

The identification of antibodies in the absence of clinical symptoms does not, at present, justify any specific treatment. The occurrence of symptoms calls for anti-platelet or anticoagulant treatment. The risk of miscarriage makes pregnancy in these patients "high risk," and they should be monitored by specialists.

## ADDITIONAL PRACTICE
### SYSTEMIC SYNDROMES

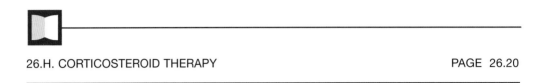

26.H. CORTICOSTEROID THERAPY                    PAGE 26.20

# OSTEOPOROTIC SYNDROME
## OSTEOPOROSIS

26.

J.A.P. da Silva, A.D. Woolf, *Rheumatology in Practice*, DOI 10.1007/978-1-84882-581-9_26,
© Springer-Verlag London Limited 2010

# 26. OSTEOPOROTIC SYNDROME OSTEOPOROSIS

*TYPICAL CASES*

**26.A. ACUTE CHEST PAIN**

Since he was a young man, Carlos Silvestre aged 56 had suffered from severe bronchial asthma, which had progressed to respiratory insufficiency. The severity of his condition had led to the chronic use of inhaled and oral corticosteroids. His physical activity was extremely limited and he rarely left home. We were called to see him after an emergency admission with violent chest pain and flail chest caused by multiple rib fractures that had occurred, according to the patient, during a recent coughing attack. Marked dorsal kyphosis reflected the presence of multiple vertebral fractures (confirmed by x-ray.), facilitated by the high pillows that he used.

Mr. Silvestre died a few months later after a pulmonary thromboembolism in a context of uncontrollable respiratory insufficiency.

If only we had prevented or treated his osteoporosis…

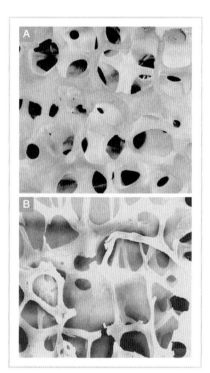

**Figure 26.1.** Osteoporosis starts by cancellous bone which is metabolically more active. Bone trabecullae become thinner and may be interrupted (microfractures), thus making the whole structure more fragile. Cortical bone is also lost. (**A.** Normal bone. **B.** Osteoporosis). © 2000 David W. Dempster, PhD.

## INTRODUCTION

"Osteoporotic syndrome" requires a particular mental attitude from the physician, as s/he should ***recognize the risk of disease*** and take action ***before any symptoms appear.***[1]

The manifestations of osteoporosis are fractures sustained after low impact trauma. They appear late and indicate that we have missed the optimal time for preventive action.

### Concept

> Osteoporosis: a systemic skeletal disease characterized by low bone mass and microarchitectural deterioration of bone tissue, with a consequent increase in bone fragility and susceptibility to low-impact fractures.

Bone owes its mechanical strength to a dense layer of cortical bone and to the bone trabeculae making up the cancellous bone that act as a support network. In osteoporosis, loss of bone mass begins with the cancellous bone, which is metabolically more active. The trabeculae become thinner and can even break (microfracture), leaving the whole structure more fragile. The cortical bone also becomes demineralized (Figure 26.1.). The process is generalized, although some parts of the skeleton are more susceptible than others.

[1]So it is not really a "syndrome" …

This weakening progresses silently without symptoms until there is a fracture. Osteoporotic fractures occur mainly in the elderly, but the process may have been developing since childhood.

- Osteoporosis is important exclusively because of the risk of fracture.
- Fractures are the complication that makes loss of bone mass relevant.
- Preventing fractures is the key goal of treating osteoporosis.

## Most common fractures and their consequences

The fractures most often associated with osteoporosis are those of the proximal femur, forearm (Colles fracture) and spine.

Fractures of the femur and forearm are usually obvious as they cause severe pain and functional disability. Fractures of the hip are accompanied by marked mortality, as about 20% of patients who suffer an osteoporotic fracture of the femur die in the following 12 months. Hip fractures alone cause more deaths than carcinoma of the cervix or ovaries and as many as breast cancer. Many of those who survive are left seriously disabled, needing help with activities of daily living, with resulting additional costs and suffering.

Spinal fractures are often asymptomatic and may be identified by chance in x-rays. In other patients, they can cause sudden, incapacitating pain, sometimes with nerve root compression. Because of the shape of vertebral bodies, there is no separation of the edges of the fracture; instead the tops of the bones become compressed resulting in a biconcave wedge- or cookie-shaped deformity (Figure 26.2.). The accumulation of vertebral deformities leads to progressive kypho-

**OSTEOPOROSIS**
**MAIN POINTS**

This is the weakening of the skeleton as a result of loss of bone mass and changes in microarchitecture.

It affects women more often than men and its prevalence increases considerably with age, even in the healthy population.

Its importance lies in the increased risk of low-impact fractures.

It develops without symptoms until fractures begin to occur.

The most common locations of osteoporotic fractures are the spine, forearm, proximal femur, ribs and pelvis.

Osteoporotic fractures constitute a serious public health problem, with a strong tendency to get worse in the next few decades.

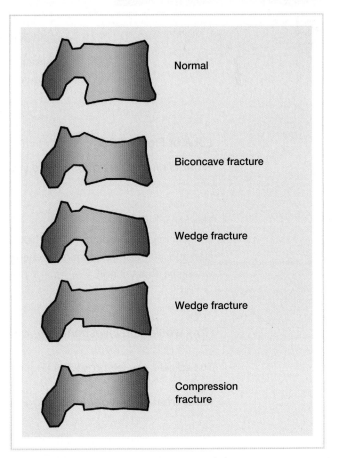

**Figure 26.2.** Different types of vertebral osteoporotic fractures.

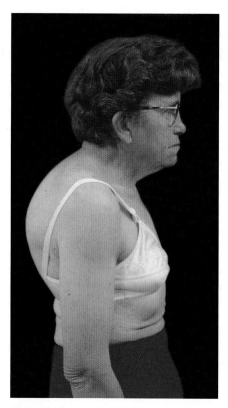

**Figure 26.3.** Clinical case "Kyphosis and back pain." Accentuaded kyphosis leading to compression of the abdomen by the chest wall.

sis, with the onset of chronic pain interspersed with exacerbations caused by new fractures. The kyphosis reduces thoracic expansion, exposing patients to respiratory insufficiency and increased risk of infection. The pressure of the thorax on the abdomen increases intra-abdominal pressure, exacerbating digestive problems and the tendency towards incontinence, which are common in the elderly. The deformity affects self-esteem, contributing further to the suffering. Even taking into account the age at which they occur, osteoporotic vertebral fractures severely affect quality of life and involve mortality similar to that of hip fractures, with a considerable reduction in life expectancy.

### TYPICAL CASES
### 26.B. KYPHOSIS AND BACK PAIN

Madalena was a charming elderly lady, whose musculoskeletal fragility contrasted with her cheerfulness at age 74. She came to us with continuous thoracic and lumbar pain that was preventing her from sleeping and leading a normal life. She also had pain in the anterior chest wall. Moreover, her "bronchitis" had worsened recently and she often "wet herself."

A simple examination of the patient made the problem clear (Figure 26.3.).

*Look at Figure 26.3.*

*What clinical clues does it give you as to the probable cause of the symptoms?*

The accentuated thoracic kyphosis was very probably due to multiple osteoporotic fractures, causing her lower ribs to rest on her abdomen, triggering pain while limiting thoracic expansion and increasing abdominal pressure. She measured a remarkable 136 cm (15 cm less than when she was young!).

*How would you investigate her condition?*

The spinal x-ray left no doubts (Figure 26.4.).

*What treatment would you suggest?*

We began analgesic and anti-osteoporotic treatment and recommended physical therapy and care with posture. We told the patient and her family to eliminate all factors that might lead to falls, which could have disastrous consequences.

## The social importance of osteoporosis

Osteoporotic fractures are recognized today as one of the largest public health problems in the developed world. They are responsible for about 1.5% of all days of hospitalization in the industrialized countries, using up far more resources than other chronic, non-transmissible diseases such as chronic liver disease, chronic obstructive pulmonary disease and many forms of cancer.

Estimates in the United States indicate that 30–50% of women will suffer at least one osteoporotic fracture in the course of their lives.[2]

The risk in men is about 20%, but it has been estimated that in around 50 years time there will be as many fractures in men as in women!

Indeed, with the progressive ageing of the population and the changes in eating habits and physical activity, we can expect the problem to grow rapidly in the next few decades, possibly doubling in the developed countries, and increasing more than sixfold in developing countries.

Osteoporosis has already been called the "silent epidemic." Only an appropriate preventive strategy based on public health measures and physicians' committed vigilance can reduce this scourge.

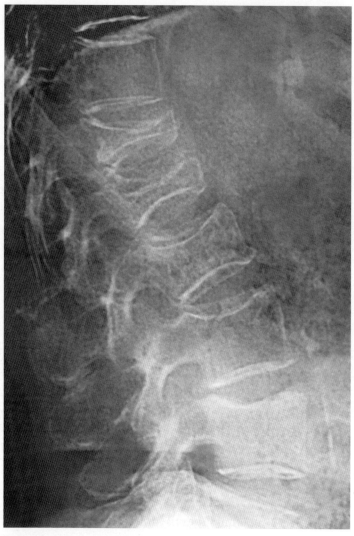

**Figure 26.4.** Clinical case "Kyphosis and back pain." Vertebral body deformities and note radiodensity of vertebral bodies barely greater than surrounding soft tissues.

# WHEN TO CONSIDER OSTEOPOROSIS

### Ideally, we should consider osteoporosis:

1. Whenever there are risk factors for developing the disease (i.e. in time to take prophylactic measures to prevent further loss of bone mass and resulting fractures).

2. Whenever a patient has suffered a fracture after minimum trauma or a spinal x-ray shows signs of accentuated osteopenia or fracture.

[2]Cauley JA. Risk of mortality following clinical fractures. Osteoporos Int 2000; 11: 556–561.

## TYPICAL CASES
## 26.C. THE "HEALTHY" PATIENT

Odete Romário, a 48-year old PA, came to our clinic with discreet, recurring pain in the lumbar and cervical region. Occasionally, she also had transient but troublesome pain in her arms. The pain was exacerbated by exercise and staying in one position for any length of time. It all seemed to have begun after the menopause, which had occurred spontaneously at the age of 46. The patient also described severe vasomotor disturbances typical of the menopause, to which she also attributed increased anxiety.

She smoked about 15 cigarettes a day. Her job meant that she led a very sedentary life. She did not do any kind of physical exercise. Her diet was varied but she avoided dairy products because of digestive problems. Where her family history was concerned, she said that her mother had suffered a wrist fracture at the age of 64.

The clinical examination found no anomalies in the painful areas. The patient weighed 47 kg (with a height of 150 cm) and her movements were easy and supple.

*Summarize the clinical problem.*[3]

*What would you do next?*

We performed a densitometry, which showed osteopenia (T score = −2.1 in the lumbar spine). Calcium and phosphate metabolism was normal. We discussed the situation with the patient, stressing the risk of developing osteoporosis and suffering fractures in the future. The patient agreed to hormone replacement treatment, to which we added calcium supplements (1 g/day). It was, unfortunately, difficult to convince her to take regular exercise and give up smoking. Two years later, the patient's bone mineral density was slightly higher and she was pleased with the general benefits of the treatment.

The main risk factors for osteoporosis are shown in Table 26.1. These factors are also the main indications for bone densitometry.

| Risk factors | Clinical manifestations |
|---|---|
| Post-menopausal woman | • Whenever a patient of any age has a history of low-impact fracture, i.e. caused by a fall of less than his or her own height from walking or standing, whether it manifests itself clinically or shows up radiologically, in a spinal x-ray for example |
| Early menopause | |
| Late menarche | |
| Low weight and stature | |
| Prolonged corticosteroid therapy | |
| Sedentary lifestyle | |
| Smoking | |
| Insufficient intake of dairy products | • Whenever an x-ray suggests low bone mass (radiological osteopenia) |
| Family history of osteoporosis | |
| Diseases causing osteoporosis: malabsorption, primary or secondary hypogonadism, gastrectomy, hyperthyroidism, hyperparathyroidism, chronic alcoholism, liver disease... | • Cases of accentuated thoracic kyphosis and/or loss of height |

Table 26.1.
Osteoporosis risk factors: indications for densitometry.

[3]Woman after early menopause, with discreet muscle pain and marked risk factors for osteoporosis: low weight and height, smoker, low intake of dairy products, sedentary lifestyle, slightly early menopause, family history suggesting osteoporosis.

Some risk factors are hard to quantify (e.g. sedentary lifestyle or low intake of dairy products) and some are more important than others. This makes it difficult to quantify the overall risk of osteoporosis in each patient and, thus, the indication for densitometry.

Several calculation methods that take into account a limited number of risk factors have been suggested for simplifying and rationalizing the selection of patients for bone densitometry.

The OST index is the simplest, as it considers only age and weight. Comparative studies[4] have shown that its specificity and sensitivity are comparable to the more complex indexes.

The calculation uses a simple formula:

$$\frac{\text{Weight (kg)} - \text{Age (years)}}{5}$$

In other words, the OST index is obtained by subtracting age from weight, dividing the result by 5 and then rounding it up or down to the nearest whole number.

For Caucasian populations, an index of less than −3 indicates a high risk of osteoporosis, indexes over 1 indicate a low risk and intermediate values (−3 to 1) a moderate risk. (Table 26.2).

| OST | Probability of osteoporosis | % Score T femur −2,5 |
|---|---|---|
| > 1 | Low risk | < 10% |
| 1 a −3 | Moderate risk | 18−23% |
| < −3 | High risk | 55−60% |

Table 26.2.
The OST index and the probability of osteoporosis in the densitometry.

Our practice is to recommend that all post-menopausal women with an OST of 1 or less should undergo a bone densitometry. This will identify over 90% of all osteoporosis sufferers and will save the need to conduct bone densitometry on about 1/3 of post-menopausal women. The use of a lower threshold (e.g. OST ≤ 0) will reduce the total cost but will leave more women undiagnosed.

Note that all these indexes have been validated only for post-menopausal women. The existence of other risk factors should also be taken into consideration. For example, a low-impact fracture justifies a bone densitometry without any other considerations.

### Radiological signs of osteoporosis

We should not place too much trust in standard radiography as an indicator of low bone mass. The bone density visible in x-rays may vary according to the dose of radiation, body mass index, etc. In addition, x-rays are not very sensitive and osteopenia only shows up after about 30% of the bone mass has been lost.

On the other hand, the presence of a vertebral fracture without apparent cause is a strong indication of osteoporosis and calls for a bone densitometry.

[4]Geusens P, Hochberg MC, van der Voort DJM, et al. Performance of risk indices for identifying low bone density in postmenopausal women. Mayo Clin Proc 2002; 77: 629–637.

We can considerably increase our sensitivity in the diagnosis of radiological osteopenia or osteoporotic fracture by conducting a methodical study of a lateral x-ray of the thoracic and lumbar spine:

1. See whether the density contrast between the vertebral bodies and the adjoining tissue is reduced.

2. Check whether the difference in radiological density between the edges of the vertebra (cortical bone) and its core (cancellous bone) has increased ("fish vertebrae").

3. Examine the transverse striation of the vertebrae – it is the first to be lost in cases of osteoporosis (Figure 26.5.).

4. If any of the vertebrae seem deformed, measure their height at the posterior and anterior edges and in the central part of the vertebral body. If these measurements differ from each other by more than 20%, this means that there is significant deformation, which is likely to be an osteoporotic wedge fracture (Figure 26.5.).

5. Rule out the possibility of focal lytic lesions that may reflect metastases or bone tumors.

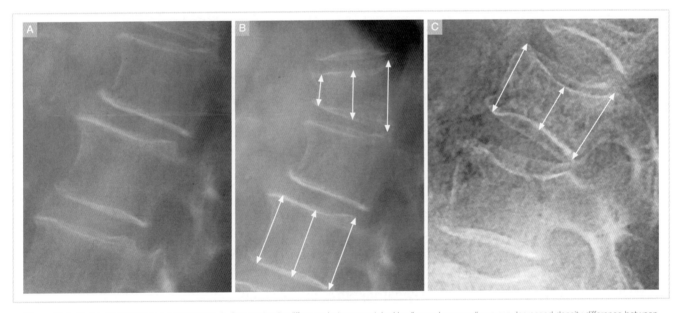

**Figure 26.5.** Radiological features of osteoporosis. **A.** Scarce density difference between vertebral bodies and surrounding areas. Increased density difference between cortical and cancellous bone. Loss of horizontal striae in the vertebral body. **B.** and **C.** Measurements to identify significant vertebral deformity. Wedege and biconcave fractures.

**A vertebral fracture of unknown cause imposes the consideration of a neoplastic disease.**

*TYPICAL CASES*

**26.D. A FRACTURE**

It was almost in passing that José Manaças, a 47-year old driver whom we saw for back pain, mentioned that he had suffered a wrist fracture 2 years before after falling while playing football with his children.

*Was this important?*

The enquiry turned up no risk factors for osteoporosis.

*Case closed?*

Even so, we decided to investigate further. A densitometry showed very low bone density in the spine and the femur (T score −2.7 in the femoral head). In view of these results, we requested a serum bone profile, which was normal, and testosterone and serum luteinizing hormone counts, both of which were very low. We began replacement treatment with two-weekly injections of testosterone. Mr. Manaças noted an immediate improvement in his general and sexual energy, though he did mention a degree of irritability. After 12 months, his BMD had gone up by 12% in the spine and 5.3% in the femoral head.

# STUDYING PATIENTS AT RISK OF OSTEOPOROSIS

If our clinical analysis of the risk factors shows a reasonable probability of osteoporosis, we have two objectives:

**1. Confirming the diagnosis and measuring bone mass:**

BONE DENSITOMETRY

**2. Assessing the existence of factors favoring osteoporosis:**

CLINICAL EXAMINATIONS AND LABORATORY TESTS

## Bone densitometry

This is the crucial test if you want to confirm osteoporosis. The most validated and widely used method is DEXA (Dual Energy X-ray Absorptiometry), which provides highly accurate, easily reproducible measurements of **bone mineral density** (BMD). The value shown is compared automatically to normal curves established for the general population of the same sex and race as the patient.

This parameter is shown in three ways in standard scans:

- **Absolute value** – This is expressed in grams of calcium per cm². This is "density" by surface unit and not by volume.

- **T score** – This describes the difference, in standard deviations, between the value measured in the patient and the average for young healthy adults of the same sex and race (which is when maximum lifelong bone mass is achieved).[5]

- **Z score** – This describes the difference, in standard deviations, between the value measured in the patient and the average for adults of the same sex and age group as the patient ("normal" value for age).

Look at Figure 26.6.

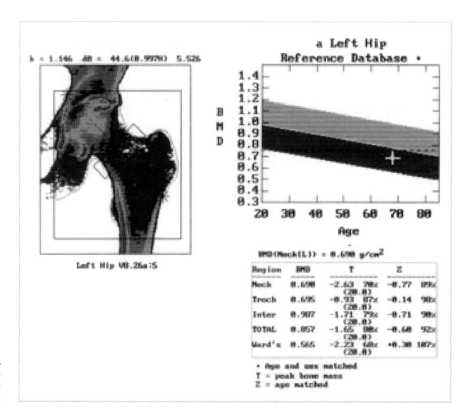

**Figure 26.6.**
Bone densitometry of the proximal femur.

### How do we interpret densitometry results?

T score is closely related to the risk of fracture. For each standard deviation lower than the young adult, the risk of fracture approximately doubles. The risk of fracture of a 70-year old women with a T score of −3 will therefore be about eight times greater than that of a woman of the same age with a T Score of 0 ($2^3$).

---

[5]The reason for expressing BMD as a T score and not as a absolute value is ordinary but unavoidable. There are different manufacturers of densitometers and the absolute values given by their machines are different for the same patient. As the error is about the same in all cases, however, including the reference population, T scores tend to be similar in different apparatuses.

The Z score indicates whether the patient's bone density is that expected in people of the same sex and age. The lower the Z score, the more likely it is that there are factors other than age and sex contributing to loss of bone mass. This warrants further investigation into secondary factors of osteoporosis requiring specific treatment.

Look at Figure 26.7. A 73-year old patient with a Z score of −0.54 (i.e. normal for her age and sex) has a T score of −2.87. This means that she has osteoporosis and an increased risk of fracture, but is perfectly normal for her age in terms of BMD. The T score of the 47-year old patient in Figure 26.8., indicates a similar increase in the risk of fracture, but the very low Z score (−2.27) shows that other factors may be contributing to the osteoporosis.

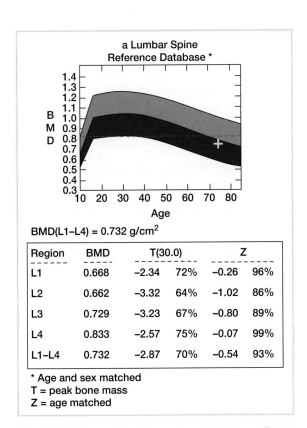

BMD(L1–L4) = 0.732 g/cm²

| Region | BMD | T(30.0) | | Z | |
| --- | --- | --- | --- | --- | --- |
| L1 | 0.668 | −2.34 | 72% | −0.26 | 96% |
| L2 | 0.662 | −3.32 | 64% | −1.02 | 86% |
| L3 | 0.729 | −3.23 | 67% | −0.80 | 89% |
| L4 | 0.833 | −2.57 | 75% | −0.07 | 99% |
| L1–L4 | 0.732 | −2.87 | 70% | −0.54 | 93% |

\* Age and sex matched
T = peak bone mass
Z = age matched

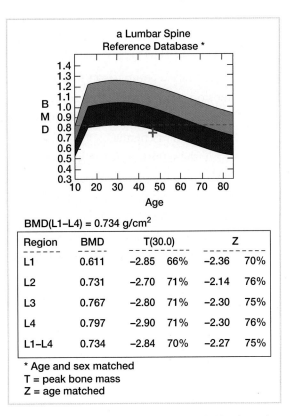

BMD(L1–L4) = 0.734 g/cm²

| Region | BMD | T(30.0) | | Z | |
| --- | --- | --- | --- | --- | --- |
| L1 | 0.611 | −2.85 | 66% | −2.36 | 70% |
| L2 | 0.731 | −2.70 | 71% | −2.14 | 76% |
| L3 | 0.767 | −2.80 | 71% | −2.30 | 75% |
| L4 | 0.797 | −2.90 | 71% | −2.30 | 76% |
| L1–L4 | 0.734 | −2.84 | 70% | −2.27 | 75% |

\* Age and sex matched
T = peak bone mass
Z = age matched

**Figure 26.7.** A 73 year old female, normal according to her age (Z score > −1), has osteoporosis (T score −2.87).

**Figure 26.8.** Z scores below −1 indicate a higher probability of secondary osteoporosis, i.e. determined by factors other than age and gender.

It is important to consider both scores at the same time, as BMD goes down progressively with age in perfectly normal people, especially after 50, and the risk of fracture increases proportionally. In other words, normal progression is to osteoporosis and fractures. If we always compared each patient with people of the same age (as we do in current definitions of normality) the risk of osteoporosis and fracture would always be the same throughout life, and this is not the case.

### Diagnosing osteoporosis

Today, the diagnosis of osteoporosis uses the WHO 1994 criteria – Table 26.3. It is based on T scores and previous fractures.

| Status | Definition |
|---|---|
| Normal | T score > –1 |
| Osteopenia | T score ≤ –1 > –2.5 |
| Osteoporosis | T score ≤ –2.5 |
| Severe osteoporosis | T score ≤ –2.5 with fractures |

**Table 26.3.** WHO criteria for defining osteoporosis.[6]

This definition is based on the relationship between T score and the risk of fracture.[7]

Note that a T score of –2.5 is a threshold of definition. It should not be regarded as a fracture threshold. The risk of fracture increases progressively as the T score goes down. A patient with a T score of –2.4 has a very similar risk of fracture to one with a T score of –2.6.

The WHO criteria should be regarded as an *operational definition of risk and not of the disease* itself. The idea is to identify patients at risk of fracture. This concept is easier to understand if we make a comparison with cardiovascular disease. In a way, a person with arterial hypertension is not sick until there are symptoms or tissue lesions. A patient with hyperlipidemia is not sick. We treat both conditions because we know that they increase the risk of disease: CVA or coronary ischemia.

In the same way, we define osteoporosis on the basis of BMD because we know that reduced BMD puts the patient at risk of disease: osteoporotic fracture and its consequences. The WHO definitions of osteopenia and osteoporosis establish a risk condition, just like hypertension or hyperlipidemia.

Note, on the other hand that, strictly speaking, a true diagnosis of osteoporosis would require a histological bone biopsy (parallel reduction in the organic matrix and mineralized bone) to distinguish it from other diseases, like osteomalacia (a reduction in mineralization only), which also involve decreased BMD. As the problem of these diseases is also the risk of fracture, however, the WHO's operational definition serves the main purpose, provided that we combine it with appropriate studies to distinguish the different metabolic conditions underlying low BMD. Idiopathic osteoporosis is, therefore, a diagnosis of exclusion.

---

[6]WHO Study Group. Assessment of fracture risk and its application to screening for postmenopausal osteoporosis. WHO Technical report Series, n° 843. WHO, Geneva, 1994.

[7]The WHO definition was established only for post-menopausal women, though its use has been extended to other groups, including men.

The concept of "severe osteoporosis" is that of a real disease, as the patient has already suffered a fracture.

> **Consideration of previous fractures is of vital importance. The simple fact that a patient has already suffered an osteoporotic fracture more than doubles the risk of new fractures, regardless of BMD.**

## Absolute risk of fracture

Ideally we should be able to base our decision to treat osteoporosis on the absolute risk of fracture for a given patient. Consideration of BMD, age and previous fracture as described above will only allow an estimate of relative risk, i.e., in comparison with someone without those risks.

Over recent years, a working group of WHO developed an extensive research program and analysis of the literature which identified several factors with a significant impact upon the risk of fracture, independently of bone density. These include: age, gender, previous fracture, a parental hip fracture, current or previous treatment with glucocorticoids, rheumatoid arthritis, smoking, low body mass index, high alcohol intake.

These factors were incorporated, together with bone mineral density, into an algorithm that allows an estimate of the risk of fracture over the ten following years for an individual patient.[8] This has also been made available as free-access tool in the internet: www.shef.ac.uk/FRAX.

The concept is that decisions on whom to treat should from now on be based on the individual's absolute risk of fracture. The threshold of risk at which medical intervention is recommended will depend on authoritative recommendations and personal choices by physicians.

In patients with osteoporosis demonstrated by densitometry, additional studies may be warranted to assess the existence of metabolic factors that favor bone mass loss and may need correcting. The tests are determined by the most common causes of secondary osteoporosis. The indication for these investigations is greater in patients with a Z score of less than $-1$.

---

*TYPICAL CASES*
### 26.E. THORACIC PAIN AND PROXIMAL MUSCLE WEAKNESS

Cândida Almeida, a charming, 66-year old retired teacher sought our help because of generalized weakness that prevented her from leaving her bed for more than a short while. She mentioned a recent episode of acute, incapacitating back pain after slipping slightly in the bath, which had further convinced her to stay in bed. She had very frequent night cramps and was visibly depressed.

She had been examined at her local hospital with no clear diagnosis.

The clinical examination showed an extremely fragile patient with highly limited movements. Muscle mass was atrophied and there was a clear reduction in proximal muscle strength, especially in the lower limbs. She had lost 7 cm in height.

*What possible explanations are there for this clinical pattern?*

*What tests would you request?*

---

[8]Kanis JA et al. FRAX TM and the assessment of fracture probability in men and women from the UK. Osteoporosis International 2008 Apr, 19(4): 385–397.

After she was hospitalized, we found very low serum calcium (7.2 mg/dl) and phosphorus (2.3 mg/dl) levels with marked elevation of alkaline phosphatase (1,232 U/ml). 24-hour urinary calcium excretion was only 22 mg. Serum parathormone was raised. Her densitometry was a "disaster": T score −4.78 in the spine and −7.08 in the femoral head. A vitamin D count and bone biopsy confirmed severe osteomalacia. Muscle enzymes were normal and a summary test for neoplasm was negative.

Intensive treatment with high doses of calcium and vitamin D with regular calcium control enabled the patient to regain her strength and resume her normal routine. After 10 months, a densitometry showed a remarkable 72% increase in BMD in the spine and 66–329% in the proximal femur (Figure 26.9.)!

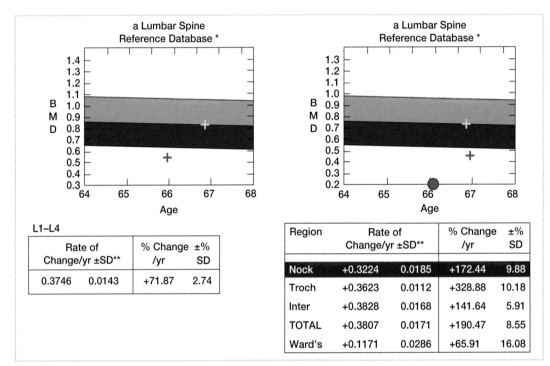

**Figure 26.9.** A case of severe osteimalacia: improvement of bone mineral density under treatment.

L1–L4

| Rate of Change/yr ±SD** | | % Change /yr | ±% SD |
|---|---|---|---|
| 0.3746 | 0.0143 | +71.87 | 2.74 |

| Region | Rate of Change/yr ±SD** | | % Change /yr | ±% SD |
|---|---|---|---|---|
| Nock | +0.3224 | 0.0185 | +172.44 | 9.88 |
| Troch | +0.3623 | 0.0112 | +328.88 | 10.18 |
| Inter | +0.3828 | 0.0168 | +141.64 | 5.91 |
| TOTAL | +0.3807 | 0.0171 | +190.47 | 8.55 |
| Ward's | +0.1171 | 0.0286 | +65.91 | 16.08 |

As a rule, we suggest that osteoporosis patients should undergo the following tests before beginning treatment (Table 26.4).

| Test | Women | Homens |
|---|---|---|
| Serum: | | |
| Calcium, phosphorus and magnesium | • | • |
| Electrophoretic protein strip | • | • |
| Alkaline phosphatase and γ-GT | • | • |
| Erythrocyte sedimentation rate | • | • |
| 24 h urine: calcium | • | • |
| Total serum testosterone and LH | | • |

**Table 26.4.** Lab tests in patients with osteoporosis.

All these tests will be normal in idiopathic osteoporosis.

Correct the level of calcium on the basis of serum albumin and compare it to the laboratory standard reference:

Corrected calcium (in mg/dl) = measured calcium – 0.8 X [albumin (in g/dl) – 4].

Corrected calcium (in mmol/l) = measured calcium – 0.2 X [albumin (in g/dl) – 4].

If there are changes in serum calcium and/or phosphate, it may be worth measuring parathormone. Joint assessment of these values makes it possible to evaluate the existence and type of anomalies in calcium/phosphate metabolism (Table 26.5.).

| Disease | Serum | | | | Urine |
|---|---|---|---|---|---|
| | Calcium | Phosphorus | Alkaline phosphatase | PTH | Calcium |
| Primary hyperparathyroidism | ↑ | ↓ | N or ↑ | ↑ | N or ↑ |
| Secondary hyperparathyroidism | ↓ or N | ↑ | ↑ | ↑ | ↓ |
| Hypoparathyroidism | ↓ | ↑ | N | ↓ | ↓ |
| Hyperthyroidism | ↑ or N | N or ↑ | N or ↑ | N or ↓ | ↑ |
| Pseudohypoparathyroidism | ↓ | ↑ | N or ↑ | N or ↑ | ↓ |
| Osteomalacia (vitamin D deficiency) | ↓ | ↓ | ↓↓ | ↑ | ↓ |
| Idiopathic osteoporosis | N | N | N | N | N |
| Paget's disease of bone | N | N | ↑↑ | N | N |

**Table 26.5.** Changes in lab tests in metabolic diseases influencing bone.

The electrophoretic protein strip measures albumin and investigates the possibility of multiple myeloma, which can involve accelerated osteoporosis. The erythrocyte sedimentation rate will be very high in these cases and also in chronic inflammatory diseases that contribute to osteoporosis. γ-GT serves mainly to confirm the bone origin of any elevation in alkaline phosphatase (γ-GT will be normal in this case but will tend to be raised if the origin is hepatic).

The need for a testosterone and LH (luteinizing hormone) count in men with osteoporosis lies in the fact that hypogonadism, which is often asymptomatic, is one of the main causes of male osteoporosis.

The clinical particularities of each patient may also warrant other studies, such as an evaluation of thyroid hormones or of 24-hour urine cortisol, among others.

# PREVENTION AND TREATMENT OF OSTEOPOROSIS

### Basic reasoning

The strategies for preventing osteoporosis are based on our knowledge of the development of BMD throughout life and the factors that influence it. Densitometry has made a decisive contribution to this knowledge (Figure 26.10.).

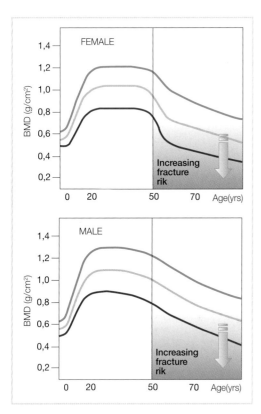

**Figure 26.10.** Normal evolution of BMD throughout life. Orange line: mean. Gree: +2 sd. Red: -2 sd.

Bone mineral density increases progressively during childhood and adolescence to reach its maximum level (peak bone mass) between the ages of 20 and 30. At this time, we have in our skeleton the calcium with which we are going to have to make do for the rest of our lives. In normal conditions, BMD remains more or less constant until the menopause in women and the age of 50 in men. In women, the lack of estrogen that sets in with the menopause causes a period of accelerated bone loss (2–3% a year) lasting about 10 years, after which it stabilizes to an annual rate similar to that of men (0.5–1% a year). We accumulate more calcium in our skeleton in childhood and adolescence than we lose in old age.

Bone mineral density (BMD) at any particular time of life is the result of the difference between bone mass achieved during the maturation of the skeleton (peak bone mass) and the loss over the subsequent years. Obviously, the higher the peak bone mass, the more protected we are against the risk of osteoporosis.

Now, the peak bone mass achieved by different people varies substantially from 20% above to 20% below the average. This means that a young man in the 5th centile of BMD has about 33% lower bone mass than one on the 95th centile. This variability is just as great, if not greater, than that found between people who do and those who do not suffer osteoporotic fractures after the age of 60.

In other words, osteopenia or osteoporosis in adults may be fully explained by deficient acquisition of bone mass in childhood, even if there has been no accelerated loss of bone mass after achieving skeletal maturity. Osteopenia in a healthy, pre-menopausal woman is more likely due to deficient acquisition of bone mass in her youth than to accelerated loss.

---

**Peak bone mass is at least as important as loss rate in determining BMD in older patients.**

**The interpretation of densitometry results must consider these two factors.**

---

**TYPICAL CASES**

**26.F. OSTEOPENIA**

Ivete Simões, a 43-year old teacher, was referred to us by her GP because of lumbar osteopenia (T score −2.1, Z score −1.7) detected in a densitometry that he had requested because
of back pain. He had prescribed treatment with biphosphonate.

Our thorough questioning of the patient was reassuring, except for her low intake of dairy products and very limited physical activity. She described a recent weight loss of 5 kg, which she
attributed to stress. She smoked about 20 cigarettes a day and was not taking any other medication. She had had her menarche when she was 11, her menstruation was still regular and
she had never had any significant diseases. She knew that her mother had osteoporosis, but
with no fractures yet.

*What do you think of this clinical pattern?*

*Do you think a densitometry should be requested for this patient?*

*What would you do?*

We suggested that she suspend treatment with bisphosphonate for at least a week before
the tests that we were requesting for calcium and phosphate metabolism and thyroid function. The results were normal.

We reassured the patient, explaining that the osteopenia was most likely due to her genetic her-
itage, exacerbated by poor diet, smoking and lack of physical activity. We encouraged her to
give up smoking, take more weight-bearing physical exercise (running or walking) and increase
her intake of dairy products (at least four doses a day). We suggested that she give serious consideration to hormone replacement treatment as soon as she reached the menopause.

## PREVENTION STRATEGIES

### Maximizing peak bone mass

The prevention of osteoporosis begins in childhood.

Several studies have shown that **60–80% of the variation in peak bone mass is determined
genetically.** Taken together, these studies suggest a polygenic hereditary influence with the
simultaneous involvement of a large number of different genes in the complex regulation of
bone formation and reabsorption. Among them are polymorphisms in the vitamin D receptor, several cytokines and growth factors, and type 1 collagen.

The non-hereditary factors that can affect peak bone mass are sex (higher values in men) and
endocrine factors, like late puberty and low levels of growth hormone or vitamin D. Low body
weight and lack of physical exercise can also contribute to deficient acquisition of bone mass.
A diet that is over-rich in proteins or poor in calcium, smoking and excessive alcohol intake also
have harmful effects.

*To maximize peak bone mass, action must be taken with young people:*

Encourage physical exercise.

Ensure sufficient calcium intake (≥ 1 g/day).

Ensure sufficient vitamin D intake.

Discourage smoking in young people.

Identify and correct conditions that limit bone mineralization (late menarche or adrenarche, malabsorption syndromes, endogenous or exogenous hypercortisolism, severe liver diseases, hemochromatosis, and hypogonadism).

**Table 26.6.** Prevention of osteoporosis in childhood and adolescence: maximizing peak bone mass.

Of the modifiable factors, smoking, calcium intake and physical exercise warrant particular attention (Table 26.6.).

Exercise plays an essential role. Some studies suggest that physical activity is actually more important in relative terms that calcium intake and can explain up to 17% of variations in BMD in people aged 25–30. Generally speaking, this beneficial effect is more marked in the peripheral than axial skeleton. The type of exercise is decisive, as only the areas placed under mechanical stress gain bone mass. Therefore, weight-bearing exercise such as walking and running are considerably more effective than swimming or cycling, where BMD is concerned.

Note, on the other hand, that excessive exercise as in championship-level sports, can sometimes have harmful effects, by inducing prolonged amenorrhea or delay puberty.

It has been demonstrated that calcium intake is decisive in increasing bone mass in children and adolescents. Consuming dairy products and other calcium-rich foods at this stage of life is therefore an essential pillar in preventing osteoporosis.

For practical purposes, we can consider that a regular dose of dairy products provides 200–250 mg of elementary calcium. In general, firm cheeses are richer in calcium than soft ones.

These factors are even more important in young people than in the elderly, as the calcium mass acquired during growth is much greater than that lost during ageing and a deficient peak bone mass cannot be corrected and will be a lifelong factor in the risk of osteoporosis.

*TYPICAL CASES*
**26.G. OSTEOPOROSIS AND CHILDHOOD**

We prescribed the appropriate treatment, when we identified osteoporosis in 53-year old Sara. Knowing that she had children, we strongly urged her to recommend to them the same as we recommended to her: abundant intake of dairy products, regular physical exercise, no drinking or smoking, and prevention of osteoporosis caused by any disease or intercurrent therapy.

### Preventing loss of bone mass in adults

These preventive measures are suitable for the whole population, but especially for those with densitometric osteopenia at a relatively young age.

Preventive measures involve ensuring sufficient calcium intake, normal vitamin D production, reasonable levels of physical activity and correction of osteoporosis-inducing diseases or treatments.

Hormone replacement therapy is the physiological medication for preventing accelerated bone loss in the postmenopausal years. Its efficacy is well established. However, its association with an increased risk of breast cancer and thromboembolic events has vastly reduced its indications.

In spite of these doubts, it is generally agreed that the overall balance of risk and benefit of hormone replacement is favorable to women undergoing early menopause (before 45 years). This benefit is greater if the patient suffers significant menopausal vasomotor manifestations.

Other medications for the prevention of osteoporosis should only be considered in cases of osteopenia in people under the age of 65 associated with other risk factors for osteoporosis, as this makes the disease sufficiently probable to justify medication. This is the case, for example, of someone aged 50 with a T *score* of −1.7 to whom we are going to prescribe prolonged corticosteroid therapy. Knowing that corticosteroids can cause massive loss of bone mass in a very short time, it is advisable to prescribe a vitamin D supplement and introduce biphosphonate or calcitonin early on as a preventive measure.

---

**_To prevent loss of bone mass in adults:_**

Encourage physical exercise.

Ensure sufficient calcium intake (≥ 1 g/day).

Prescribe a vitamin D supplement (~800 U/day) if you suspect vitamin deficiency.

Discourage smoking, excessive alcohol.

Consider hormone replacement treatment in early postmenopausal women.

Reduce corticosteroids and thyroxine to the minimum necessary dose.

Identify and correct conditions that obstruct bone mineralization (late menarche or adrenarche, malabsorption syndromes, endogenous or exogenous hypercortisolism, severe liver diseases, hemochromatosis, and hypogonadism).

Consider other preventive medication if the patient has osteopenia and other important risk factors for osteoporosis.

Table 26.7.
Preventing loss of
bone mass in adults.

---

### Preventing corticosteroid-induced osteoporosis

Corticosteroid treatment in moderate and high doses (over 5 mg/day of prednisone equivalent) is associated with accelerated loss of bone mass and an increased risk of fracture. This loss is faster in the first 6 months of treatment, and the cancellous bone is more susceptible than cortical bone. For this reason, any steroid therapy that is expected to last more than 3 months should be associated with osteoporosis prevention from the start.

---

*TYPICAL CASES*

**26.H. CORTICOSTEROID THERAPY**

Sandra Antunes was 27 when we diagnosed systemic lupus erythematosus with renal involvement, which would oblige us to prescribe long-term corticosteroid treatment. The patient had no osteoporosis risk factors other than a family history of the disease. Her densitometry showed a T score of −1.7 in the spine and −1.2 in the femoral head.

---

***What care would you recommend in addition to the treatment of the basic disease?***

We associated 70 mg/week of alendronate and 800 U/day of cholecalciferol, and encouraged the patient to follow a calcium-rich diet and do 30–60 minutes' exercise a day.

The rules for preventing corticosteroid-induced osteoporosis can be summarized as follows.[9]

- *Minimum essential dose of corticosteroids*
  Administration on alternate days is not enough to prevent bone mass loss.
  Preference should be given to topical or inhaled forms whenever possible.

- *No smoking, limited alcohol intake,* and *weight-bearing exercises* for 30–60 minutes a day.

- *Daily calcium intake of 1.5 g* in food or supplements unless there is a contraindication.

- *800 U/day of vitamin D or 0.5 µg/day calcitriol.*

- *Associated alendronate, risedronate* in high-risk cases or if the above measures are not applicable or sufficient.

### TREATING OSTEOPOROSIS

Here we are assuming that the patient has demonstrable osteoporosis, i.e. a bone densitometry has shown a T score of < −2.5 in one or more sites. According tom the new WHO paradigm, treatment is also justified if the absolute risk of fracture is significantly increased, even if T score is above the diagnostic threshold.

Ideally, a densitometry should be performed before starting pharmacological treatment, as this will allow a better estimate of fracture risk and assist in the evaluation of treatment efficacy.

### A. General measures

Treatment obviously requires correcting all modifiable risk factors (Table 26.7.). If in doubt as to your patient's vitamin D concentration, administer 800 U/day of cholecalciferol, as the iatrogenic risk is minimal. On the other hand, all specific drugs for osteoporosis are only demonstrably effective in the presence of sufficient levels of calcium and vitamin D.

---

[9]Recommendations for the prevention and treatment of glucocorticoid-induced osteoporosis. American College of Rheumatology task force on osteoporosis guidelines. Arthritis Rheum 1996; 39: 1791–1801.

Devogelaer et al. Evidence-based guidelines for the prevention and treatment of gulcocorticoid-induced osteoporosis: a consensus document of the Belgian Bone Club. Osteoporos Int 2006; 17: 8–19.

## B. Pharmacological treatment

Most products used in the treatment of osteoporosis inhibit bone resorption. Their administration to osteoporotic patients causes a slight increase in BMD (2–10% in the spine and less at other sites) in the first 2 or 3 years, stabilizing after that. This increase is not usually enough to restore a normal level. In spite of relatively modest increases in BMD, however, some anti-resorption medications have proved to be more effective in preventing fractures than the change in BMD would suggest. This means that bisphosphonates, in particular, act to reduce fractures in ways other than through bone mass.

### Bisphosphonates

Alendronate has been the subject of extensive, conclusive studies. Administered in a continuous dose of 10 mg/d it increases bone mass from 5–8% in the spine and 3–5% in the femoral head and reduces the incidence of vertebral and non-vertebral fractures by about 50%. Administration of 70 mg a week has a similar effect on BMD.

Risedronate is recommended in a dose of 5 mg per day or 35 mg once a week, with which it has been possible to achieve significant increases in BMD and reduce the vertebral fracture rate by about 50% in good-quality studies. Risedronate is also efficacious in the prevention of non-vertebral fractures.

Zoledronic acid administered at the dose of 5 mg in intravenous infusion at yearly intervals has also demonstrated efficacy in the prevention of both vertebral and non-vertebral fractures.

Other bisphosphonates, such as etidronate and ibandronate have less solid evidence of efficacy upon non-vertebral fractures. Digestive absorption of all bisphosphonates is poor and is reduced to zero in the presence of food. They should therefore be administered far away from mealtimes, preferably in a fasting state, with water only, and at least half an hour before eating. The most common side effects include irritation of the proximal digestive tract. Rarely, they can cause hypercalcemia.

### Raloxifene

Raloxifene is a selective estrogen receptor modulator. It acts on the bone and vascular receptors, preventing and treating osteoporosis, but does not stimulate the breast or endometrium, thus avoiding the risk of carcinoma in these sites that is found with long-term administration of natural estrogens. It is, however, associated with a high degree of recurrence of the vasomotor manifestations of the menopause. A large prospective, randomized study has shown that long-term administration of raloxifene (60 mg/day) prevents about 50% of osteoporotic vertebral fractures. Unfortunately, it showed no efficacy in preventing non-vertebral fractures, including hip fractures.

---

**TREATMENT OF OSTEOPOROSIS**
**MAIN POINTS**

**General measures:**

- Correcting risk factors
- Diet
- Physical exercise

**Medication**

- Biphosphonate
- Raloxifene
- Strontium Ranelate
- Calcitonin
- Estrogen

**Preventing falls**

### Strontium

A large randomized controlled trial of strontium ranelate in the dose of 1 g twice daily over 3 years demonstrated that this medication may approximately halve the incidence of vertebral fractures in osteoporotic women. Data suggests the extravertebral fractures can also be significantly reduced in certain subgroups of patients. All patients were given supplements of calcium and vitamin D. This medication was well tolerated.

### Hormone replacement treatment

Hormone replacement treatment (HRT) is effective in preventing loss of bone mass in post-menopausal women. Retrospective studies have shown that it significantly reduces the incidence of fractures of the vertebrae and probably also of the proximal femur. A large prospective study of unselected women also showed that HRT (conjugated equine estrogen 0.625 mg, with 2.5 mg of medroxyprogesterone acetate, in this case) is associated with a significant reduction in the incidence of osteoporotic fractures of the femur. The same study also demonstrated that this treatment is, however, associated with an increase in the risk of breast cancer and cardiovascular events, which questions its overall utility.[9] Although many points of this issue still have to be clarified, **in the light of present evidence the use of HRT is not justified in the treatment of osteoporosis.**

### Calcitonin

Nasal spray salmon calcitonin prevents loss of bone mass. Its effect on the occurrence of fractures with long-term administration was the subject of a study that showed efficacy in the prevention of vertebral fractures (a reduction of about 33%) but not non-vertebral fractures. The efficacious dose is 200 U/day, on a continuous basis. There is no demonstration of efficacy on fractures with lower or higher doses. Calcitonin also has analgesic properties independent of its anti-osteoporotic effect which makes it useful when treating the acute, painful phase of vertebral fractures.

### Other agents

Replacement doses of testosterone are the basis for treatment of male osteoporosis due to hypogonadism, where it can induce substantial increases in bone mass. Its effect on BMD has also been demonstrated in osteoporotic men without hypogonadism. It requires monitoring of the risks of prostate hyperplasia and neoplasm, and dyslipidemia.

In rare selected cases of osteoporosis with general muscle fragility, careful use of anabolic androgens, like nandrolone, may be considered.

Tibolone is a synthetic derivative with estrogenic, progestational and slightly androgenic properties. It has a beneficial effect on several symptoms of the menopause and does not cause endometrial proliferation or hemorrhage. It increases bone mineral density but its effects on the incidence of fractures have not yet been described and its long-term impact on cardiovascular mortality has not been evaluated.

Recent studies of parathormone derivatives (Teripatide) have shown a marked increase in BMD and an accentuated decrease in the risk of fracture in post-menopausal women with osteoporosis and previous fractures, opening up new prospects in the treatment of severe fracturing

[9]Writing Group. Risks and benefits of estrogen plus progestin in healthy postmenopausal women. Principal results from the Women's Health Initiative randomized controlled trial. JAMA 2002; 288: 321–333.

osteoporosis. A extensive evidence-based guideline for osteoporosis diagnosis and treatment has been recently published.[10]

### C. Preventing falls

Even when fragile, osteoporotic bones only usually fracture with trauma. Falls at home are the main cause of osteoporotic fractures. Preventing them can be as, or even more, effective than pharmaceutical treatment to prevent fractures.

When possible, avoid using psychotropic or other agents that can reduce your patient's alertness. Advise against alcohol. Compensate for disturbances in sight and balance. Encourage patients to remove any risk factors from their homes: loose rugs, wires, poor lighting, etc. Advise them to wear firm, adherent footwear and install support handles in the bathtub. Encourage the elderly to take exercise (dancing, for example). Even if it does not increase bone mass it will improve balance and stability.

### *Monitoring treatment*

Clinical evaluation should include weight, height, risk factors, medications and previous fractures. In cases of acute vertebral pain or significant loss of height (> 1 cm), the comparison of a lateral x-ray of the thoracic and lumbar spine with recent radiographs enables us to identify new fractures. In case of doubt as to whether they are old fractures, local hyperfixation in bone scintigraphy identifies recent fractures (Figure 26.11.).

Assessment of BMD response is currently the basis for evaluating the efficacy of treatment. Given that the reproducibility error in densitometry is 1–2%, there must be a minimum difference of 3–6% in the same patient to guarantee that there has been a significant change in bone density. As a rule, it is therefore no use in repeating the densitometry less than 2 years after beginning a treatment regimen, unless we expect a more dramatic change (Figure 26.9.).

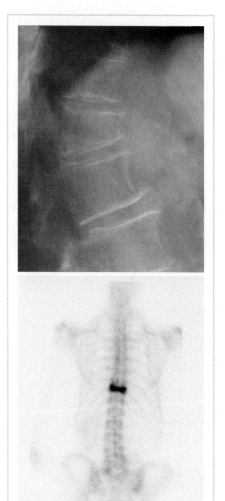

**Figure 26.11.** Bone scintigraphy in osteoporosis. Increased radiotracer fixation indicates that the fracture is relatively recent (< 1 year).

### *Treating acute fractures*

The treatment of vertebral pain associated with fractures involves general measures and not anti-osteoporotic treatment. Acute pain: bed rest (several days), analgesics, local heat and massage. Calcitonin is quite useful in this phase. The *temporary* use of a spinal support may be useful. Physical therapy should begin as soon as possible.

Chronic pain associated with multiple fractures: analgesics, physical therapy, intermittent use of a spinal support for certain activities, a regular exercise program and loss of excess weight.

In most patients, fracture of the proximal femur requires surgery with internal fixation or a total hip prosthesis. Early mobilization and proper diet after fractures are important.

Always begin appropriate osteoporosis treatment if the patient is not already taking it.

[10]Kanis et al. European Guidance for the diagnosis and management of osteoporosis in postmenopausal women. Osteoporos Int 2008; 19: 399–428.

## ADDITIONAL PRACTICE
### OSTEOPOROSIS.

# BONE SYNDROME
## BONE DISEASES

**27.**

J.A.P. da Silva, A.D. Woolf, *Rheumatology in Practice*, DOI 10.1007/978-1-84882-581-9_27,
© Springer-Verlag London Limited 2010

# 27. BONE SYNDROME BONE DISEASES

### *When to consider bone disease*

Essentially in two circumstances:

1. Deep, ill-defined, continuous pain, unrelated to movement, confined to one area of the skeleton, after excluding pain referred from the internal organs.

2. Whenever a pathological fracture occurs, i.e. with no significant trauma (see Chapter 4).

Pain originating exclusively in the bone is rare in clinical practice. Table 27.1. lists the most common bone diseases. It may appear in association with bone tumors (primary or secondary/metastatic), metabolic diseases (e.g. osteoporosis, Paget's disease of bone or hyperparathyroidism) or inflammation of the periosteum. It is most common in the spine and pelvis and proximal segments of the limbs. In malignant lesions and osteomyelitis there is often fever. The local examination is usually normal.

| |
|---|
| Osteoporosis |
| Primary and metastatic bone tumors |
| Osteomalacia |
| Hyperparathyroidism |
| Paget's disease of bone |
| Osteonecrosis |
| Osteomyelitis |

**Table 27.1.**
The most common bone diseases.

Osteoporosis is, by far, the most common of the bone diseases, causing more fractures than all the others together. Its clinical context is quite different, however. Unlike the other conditions, we must act before any symptoms appear. This is why it has been discussed separately in Chapter 26. The other bone diseases may also be asymptomatic for a long time and are detected by chance in x-rays.

When the patient's condition suggests bone disease and we can find no suggestion of referred pain, we must look for signs and symptoms of systemic neoplastic disease and request the appropriate diagnostic tests.

The most important is an ordinary x-ray which, in most cases, indicates the type of lesion. Calcium/phosphate metabolism, erythrocyte sedimentation rate and electrophoretic protein strip can be very useful (Table 26.5.). Scans such as MRI and bone scintigraphy can also be helpful.

### *Diagnostic strategy*

1. *"Bone" pain or pathological fractures*

   As we have already mentioned, pain is rare in primary osteoporosis except when there is a fracture. Intense, unrelenting pain suggests a neoplastic lesion. Paget's bone disease is often asymptomatic but can also cause continuous dull pain or a sensation of deep heat in the affected area. All bone diseases can lead to pathological fractures.

2. *Assess signs and symptoms of systemic disease (neoplastic, metabolic)*
Ask the patient about weight loss, fever and any symptoms suggesting the most common forms of neoplasm for their risk group. Evaluate possible causes of pain referred to the region in question (Chapters 4 and 5, Table 5.1.). Recent infection may, rarely, herald osteomyelitis. Osteomalacia and hyperparathyroidism can cause generalized pain and proximal muscle weakness. Look for signs of finger clubbing and risk factors for hypertrophic osteoarthropathy. Conduct a thorough general investigation, including a neurological examination.

3. Request *x-rays of the painful region* and neighboring areas if the pain is localized, *and/or*
*bone scintigraphy* if you suspect disseminated disease.
X-rays may be informative but are rarely diagnostic.

4. *Ask for additional diagnostic tests, if appropriate, or immediately refer the patient to a specialist.*

## PAGET'S DISEASE OF BONE

This is a local disturbance of bone remodeling that leads to profound changes in tissue structure. It can affect only one or several separate areas of the skeleton. Localized high volume circulation of the blood can cause pain and local heat. The weakened bone may fracture. Bone deformities may cause symptoms by compressing adjacent structures or involving the joints. In severe cases, the bone deformities can be obvious on mere inspection. X-rays and bone scintigraphy show the site of the lesion (Figure 27.1.).

The geographical distribution of Paget's is strange, as it is more prevalent in certain areas. This characteristic led to the suspicion of

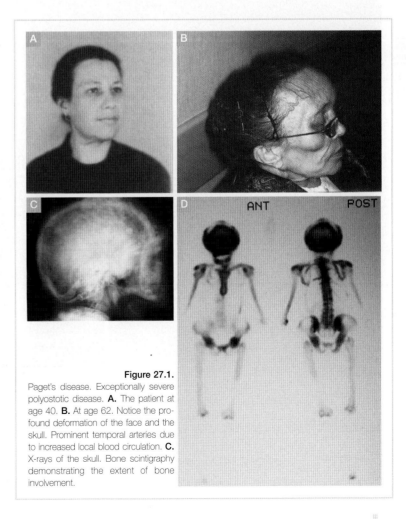

**Figure 27.1.**
Paget's disease. Exceptionally severe polyostotic disease. **A.** The patient at age 40. **B.** At age 62. Notice the profound deformation of the face and the skull. Prominent temporal arteries due to increased local blood circulation. **C.** X-rays of the skull. Bone scintigraphy demonstrating the extent of bone involvement.

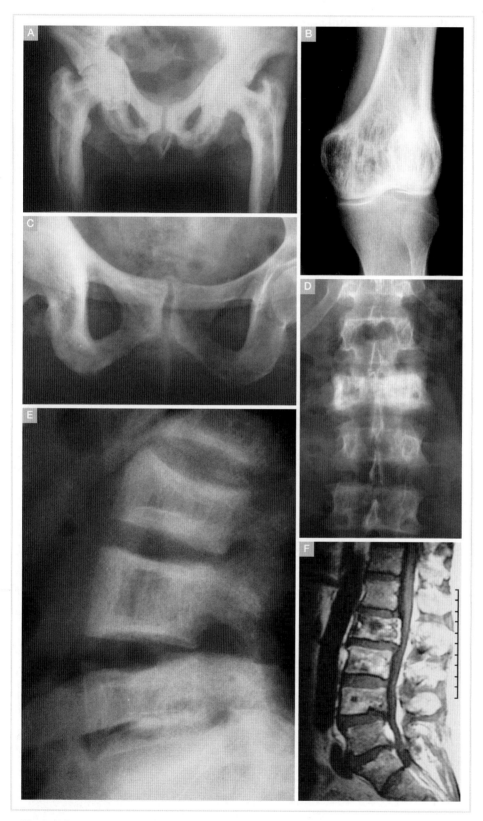

**Figure 27.2.** Radiological features of Paget's disease. **A.** and **B.** Trabecullar disorganization with and "cotton-wool" look. **C.** and **D.** Increased dimensions of affect structures. **E.** "Picture frame" vertebrae. F. CT scan. Disorganization of bone structure and enlargement of the vertebral body.

a source of infection, though this was never proved.

We should consider the possibility of Paget's disease of bone in patients with bone pain unrelieved by rest or with progressive bone deformities. The most common forms of presentation are the chance detection of high levels of alkaline phosphatase, in the absence of other indicators of a biliary or hepatic condition, or the findings of typical radiographic changes.

The radiographic features are, in fact, highly suggestive. There is marked disorganization of the trabecular structure with alternating osteopenic and osteosclerotic areas, looking like cotton wool. The bone increases in size. The vertebrae may gain the characteristic "picture-frame" appearance. In the skull, the disease may look like circumscribed osteopenia. The bones can become severely deformed (Figure 27.2.).

## TYPICAL CASES
## 27.A. ELEVATED ALKALINE PHOSPHATASE AND BACK PAIN

Fernanda was sent to us by her GP with back pain that was unresponsive to analgesics. He had noticed clear deformity of the 10th thoracic vertebra in an x-ray.

*Look at Figure 27.3. What is your interpretation?*

*What additional tests would you run?*

We found these images highly suggestive of Paget's disease of bone: coarse disorganization of the trabeculae, and an increase in size of the vertebral body. We requested lab tests, which showed 736 U/ml alkaline phosphatase, while the other liver enzymes were normal. This information confirmed our diagnosis. We requested an isotope bone scan to check for other sites of the disease. The 10th dorsal vertebra showed marked uptake of radioisotope. The scan revealed another area of increased uptake involving the sacrum. A local x-ray also found changes compatible with Paget's disease (Figure 27.4.).

We began treatment with alendronate (10 mg/day). The patient's alkaline phosphatase went back to normal in the following months and her pain at rest disappeared progressively.

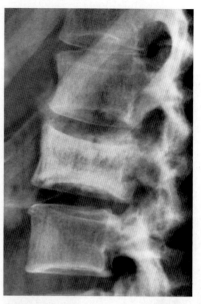

**Figure 27.3.** Clinical case "Elevated alkaline phosphatase and back pain".

## PAGET'S DISEASE OF BONE
## *MAIN POINTS*

This is a profound but localized bone remodeling disturbance.

Its cause is unknown.

It usually appears after the age of 50.

Its most common locations are the pelvis, spine, femur, skull, humerus and tibia.

It can be mono- or polyfocal.

Only about 30% of patients have symptoms: bone pain, local sensation of heat and deformities.

It may cause arthropathy in the neighboring joints and neurological and vascular complications due to pressure.

X-ray images are typical.

Alkaline phosphatase is elevated and its levels enable us to assess response to treatment.

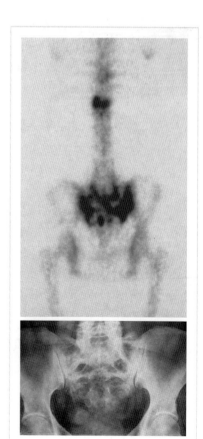

**Figure 27.4.** Clinical case "Elevated alkaline phosphatase and back pain." Paget's disease.

Although they are typical, these images require differential diagnosis from other conditions, such as prostate cancer metastases (Figure 27.5.). The study of these patients should therefore include a search for possible neoplasm. Isotope bone scanning is extremely useful in assessing local lesions and their extent.

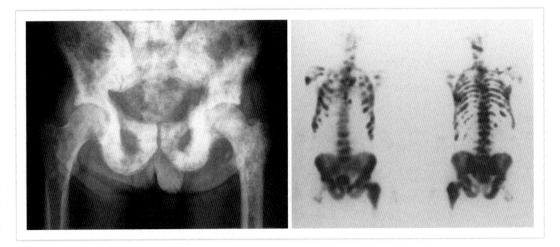

**Figure 27.5.**
Massive bone metastases from prostate cancer, simulating Paget's disease.

Mild forms can be treated in outpatient clinic with oral calcitonin or biphosphonates. More extensive forms or those affecting sensitive areas (the spine, temporal bone or around the joints) are better treated with intravenous 3rd generation biphosphonates (pamidronate or zoledronic acid, for example), in order to prevent osteoarthritis and pressure complications (compression myelopathy, deafness, etc.). The efficacy of the treatment is assessed by the reduction in alkaline phosphatase. The goal is to normalize it.

Follow-up of these patients should take into account the risk of these pagetic lesions developing into sarcoma.

All patients with suspected Paget's disease should be examined at least once by a specialist.

## OSTEOMALACIA

Osteomalacia should be suspected in elderly patients with a poor diet and little exposure to sunlight. Institutionalized patients are particularly at risk. Other high-risk patients are those with malabsorption syndromes (chronic pancreatitis, for example), gastrectomy or renal disease. Today many patients are diagnosed during densitometry for osteoporosis.

This is a general impairment of bone mineralization caused by vitamin D deficiency.

For a typical case, see "thoracic pain and proximal muscle weakness" (Chapter 26).

The patient may present with ill-defined axial and proximal pain and pain on pressure on the bone. More severe forms are accompanied by proximal myopathy, with sometimes incapacitating weakness. There may be spontaneous fractures of the femur, pelvis and other sites. The fractures are often "green stick" fractures with pain but only limited functional disability. In x-rays they may show up as the so-called Looser lines (Figure 27.6.).

A study of calcium/phosphate metabolism shows low serum levels of calcium, phosphorus and vitamin D. PTH is usually elevated (secondary hyperparathyroidism). Bone mineral density is often very low. If in doubt, a bone biopsy confirms the diagnosis.

Treatment involves vitamin D2 or D3 in doses of 800 to 4,000 UI/day for 8 to 12 weeks, followed by 200 to 400 UI/day. A calcium supplement should be added, depending on the patient's diet. The response to treatment is marked by a rapid rise in phosphorus levels. If there is none, this indicates resistance to vitamin D.

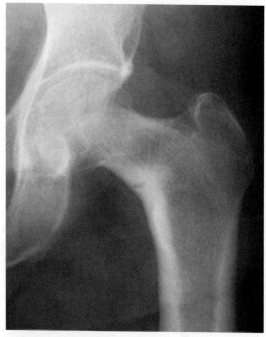

**Figure 27.6.** Insufficiency fracture – Looser zone. Patient with osteomalacia. (Courtesy: Dr. Pratas Peres. Coimbra.)

## PRIMARY HYPERPARATHYROIDISM

The frequency of hyperparathyroidism varies considerably from one population to another, though it mainly affects people over 60. Widespread measurement of serum calcium means that many patients are identified in the early stages before any symptoms appear. In severe forms, the symptoms can include diffuse pain, kidney stones and neuropsychiatric disturbances, such as depression ("bones, stones, groans and moans"). Pathological fractures may occur. The so-called brown tumor is rare these days.

Diagnosis is based on high calcium levels (corrected for albumin), generally associated with hypophosphatemia. The association of high serum PTH makes the diagnosis (Table 26.5.). In the other causes of hypercalcemia (e.g. sarcoidosis and bone metastases), PTH is low.

Radiographic changes (Figure 27.7.) appear late and are inconsistent.

Ultrasound and CT scans of the parathyroid glands almost always show a nodule or hypertrophy of one or more parotids. Basic treatment involves their surgical removal.

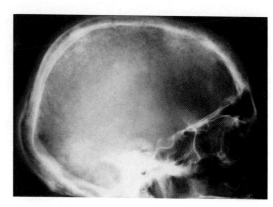

**Figure 27.7.** Hyperparathyroidism. Patchy resorption of cortical bone leading to a suggestive "salt and pepper" appearance in the X-ray of the skull.

## METASTATIC BONE DISEASE

In many cases, bone metastases and the associated symptoms appear in patients with known neoplasm or with suggestive systemic symptoms. It is not, however, uncommon for bone metastases to be the first sign of asymptomatic neoplasm, especially of the breast or prostate. Continuous bone pain and pathological fractures are the usual signs. A pathological fracture should always raise this suspicion, even in patients with risk factors for osteoporosis.

Lab tests may reveal hypercalcemia and elevated alkaline phosphatase.

Metastases occur most frequently in the spine, hips and proximal bones in the limbs. Most of the lesions are radiographically osteolytic, but breast and prostate metastases can be osteosclerotic (Figure 27.5.).

Isotope bone scanning is the technique of choice for locating the lesions (Figure 27.8.). A specific biopsy may be necessary to identify the nature of the tumor and orient the search for the primary lesion.

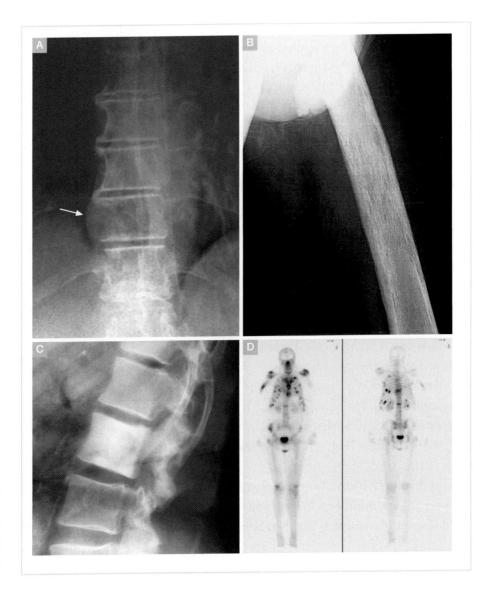

**Figure 27.8.**
Bone metastasis. **A.** Lytic lesions in the spine (Gastric carcinoma). **B.** Lytic lesions of the humerus (Lung cancer). **C.** Sclerotic metastasis – Ivory vertebra (Breast cancer). **D.** Bone scintigraphy showing multiple bone metastasis (lung cancer).

# PRIMARY BONE TUMORS

These are relatively rare. A large number of benign tumors are found by chance in x-rays or scintigraphy. The existence of pain seemingly of the bone should suggest this possibility and is often accompanied by weight loss and fever in malignant tumors.

They can originate in the bone, cartilage or bone marrow. Some come from cartilaginous residue inside the bone.

The most common forms are described briefly below.

## Multiple myeloma

This is the most common form of primary bone tumor. It generally affects men aged between 40 and 60. It consists of monoclonal proliferation of B lymphocytes. The patient usually suffers weight loss and fever. An accelerated form of "osteoporosis," with multiple fractures, may be a misleading presentation, but it should still undergo the investigation recommended for all patients with osteoporosis. Erythrocyte sedimentation rate is usually very high and, in most patients, the protein strip shows a monoclonal peak in the gamma fraction.

X-rays may show osteolytic lesions (Figure 27.9.), though in some cases there is nothing more than diffuse osteopenia, indistinguishable from idiopathic osteoporosis.

The diagnosis is confirmed by a bone marrow biopsy. The treatment involves chemotherapy.

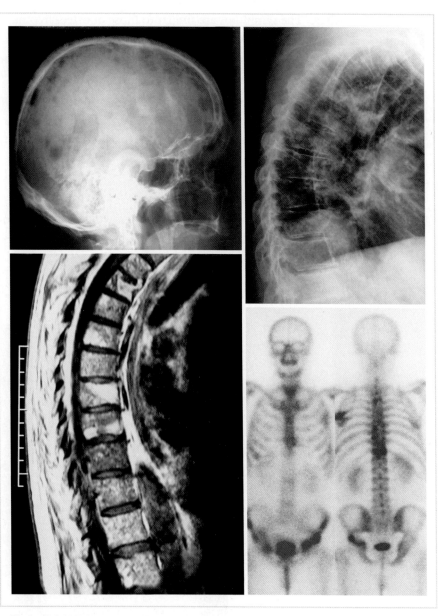

**Figure 27.9.** Multiple myeloma. All images refer to the same patient. Round lytic lesions affecting the skull are very suggestive of this diagnosis. X-rays of the spine may suggest simple osteoporosis, occasionally with associated fractures. Bone scintigraphy can be quite discrete even in cases of massive plasma cell infiltration, as demonstrated by MRI.

## Osteosarcoma

This is a malignant, aggressive tumor that mainly affects males aged from 10 to 30 with an affinity for the distal end of the femur and proximal tibia. Pain, bone swelling, fever and sensitivity to local pressure are the main symptoms. X-rays may show a characteristic spiky appearance of the bone (Figure 27.10.).

## Ewing's sarcoma

This is a malignant tumor of the bone marrow almost exclusively affecting children and young people (up to the age of 25). It appears most frequently in the long bones but can be located anywhere. The symptoms are similar to those of osteosarcoma, though it may be accompanied by high fever and leukocytosis, suggesting osteomyelitis. Its radiographic appearance can vary considerably but, in its initial phases, sclerotic lesions predominate with areas of internal bone destruction and enlargement of the cortex, with a periostic reaction (Figure 27.10.). Erosion of the cortex underscores the malignancy. In advanced stages, the bone may be completely destroyed.

Treatment involves chemotherapy followed by radical surgery.

## Osteoid osteoma

These are benign bone-forming, slow-growth tumors. They occur most often in the long bones and are most commonly in young adults. Occasionally, they may be located in the foot or in joints, suggesting other diagnoses, including arthritis.

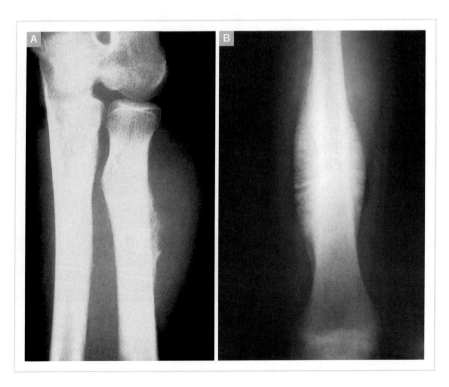

**Figure 27.10.**
Primary malignant bone tumors. **A.** Osteosarcoma. The radiological appearance can be quite varied, from purely osteolytic to purely sclerosing forms. In same cases (picture) cortical thickening and periosteal proliferation predominate. **B.** Ewing sarcoma. Suggestive radiological features include periosteal proliferation, cortical erosion and tumor infiltrating the surrounding soft tissues. (Courtesy: Prof. José Casanova.)

The predominant symptom is continuous pain unrelated to exercise. The pain may be exacerbated by drinking alcohol and is noticeably relieved by aspirin.

Scintigraphy and CT are the scans of choice for diagnosis (Figure 27.11.). Treatment is surgical.

### Enchondroma

This is a benign tumor characterized by the formation of mature cartilage. It is generally asymptomatic, but can cause pain if located in small bones or close to the periosteum.

On x-rays, it is characterized by round or oval osteolytic lesions, with no reaction from the surrounding bone, sometimes with heterogeneous interior calcifications (Figure 27.11.). Treatment is surgical, though it is only justified in symptomatic forms.

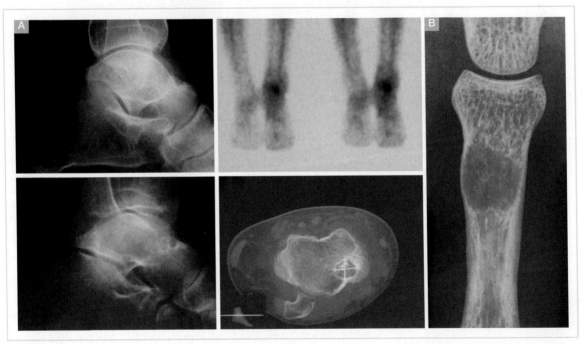

**Figure 27.11.** Benign bone tumors. **A.** Osteoid osteoma. (Courtsey: Dr. Manuel Salgado). **B.** Enchondroma.

## OSTEONECROSIS

The most common forms of osteonecrosis (aseptic necrosis or avascular necrosis) occur in the femoral head or in the tibial plates causing a regional articular syndrome (Chapters 12 and 13, respectively).

Osteonecrosis can, however, occur in other parts of the skeleton, with a variety of symptoms. While it is asymptomatic in most cases, it may cause bone-type pain and pathological fractures. In many cases, it is found by chance in x-rays (areas of intraosseal sclerosis with no perilesional reaction).

The most important thing is to recognize and treat risk factors for this condition: corticosteroid therapy, alcoholism, hyperlipidemia, sickle cell anemia, antiphospholipid syndrome and HIV infection (Figure 27.12.). The treatment of the lesion depends on the location and symptoms.

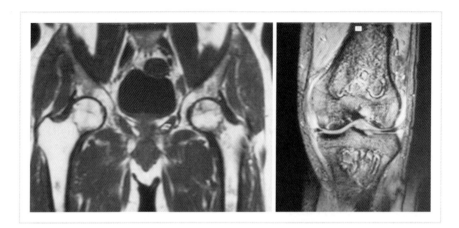

**Figure 27.12.** Aseptic avascular necrosis. Multiple extensive lesions in a patient with AIDS.

## OSTEOMYELITIS

We should suspect acute osteomyelitis whenever a patient presents with fever and localized bone pain. It is not uncommon in very small children, and we should consider this possibility in cases of high fever and signs of septicemia. In adults it appears most often in diabetics and immunosuppressed patients.

The knee and humerus are the areas most commonly affected. There may be swelling and intense local pain on palpation. The infection can spread to a neighboring joint. It only shows up late on plain films (Figure 27.13.). It can be detected earlier by scintigraphy, which is more sensitive. MRI is very useful in investigating more difficult cases.

If we suspect osteomyelitis, it is important to perform repeated bacteriological blood cultures to identify any possible source of sepsis and begin immediate intravenous antibiotic treatment, which will be adapted according to the antibiogram. The most frequent agent is *Staphylococcus aureus.* In children *Hemophilus influenza* and *Escherichia coli* are also common. Surgical exploration of the lesion is sometimes necessary.

Osteomyelitis can sometimes be subacute or chronic, with an intermittent or continuous course. It almost always appears after open trauma or a surgical procedure. The symptoms are the same as in the acute form but more moderate. There may be intermittent purulent drainage due to a fistula. A special forma of subacute osteomyelitis, Brodie's abscess, involves pain, with no inflammatory signs. Tests and treatment are along the same lines as for the acute form.

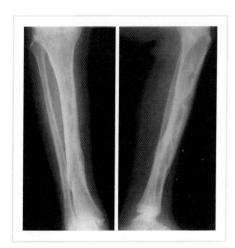

**Figure 27.13.** Extensive chronic osteomyelitis following fracture. Note the presence of lytic lesions surrounded by sclerotic areas (abscesses). Sometimes a dense structure can be found within an abcess (bone sequester). Periosteal reaction may be quite intense leading to the formation of abundant new bone.

# RHEUMATIC SYMPTOMS IN CHILDREN AND ADOLESCENTS

## 28.

J.A.P. da Silva, A.D. Woolf, *Rheumatology in Practice*, DOI 10.1007/978-1-84882-581-9_28,
© Springer-Verlag London Limited 2010

# 28. RHEUMATIC SYMPTOMS IN CHILDREN AND ADOLESCENTS

Musculoskeletal signs and symptoms are common in childhood and adolescence but, fortunately, rarely represent a severe rheumatic disease. The principles of the diagnostic approach are similar to those for adults. Many rheumatic conditions arising in children have already been described in previous chapters, to underline the syndrome pattern in which they appear.

The study of rheumatic manifestations of childhood does, however, requires a special attention for several reasons. One of them is the relative absence of pain even in conditions like juvenile idiopathic arthritis. The physician has to pay attention to changes in function (limping or reduced activity) rather than pain. It is not possible to count on the diagnostic support provided by the nature of pain that is so valuable in adults. The clinical examination is therefore even more important and requires a particular technique. In addition, the physician has to be able to deal with the clear anxiety often affecting the patients and, above all, their parents.

### General strategy

Most rheumatic complaints in the young are limited to a single joint and are due to small developmental defects in young children or to a traumatic condition in older ones. The clinical examination should focus on whether or not there is articular swelling. Generalized pain is not unusual and, in most cases, is due to non-organic causes, including fibromyalgia, growing pains, emotional stress and attention seeking.

Systemic signs like fever and rash flag up a potentially serious rheumatic disease.

With these considerations in mind, we suggest that you answer the following questions before going on to a specific diagnosis when dealing with a child with rheumatic symptoms:

1. Is the symptom local or general?
2. Is there any articular swelling?
3. Are there any systemic signs? (fever, rash, weight loss?)

Look at the algorithm in Figure 28.1.

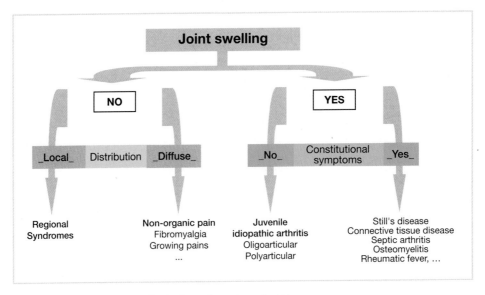

**Figure 28.1.** Basic diagnostic algorithm for rheumatic syndromes in children.

# REGIONAL SYNDROMES IN CHILDREN

### Deformities of the feet

*Equine foot* (characterized by dorsal flexion of the hindfoot) is a common condition (Figure 28.2C.). Caused by intra-uterine pressure, it generally resolves spontaneously. *Pes equinovarus*, characterized by an association of the above deformity with a fixed inversion of the foot (Figure 28.2D.), is a complex condition with considerable functional disability. Early treatment by a specialist is essential and requires corrective braces or surgery.

*Flat foot* is common and usually asymptomatic (Figure 28.2A.). In most case, the foot maintains flexibility (the arch forms when the patient stands on tiptoe). Rigid flat foot, due to deformities of the tarsus, may cause symptoms and require the use of insoles or surgery.

### Genu varum and genu valgum

Genu varus and genu valgus malalignment of the knee is common in children. In most cases there are no symptoms and the condition resolves spontaneously before adolescence. In the appropriate setting, genu varus may be caused by rickets.

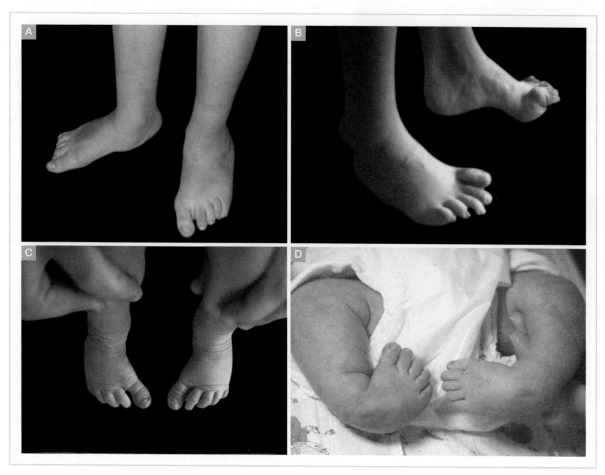

**Figure 28.2.** Pediatric foot deformities. **A.** Pes planus. **B.** Pes cavus. **C.** Equine foot. **D.** Pes equinovarus. (Courtesy: Dr. Manuel Salgado and Dr. Jorge Seabra. Coimbra.)

### Limping – hip conditions

**Congenital dislocation of the hip** (CDH) affects one in every 1,000 children. At present, most cases are identified in the maternity hospital. Cases that have gone unnoticed may result in late walking or limping. Asymmetry of the gluteal folds and of the legs are clues for the diagnosis. Suspicion warrants sending the patient to a pediatrician.

The epiphysis of the femoral head is particularly susceptible to interruption of the circulation between the ages of 3 and 12 years. This results in osteonecrosis, with fragmentation and deformity of the femoral head (**Legg-Perthes disease**), reflected by the progressive onset of limping, with relatively little pain. The pain may be referred to the knee, thus making diagnosis difficult. Its appearance on x-ray films is typical (Figure 28.3.). Diagnosis and treatment by specialists should be as early as possible.

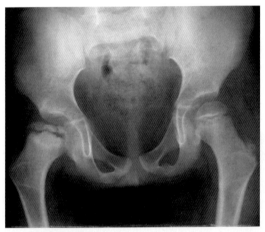

**Figure 28.3.** Legg-Perthes' disease. Radiology shows fragmentation of the right femoral epyphisis (Courtesy: Dr. Jorge Seabra. Coimbra.)

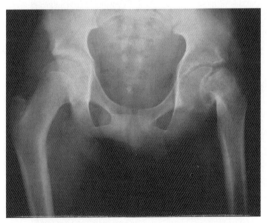

**Figure 28.4.** Slipped upper femoral epiphysis. Note the postero-inferior dislocation of the upper left femoral epiphysis. The continuation of the upper border of the femoral neck does not cross the epiphysis. Always compare with the contralateral joint. (Courtesy: Dr. Jorge Seabra. Coimbra.)

**Slipped femoral epiphysis** occurs when the femoral head glides back and down over the neck. This leads to varus deformity, which can cause acute or subacute pain and leads later to osteoarthritis. It occurs in boys more than girls, and can appear after trauma or for no apparent cause. Anteroposterior and oblique x-rays of the hip provide the diagnosis (Figure 28.4.). Treatment is surgical.

**Transient synovitis of the hip** (toxic synovitis) is a condition of unknown origin and is the most common cause of hip pain and limping in children (in boys more than girls). It sometimes involves low-grade fever and a discreet increase in erythrocyte sedimentation rate, which may require differential diagnosis from osteomyelitis and septic arthritis. The latter are suggested by fever >38°C and ESR>20 mm/h but in view of their seriousness, it is often necessary to aspirate and test synovial fluid.

Generally unilateral, it resolves without sequelae in a few weeks or months. Treatment involves rest and analgesics. Rarely, it is necessary to use anti-inflammatory drugs or traction.

### Limping – knee conditions

This is a rare complaint before the age of 12 and is usually significant. **Pain originating in the knee in children is often referred to the hip**. The causes include meniscal lesions, pulled ligaments, or osteochondritis dessicans. Swelling in the joint suggests juvenile idiopathic arthritis. Systemic signs, like fever, suggest septic arthritis or osteomyelitis.

***Osgood-Schlatter's disease*** is relatively common in adolescents, especially boys. It consists of traction enthesitis of the tibial tuberosity where the patellar tendon inserts. Intensive sports are a predisposing factor. It is reflected by local pain exacerbated by exercise. The tibial tuberosity is elevated, swollen and highly painful on palpation. The tibial tuberosity has a fragmented appearance on x-ray (Figure 28.5.). Larsen-Johannson's disease is a similar condition affecting the lower end of the patella.

Treatment is conservative and based on rest and, possibly, anti-inflammatory drugs. It generally disappears when the growth plate of the tibial tuberosity closes.

In ***osteochondritis dessicans*** a fragment of bone and cartilage detaches itself resulting in recurring pain and episodes of articular block (when knee can be neither flexed or extended) sometimes with effusion, due to the presence of a loose body. It most commonly affects adolescents of low height. The femoral condyle is the most frequent detachment site (Figure 28.6.).

Rest helps to relieve the pain and fix the bone fragment spontaneously. Rarely, surgical fixation is necessary.

***Anterior knee pain syndromes***, described in Chapter 13, are common in adolescent girls.

### Shoulder pain

The most common causes of shoulder pain in children and adolescents are tendonitis of the rotator cuff and instability of the shoulder (see Chapter 8).

### Back pain

Axial pain in children and adolescents always requires attention, especially if it appears before the age of 4 years, or persists for more than 4 weeks.

About 50% of cases of back pain in children have some significant underlying condition. Bear in mind the possibility of a local infection or tumor. Spondylolisthesis can cause pain, especially in athletic children. Ankylosing spondylitis and other seronegative spondyloarthropathies can cause inflammatory back pain.

The development of deformity (kyphosis or scoliosis) warrants referring the patient for further investigation.

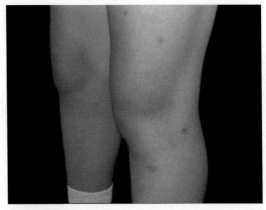

**Figure 28.5.** Osgood-Schlatter disease. Painful swelling around the tibial tuberosity. (Courtesy: Dr. Manuel Salgado. Coimbra.)

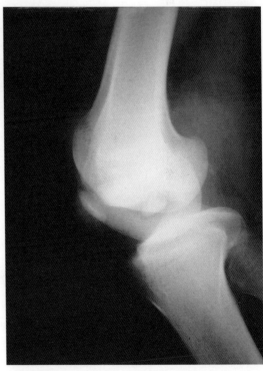

**Figure 28.6.** Osteochondritis dissecans. A bone fragment is detached from the surface of the condyle. (Courtesy: Dr. Manuel Salgado. Coimbra.)

Scoliosis is usually idiopathic. Rule out lower limb length inequality requiring correction and monitor all other cases. There may be a rapid deterioration justifying referral to a specialist.

Kyphosis may be merely postural but is often associated with Scheuermann's disease. This is osteochondrosis of the vertebral plates that can involve discreet but persistent pain and has a tendency towards progressive, generally moderate kyphosis. The intervertebral spaces may assume a typical vase-shaped deformity (Figure 28.7.). Treatment is based on analgesics, if necessary, care with posture and physical therapy.

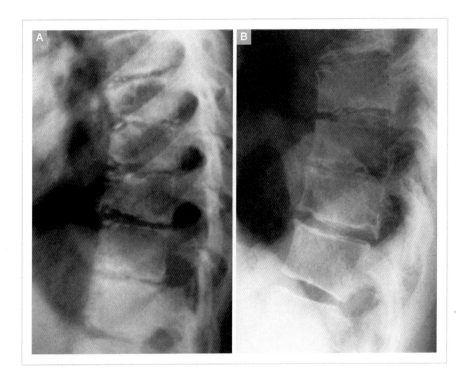

**Figure 28.7.**
Scheuermann's disease.
Deformity of the vertebral
endplate without bone
reaction in the vicinity. **A.**
Severe form, in a child
(Courtesy: Dr. Jorge
Seabra. Coimbra.) **B.**
Coincidental radiological
finding in an adult.

## DIFFUSE OR GENERALIZED PAIN SYNDROMES

Patterns of musculoskeletal pain with no identifiable organic cause appear in 5–15% of all children. The main clinical goal is to look for significant causes.

Fibromyalgia and even hysterical conversion can occur at this age with the same characteristics as those described for adults. Other cases are caused by attention seeking related to emotional stress resulting from family, school or some other conflict that must be looked into and resolved. It is naturally essential to conduct a careful enquiry and physical examination before attributing the symptoms to these causes.

So-called *growing pains* appear in about 5% of all children, generally between the ages of 6 and 13 years. The distribution is the same for both sexes. They are characterized by intense pain in the lower legs and thighs that wake the child up at night, but are relieved by local massage. About one third of these children also mention pain in the torso and upper limbs, and associated headache and abdominal pain are not uncommon. The physical examination is normal. Explore the possibility of stress factors in the child. Reassure the child and the parents.

In all cases of non-organic pain, the sensitivity of the doctor-patient-family relationship is key. We should avoid saying that there is nothing wrong, but also discourage any conviction of a serious organic disease. Exploration of the family dynamics is important, with referral to specialists in more complex cases. Generally, this approach is successful when combined with physical therapy and the child's gradual return to his or her normal activities.

## JUVENILE IDIOPATHIC ARTHRITIS

Children can be affected by practically all types of adult arthritis. Their presentation and course in childhood and adolescence are similar to those in adults, with a few differences that do not fall within the scope of this book. We can therefore find juvenile psoriatic arthritis, juvenile anky-losing spondylitis, juvenile lupus, etc. (Figure 28.8.)

Excluding these diseases, there are, however, some chronic arthritic conditions that are found only in children. They are called juvenile idiopathic arthritis.

Juvenile idiopathic arthritis is rare, but is still the most common rheumatologic diagnosis in children.

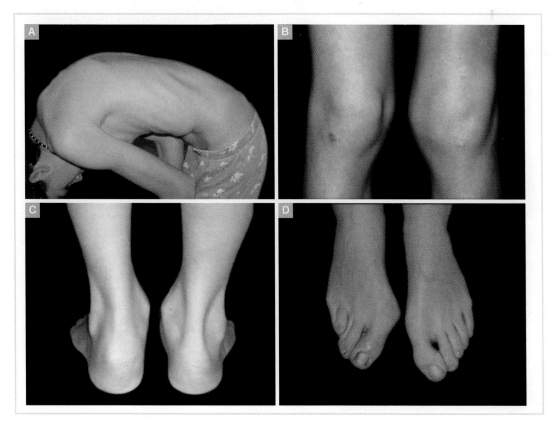

**Figure 28.8.**
Clinical aspects in a case of juvenile seronegative spondy-larthropathy affecting a HLA-B27 positive boy. **A.** Reduced lumbar flexion. **B.** Swelling of the left knee. **C.** Achilles tendonitis (Enthesitis). Hallux val-gus and secondary pes planus. (Courtesy: Dr. Manuel Salgado. Coimbra.)

## Diagnostic criteria

**Onset before the age of 16 years**

**Duration > 6 weeks**

**Arthritis** (articular swelling or effusion observed by the physician)

**Exclusion of other childhood forms of arthritis** (viral arthritis, reactive arthritis, psoriatic arthritis, ankylosing spondylitis, lupus, etc.)

## Subtypes

- Oligoarticular (1–4 joints) – 55 to 75% of cases

- Polyarticular (> 4 joints) – 15 to 25% of cases

- Systemic – Still's disease – <20% of cases

**Table 28.1.** Diagnostic criteria and subtypes of juvenile idiopathic arthritis.

To consider it, we have to find arthritis in one or more joints for more than 6 weeks. By this time, the distribution of the affected joints and associated manifestations will, as a rule, make it possible to classify the case into one of the subtypes of JIA (Table 28.1.).

The systemic form, which involves high fever, rash and other general manifestations, is the rarest and also the most serious. It is associated with considerable long-term morbidity and mortality. It is dealt with in Chapter 23.

The polyarticular form may also be profoundly destructive. It presents as chronic, symmetrical, peripheral polyarthritis, similar to rheumatoid arthritis in adults. Indeed, a high percentage of these children present positive tests for rheumatoid factor. The course of the disease and its treatment are similar to those of rheumatoid arthritis in adults (Figure 28.9.).

Either condition requires urgent, appropriate treatment and requires early referral to a specialist.

In this section, we will discuss the oligoarticular form.

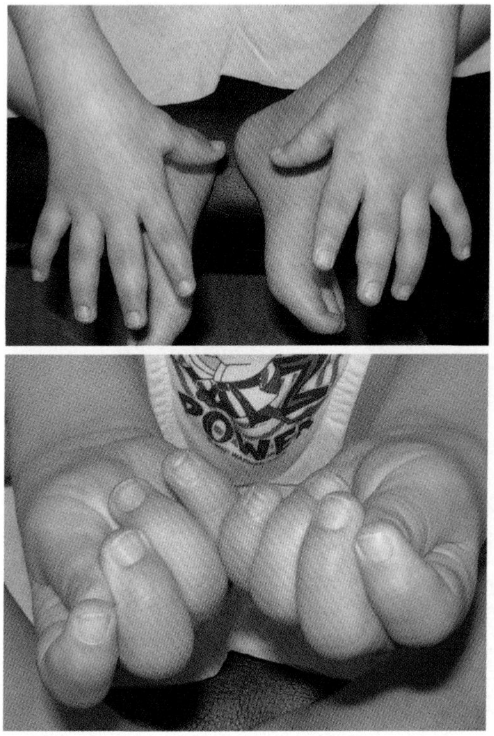

**Figure 28.9.** Juvenile chronic arthritis – polyarticular onset. (Courtesy: Dr. Manuel Salgado. Coimbra.)

## JUVENILE IDIOPATHIC ARTHRITIS
### MAIN POINTS

Chronic arthritis sets in before the age of 16 and does not adapt to the patterns that are common in adults.

It affects particularly girls aged between 2 and 6 years.

It can take an oligoarticular (the most common), polyarticular or systemic pattern.

Persistence of the inflammation may lead to irreversible sequelae.

The oligoarticular form associated with antinuclear antibodies has a high risk of eye complications.

Most cases resolve before the age of 15, but about 10% persist in adulthood.

# JUVENILE IDIOPATHIC ARTHRITIS – OLIGOARTICULAR FORM

---

### TYPICAL CASES
### 28.A. OLIGOARTICULAR ARTHRITIS IN A CHILD

Joana, a 5-year old girl, was taken to her family doctor by her parents who had noticed that she had begun to limp and was less active than usual. Her mother thought that her left knee was swollen. After examining the child, the doctor sent her to our ER. We confirmed the presence of swelling and effusion in the left knee and both ankles. There were no other abnormalities such as fever or rash. There had been no intercurrent health conditions in the weeks preceding the symptoms. The general clinical examination was normal.

---

*What possible diagnoses would you suggest?*

*What action would you take?*

Her sedimentation rate was elevated. Rheumatoid factor was negative. We began treatment with an anti-inflammatory drug. During the consultation, we confirmed positive antinuclear antibodies. Although there were no ocular symptoms, we asked for an ophthalmologic examination, which detected asymptomatic iridocyclitis, which responded to topical treatment. The inflammation of the knee persisted in spite of the anti-inflammatory drugs. After a few months, there was a slight but appreciable increase in length of the left leg compared to the right. We administered under anesthesia a local injection of glucocorticoid.

This form of arthritis usually presents with limping and a reduction in the child's physical activity. The parents may have noticed swelling of the joints, but, PLEASE NOTE that pain is unusual.

It appears most often in children between the ages of 1 and 6 years and affects girls more than boys. The joints affected most are the knees, ankles and wrists (Figure 28.10.). As a rule, there are no systemic manifestations. The condition is chronic and persistent if left untreated. The increase in blood circulation induced by the inflammatory process affects the surrounding growth cartilage, resulting in excessive growth of the affected bone and therefore

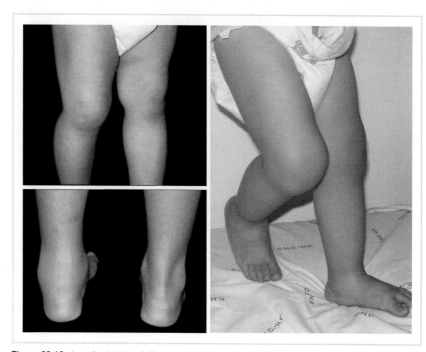

**Figure 28.10.** Juvenile chronic arthritis – oligoarticular onset.

asymmetry (Figure 28.11.). The arthritis may, in time, progress to a distinct pattern (polyarthritis, spondyloarthropathy, etc.) requiring reclassification and a review of the treatment.

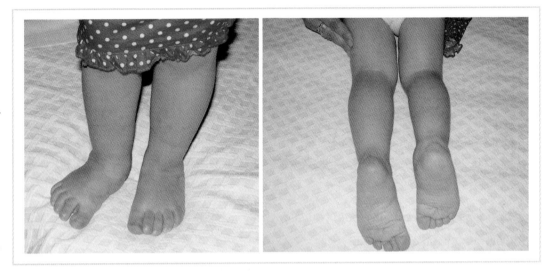

**Figure 28.11.** Juvenile chronic arthritis. Leg length discrepancy due to chronic arthritis of the left knee.

About 40% of these children have antinuclear antibodies, whose presence indicates a high risk of anterior uveitis, which is often asymptomatic and can lead to blindness (Figure 28.12.). Regular ophthalmologic monitoring and early treatment are therefore essential.

With the right treatment it is possible to prevent the destruction of the joints and leg length inequality, increasing the child's quality of life and opportunities for all-round development. Anti-inflammatory drugs, intra-articular injections and physical therapy are the basis of the treatment. Immunosuppressant therapy is occasionally necessary.

Most cases will have no manifestations before the age of 15 years, though about 10% will maintain chronic arthritis of varying intensity.

## Treatment

**In cases of juvenile arthritis persisting for more than 6 weeks**

**REFER THE PATIENT TO A SPECIALIST AS SOON AS POSSIBLE**

**with no treatment other than anti-inflammatory drugs in a weight-adjusted dose.**

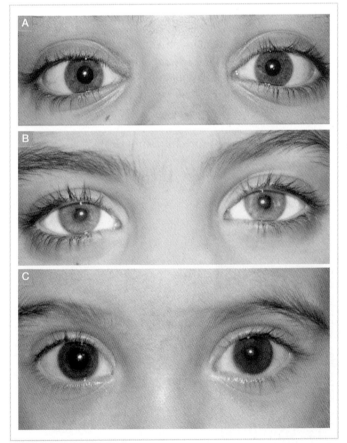

**Figure 28.12.** Anterior uveitis in children with oligoarticular juvenile chronic arthritis. **A.** Normal. **B.** Bilateral crenelated iris due to synechiae. **C.** Anisocoria can be a clue to the diagnosis. (Courtesy: Dr. Manuel Salgado. Coimbra.)

## VIRAL ARTHRITIS

These forms are particularly common in childhood and adolescence. Onset is usually acute with peripheral, polyarticular distribution. They are accompanied by fever and rash, associated with other symptoms of viral disease. In some cases, the manifestations are limited to polyarthralgia, falling into a context of differential diagnosis of diffuse pain with no apparent organic cause.

The specific aspects of viral arthritis are addressed in Chapter 23.

## RHEUMATIC FEVER

This is an acute, systemic, inflammatory disease that sets in two to 4 weeks after a pharyngeal infection by group A -hemolytic Streptococcus. It is rare these days in industrialized countries but is still a frequent problem in other areas of the world.

Peak incidence is between 5 and 10 years of age, although it can appear at other ages.

It is a form of reactive arthritis. The pathogenesis is thought to be rooted in immunological cross-reactions between antigenic determinants of the infectious agent and different tissues of the host, including the joints, heart, skin and nervous system. The disease is generally self-limiting, though the risk of cardiac and neurological involvement requires early diagnosis and long-term prevention.

The clinical pattern is dominated by the following manifestations:

- **Fever**, persisting or reappearing with the onset of the systemic disease

- **Arthritis**, which is polyarticular, but typically migrates from one joint to another. Erythema of the skin overlying the joint is common.

- **Subcutaneous nodules**, which may appear, especially in the elbows, ankles and occipital region

- **Rash**, erythema marginatum (Figure 28.13.), which is more accentuated on the torso and proximal part of the arms, usually exacerbated by bathing

- **Sydenham's chorea**, characterized by uncoordinated, involuntary movements. It appears later, or may be absent in many cases

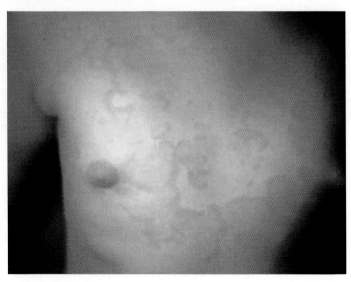

**Figure 28.13.** Erythema marginatum in rheumatic fever. (Courtesy: Prof. Odete Hilário. S. Paulo, Brasil.)

- **Pancarditis**, in which the inflammation may be limited to the valves, leaving frequent chronic sequelae, though it can also affect the pericardium and myocardium, causing cardiac dysfunction. Conduction anomalies (prolongation of the PR interval) are common.

A prior throat infection is obvious in almost all patients.
Sedimentation rate and reactive-C protein are very high.

---

### TYPICAL CASES
### 28.B. MIGRATORY ARTHRITIS

10-year old Susana was taken to the doctor by her parents because of the recent appearance of fever and migratory joint pain, affecting the left knee, ankle, right elbow and wrists, successively. The doctor confirmed articular swelling of the wrists. The systematic examination suggested a mitral systolic murmur, which the doctor thought might be due to the fever. When asked about her recent history, however, Susana's parents mentioned that she had had a sore throat about three weeks before, which they had treated with an antibiotic, as usual.

---

*How would you assess this clinical pattern?*

*What lab tests would you request and what treatment would you opt for?*

The doctor recommended an urgent visit to our hospital, where we confirmed migratory febrile arthritis. The systolic murmur seemed quite harmless but an ECG showed prolongation of the PR interval. Her sedimentation rate was 52 mm/h and there was leukocytosis with neutrophilia. We conducted a pharyngeal swab and an anti-streptococcus antibody count and immediately began treatment with aspirin, corticosteroids (1 mg/kg/day) and benzathine penicillin G (an intramuscular injection of 1.2 million U). The lab tests confirmed infection by group A -hemolytic Streptococcus. The patient's pain resolved rapidly. The heart murmur was inaudible about 3 weeks later. Her sedimentation rate went back to normal in 6 weeks, when we discontinued treatment. A control echocardiogram ruled out any valvular sequelae.

We then began preventive treatment: (oral penicillin, 250,000 U once a day), which we asked the GP to continue for at least 5 years. Given that the patient's parents described recurrent sore throats with fever, we asked for an examination by an ear, nose and throat specialist, who identified chronic tonsillitis and suggested a tonsillectomy.

This diagnosis should only be confirmed if there is clinical evidence of prior infection by the above agent or a positive throat swab culture. A demonstration of elevated antistreptolysin O (or antiDNAse B, antistreptokinase or antihyaluronidase) serves the same purpose.

It is worth remembering that only a small minority of patients suffering from this infection will develop rheumatic fever. On the other hand, many patients maintain elevated levels of antistreptolysin O as a chronic immunological scar, with no infection. In the absence of compatible clinical symptoms, this lab test is meaningless.

Diagnosis of rheumatic fever should follow the Jones' criteria (Table 28.2.).

| Major criteria | Minor criteria |
|---|---|
| Polyarthritis | Arthralgia or fever |
| Carditis (valvulitis or pancarditis) | Elevated sedimentation rate or reactive C protein |
| Chorea | Prolonged PR interval in an ECG |
| Erythema marginatum | |
| Subcutaneous nodules | |

**Evidence of a recent group A streptococcal infection:**

• Oropharyngeal culture or

• Elevated anti-streptococcal antibodies in successive tests

The diagnosis is highly likely if the patient presents:

- two major criteria + evidence of a prior group A streptococcal infection, or

- one major and two minor criteria  + evidence of a prior group A streptococcal infection.

**Table 28.2.** Jones' criteria for the diagnosis of rheumatic fever, modified in 1992.[1]

### TYPICAL CASES
### 28.C. PAIN AND ELEVATED ANTI-STREPTOLYSIN

Maria, an active 13-year old, described occasional, migratory pain affecting different joints. As a rule, it appeared after more strenuous exercise, such as sports, and resolved spontaneously in about 2–3 days. She had never noticed any swelling, or redness of the joints.

She had been examined by her doctor 2 years before. The tests had shown that she had rheumatic fever. Since then, she had been having a monthly injection of penicillin, and it was the pain that led Maria to insist on another visit to the doctor. She had been advised to avoid doing sport, which also made her sad.

*Think about this case. What is your assessment of the diagnosis?*

*What other information would you try to get?*

A thorough enquiry excluded skin lesions of any kind or any significant neurological manifestations. The girl maintained normal physical activity and denied dyspnea with exercise. She also denied any fever, except in association with the many episodes of tonsillitis that she had had until the age of 10, when she had undergone a tonsillectomy. She also said that the articular complaints had not improved since she had begun antibiotic treatment and that there was no connection between the throat infections and the pain.

The clinical examination found nothing unusual, except for clear signs of hypermobility, which contributed to her love of gymnastics. The heart auscultation was normal.

[1]Special writing group of the committee on rheumatic fever of the Council on Cardiovascular Disease of the Young, American Heart Association. Guidelines for the diagnosis of rheumatic fever: Jones criteria, updated 1992. JAMA 1992; 268: 2069–2073.

*What is your diagnosis?*

*What would you do next?*

We ruled out rheumatic fever because the patient did not meet the diagnostic criteria. We explained that the pain was probably due to the hypermobility and recurring subluxations. We paid little attention to the antistreptolysin levels, which were consistently high in the several test results that she had with her. This was probably a sequela of the episodes of tonsillitis that they described. We advised her to wear an elastic support on the most exposed joints and suggested that she avoided physical exercises in forced or unusual positions. We discontinued the antibiotic treatment and said that she could do sport. We explained these points in a letter to her GP.

### Treatment

There are four objectives in the treatment of acute rheumatic fever.

**Relieving the fever and articular pain.** Salicylates are the drugs of choice and achieve results in about 12–24 hours after reaching the effective dose. The initial recommended dose is 80–100 mg/kg/day in divided doses. Other anti-inflammatories are also effective. They should be continued until the patient is completely asymptomatic and acute phase markers are back to normal.

**Treating the carditis.** When present, glucocorticoids are warranted (prednisolone 1–2 mg/kg/day) with rest.

**Treating infection.** Antibiotic therapy is indicated if the throat infection still persists at the time of diagnosis (oral penicillin or erythromycin for 10 days, or a single intramuscular injection of benzathine penicillin G).

**Preventing recurrences.** Antibiotic prophylaxis should begin as soon as the initial attack resolves. The recommended regimens include intramuscular injections of benzathine penicillin G (1.2 million U every 4 weeks) or continuous treatment with phenoxymethylpenicillin (250 mg once a day in children, twice a day in adults) or erythromycin (250 mg/day).

Prophylaxis should be maintained for at least 5 years or for ever in patients with confirmed rheumatic cardiac disease. We must therefore be very sure of the diagnosis.

All patients with cardiac or neurological involvement should be urgently referred to a specialist.

# TREATING RHEUMATIC DISEASES
## GENERAL PRINCIPLES

J.A.P. da Silva, A.D. Woolf, *Rheumatology in Practice*, DOI 10.1007/978-1-84882-581-9_29,
© Springer-Verlag London Limited 2010

# 29. TREATING RHEUMATIC DISEASES GENERAL PRINCIPLES

### *Introduction*

Physicians are faced with a variety of challenges when treating rheumatic diseases. Such conditions are generally chronic, meaning that, with rare exceptions, they will persist for the rest of the patient's life and may involve considerable suffering. The limitations they impose on leisure and work activities may have a profound psychosocial impact. The need for effective, sometimes aggressive treatment resulting from the severity of the symptoms and the risk of progressive disability must be weighed against the cumulative risk of toxicity.

No treatment can therefore be considered in isolation, but rather as part of a global, integrated intervention over time whose final aim is to maintain and improve of the quality of life of the patient, in its many dimensions. The family physician is responsible for coordinating the contributions of a variety of specialists, guiding the patient's choices and safeguarding his or her short and long-term interests.

A comprehensive diagnosis should therefore include not only a functional and psychosocial assessment but also the prognosis. The treatment strategy should be guided by clearly defined goals.

Assessment of the patient at each appointment should include an evaluation of the disease activity and response to treatment. The physician must be able to identify and measure the appropriate parameters for each particular condition and assess them consistently and repeatedly. Treatment should be regularly adjusted according to adequate disease activity assessment and this is only possible if you know *what* to evaluate and *how* to evaluate it.

Rheumatic diseases are often unpredictable, with flares and remissions, which you must know how to deal with. Their relationships with other aspects of life are complex and bi-directional, demanding the consideration of such diverse factors as ageing, comorbidity, education, job, school activities, social resources and networking, etc. Appropriate holistic treatment requires the integrated consideration of most of these factors and dimensions.

We would like to stress the demands that this places on your ability to communicate and empathize with the patient, and the need for a special mental attitude and consistent strategy.

## OBJECTIVES OF THE TREATMENT

Let us give a little thought to the goals of treating a patient.

Whatever the medical condition in question, the overall objectives of treatment fall into two basic categories: improving quality of life and prolonging life.

Biological or apparent normality will only be one of your goals if they contribute to the other two. These obvious truths should be always present in our choices of treatment.

The goals of treatment of most rheumatic diseases can be organized as follows.

### *1. Relieving suffering and improving quality of life*

No patient goes to the doctor because s/he has a disease; s/he goes because it causes symptoms or concern. Pain is the main cause of suffering in rheumatic diseases and treating it should one of our priorities, even when its cause is not evident or accessible to etiological treatment. We feel that it is as inappropriate to take painkillers for the smallest pain without considering the risks of treatment, as it is to suggest that the patient should bear the pain to the limit. Limited mobility caused by the pain, stiffness, articular limitations and weakness are dominant causes of suffering. Movement is one of the main contributions to our quality of life, as social creatures. Preserving function is therefore also essential in relieving suffering.

We should also realize that the psychological suffering caused by

> **TREATMENT STRATEGY IN RHEUMATIC DISEASES**
> *MAIN POINTS*
>
> - Diagnosis should include a functional, prognostic and psychosocial assessment, and establish concrete goals.
>
> - Regular reassessment is essential and should be based on appropriate parameters of activity, function, psychosocial impact and structural progression.
>
> - Coordination of multidisciplinary resources and the re-adaptation of treatment on the basis of reassessment are essential.
>
> **The objectives of treatment include:**
>
> - Relieving suffering (from a bio-psychosocial point of view) and improving quality of life.
> - Preserving structure and function.
> - Minimizing the risk of death.
> - Minimizing toxicity.

pain, limited function, loss of social role, and the specter of a chronic inescapable, deforming disease can have more impact on the patient's quality of life than his or her strictly physical condition. The patient is a single bio-psychosocial being and his or her suffering deserves equal attention, whatever its predominant cause.

## 2. Preserving structure and, above all, function

The pursuit of this goal is based on the measures required to preserve the integrity and competence of the musculoskeletal structures responsible for movement and function. The use of disease-modifying agents in inflammatory arthropathies is intended not only to reduce articular inflammation, pain and stiffness, but also to prevent the progressive destruction of the joint, which, in time, will be the main cause of disability. Encouraging the patient to take physical exercise and maintain good muscle strength is part of this same objective. In more advanced conditions, the use of aids in daily life such as a stick, orthosis, or even surgery is also aimed at improving function, in spite of structural alterations inaccessible to pharmacological treatment.

Both doctor and patient will sometimes have to accept the irreversibility of accumulated structural damage and try to find ways of preserving function as much as possible, as this is decisive to quality of life. Making function and safety the priority (not "normalizing tests" or appearance), should always inform our management. The temptation to adopt a surgical approach to a severely deformed hand should be resisted if function is enough to satisfy the needs of the patient's everyday life. Conversely, articular arthrodesis may be the best solution for a joint whose function is limited by structural damage and extreme pain.

It is also important to consider the relative importance of each determinant of disability in the patient. For example, arthrodesis of an unstable first interphalangeal joint may have a decisive impact on the function of the hand.

Making function and quality of life a priority imposes careful consideration of the patient's psychological state and his or her way of relating to the disease. The will to do something is always a fundamental determinant of what a person can actually do, whatever the structural damage. One of your main goals is to help patients minimize the impact of their physical condition on their activities and quality of life.

### 3. Minimizing the risk of death

Many rheumatic diseases, especially the connective tissue diseases, involve a considerable risk of death. Examples are involvement of the kidneys and central nervous system in systemic lupus erythematosus, respiratory insufficiency in myositis, and hypertensive crises in diffuse systemic sclerosis, among many others. These life-threatening conditions should obviously be your main concern and will determine the priority to be given to therapeutic and prophylactic measures, as well as the follow-up plan.

### 4. Minimizing toxicity

Rheumatic diseases often require the prolonged use of potentially damaging drugs. The balance between the pursuit of short and long-term efficacy and the obligatory concern for the risks of immediate and cumulative toxicity is one of the most difficult challenges in the treatment of rheumatic diseases. For example, the temptation of "miraculous" short-term effects with high dose glucocorticoids must often be resisted because of their longterm toxicity.

In order to achieve these goals, the physician must make use of a variety of treatment modalities, which go far beyond the simple use of medications (Table 29.1.). Different forms of intervention are usually combined in each case. Choice, sequence and timing of interventions play an essential role in the quality of the treatment and its final result.

This chapter briefly addresses the non-pharmacological forms. The medications most commonly used are discussed in the next chapter.

| Treatment modalities in rheumatic diseases | |
|---|---|
| **Psychosocial support** | **Physical agents and rehabilitation** |
| Education | Exercise and rest |
| Social network | Heat and cold |
| **Pharmacotherapy** | Mobilization and manipulation |
| | Hydrotherapy |
| Analgesics | Electrotherapy |
| Non-steroidal anti-inflammatory drugs | Ultrasound |
| Corticosteroids | Surgical appliances |
| Immunosuppressants | • Splints and insoles |
| Biological agents | • Orthoses |
| Uric acid lowering agents | • Aids to daily life |
| Anti-osteoporotic agents | **Surgery** |
| Etc. | |
| | Reconstruction of tendons and ligaments |
| | Synovectomy |
| | Arthroplasty |
| | Arthrodesis |
| | Osteotomy |
| | Decompression – spinal cord, nerves and roots |
| | Etc. |

**Table 29.1.** Classification of some forms of treatment used in rheumatic diseases.

# PSYCHOSOCIAL SUPPORT

## *Educating the patient*

A well-informed patient is your best ally in achieving treatment goals. Information will help the patient understand the scope, limitations and risks of the treatment. This will not only result in more realistic expectations but also in earlier identification of significant intercurrences and a reduction in anxiety, as the patient can solve small problems alone. The intrinsic subjectivity of rheumatic complaints imposes a special need to develop a common language with the patient. This is indispensable to assure appropriate assessment and, ultimately, the success of the treatment program.

Inform the patient of the nature of the disease and its expected evolution. True professionals keep any anxieties and concerns inspired by the patient's condition to themselves unless informing the patient can change the disease's course. In our opinion, it is counterproductive to tell the patient of concerns we may have regarding possible but rare intercurrences, whose risk does not depend on his or her attitude. Discuss the benefits and risks of medications with the patient, stressing his or her role in identifying and controlling potential side effects. Explanatory leaflets in accessible language are very useful tools for this purpose.

Note that there are often great differences between the patient's and the physician's expectations, and it is important to clarify these. It is easy to understand that the patient's concerns may be dominated by immediate control of the symptoms – s/he does not know what might happen in 10 or 20 years. Patients should be informed partners in establishing the goals of the treatment and it is very important that they accept sharing responsibility in finding the best solutions, including, for example, decisions on weight and lifestyle. This attitude is not only of invaluable help to you but also a useful tool in maintaining a positive relationship between the patient and his or her disease, thus helping to reduce its psychological impact.

Patients should be encouraged to lead as active a life as possible, doing all they can, at their own speed, to try and reduce the impact of their physical condition on their quality of life. Patients should focus on what they are able to do and not dwell on the pain, the disease or lost capacities.

Many patients ask their doctor about the role of diet in triggering or treating their condition. In practice, there is little evidence that diet influences most rheumatic diseases, with rare exceptions:

- Obese patients with gout or osteoarthritis of the lower limbs should be encouraged to lose weight;

- Some studies have shown that a diet rich in fish oils (rather than animal fat) can make a small contribution to reducing pain and stiffness in inflammatory arthropathies;

- Patients with osteoporosis should be encouraged to adopt a calcium-rich diet;

- Diet plays an important role in the treatment of gout, especially abstinence from alcohol.

Many patients seem convinced that a particular food affects their symptoms. Although this has not been demonstrated scientifically, it is neither possible nor productive to contradict these convictions.

## SELF-HELP
## SELF-SUFFICIENCY
### *Principles*

Understand your disease.

Understand the role of the doctor and other practitioners and your own role in the control and treatment of your condition.

Understand the scope and limitations of the treatment.

Lead as active and fruitful a life as possible.

Adapt your tasks to your capabilities.

Try to control your disease. Don't let it control you.

Find satisfactory ways of getting round difficulties and saving energy.

Keep the focus on getting satisfaction from life and not on your body.

Watch out for and combat despondency and depression.

Make the most of the resources of your social environment.

### *Involving the family*

Rheumatic diseases can have a decisive impact on the social- and family lives. Understanding and support from friends, family and coworkers can therefore play a very important role in achieving the goals of treatment. Do not ignore the importance of these aspects.

### *Social resources and associations*

Patients should be informed of the medical and social resources at their disposal, in terms of social security, support groups and patient associations that can provide help and counseling. Patient associations play a very important role in increasing social awareness of the importance of rheumatic diseases, raising funds for research, influencing the focus of research and medical intervention goals, mobilizing patient support schemes and providing direct support to their members. For many patients, active involvement in these organizations is a substantial source of satisfaction and balance in their relationship with their disease.

| EDUCATING THE PATIENT | |
|---|---|
| **Address the patient's concerns** | It is essential to listen. Resolving or clarifying the patient's concerns is a compulsory part of the treatment. |
| **Inform the patient about his or her condition** | Use accessible language so that the patient understands the nature of the problem. Stress any aspects with potential impact on his or her relationship with the disease and its treatment. Avoid pessimism. |
| **Establish the goals of treatment** | Compare your expectations with the patient's |
| **Inform the patient about the treatment** | Discuss the scope, risks and limitation of possible treatments. Involve the patient in the decision. |
| **Inform the patient about intercurrences Maximize compliance with the** | Warn the patient about flare-ups and remissions. Explain small intercurrences with the disease, their treatment and how to deal with them. |
| **Treatment plan** | Justify it in understandable terms. Identify obstacles to compliance: preferences, fears, costs, etc. Provide written instructions. Involve family members. Underline the importance of the patient's role. Monitor compliance during successive visits. |
| **Additional resources** | Supply information about available social aid: support groups, applicable legislation, logistical and financial support, patient associations, associated practitioners (physiotherapists, orthopedists, podiatrists, etc.) |

# PHYSICAL AGENTS AND REHABILITATION

Physical medicine and rehabilitation play an extremely important role in the treatment of most rheumatic diseases, preventing lesions, helping to relieve pain and stiffness and compensating for deformities and limitations.

Specialized centers have at their disposal a variety of techniques that are only available through prescription by specialists. Nevertheless, patients can and should make use of simple tools and techniques which can help relieve suffering and preserve function and independence. Visits to physical therapy centers should always be used as an opportunity to educate and stimulate patients in this regard, but the physician can also make a important contribution by giving simple advice and continuous encouragement.

## Exercise and rest

Patients should be encouraged to remain as active as possible. In many cases, they have to accept a reduction in their ability to work, while not allowing this to become a cause of emotional stress. Organizing tasks into manageable work periods, alternating jobs of differing physical requirements, and programming periods of physical exercise and rest can be very important in optimizing our patients' capacities.

Inflammatory arthropathies warrant some special considerations here. Repeated exercise of an inflamed joint, especially if there is effusion, can exacerbate the inflammatory process thanks to ischemia/reperfusion cycles caused by variations in intra-articular pressure. Once the inflammatory process is over, however, it is fundamental to mobilize the joint in order to recover range of movement and muscle strength. During inflammatory flares, patients should therefore be instructed to perform only a limited number of full-range mobilizations of the joint. During remission, they should actively work the joint in range and resistance exercises so as to recover mobility and strength.

Note that bed rest or immobilizing inflamed joints with splints helps to relieve the inflammation and pain. Prolonged immobilization can, however, result in fixed flexion deformities and weakening of the articular and periarticular structures causing loss of mobility and resistance, in addition to general harmful effects such as osteoporosis. Immobilization is therefore used as little as possible.

## Heat and cold

The application of heat facilitates muscle relaxation, the mobilization of stiff joints and local circulation, thus helping to reduce the pain. Hot water bottles or hot, wet towels are ways of applying superficial heat that are appreciated by many patients with osteoarthritis, muscle contractures and fibromyalgia, for example. A hot bath or shower has a powerful muscle relaxing effect, which is very useful in patients with fibromyalgia, stiff neck or lumbago. Generally speaking, heat is contraindicated in acute arthritis (as in an acute gout attack), though many patients with more indolent forms of inflammation, like rheumatoid arthritis and spondyloarthropathies, get relief from wet heat.

Short wave, ultrasounds and microwave diathermy are forms of deep heat, and are generally used to treat chronically inflamed structures, like tendons and capsules (in adhesive capsulitis, for example). Their use should be reserved for qualified professionals.

Cold induces vasoconstriction and reduces nerve conduction. This produces an analgesic and anti-inflammatory effect. Superficial cold can be applied with ice packs, ice massages or cooling sprays. The use of simple domestic tricks can improve efficacy and comfort: a bag of frozen peas adapts better to the joint surface than ice cubes. The skin should be protected to prevent cold burns. Local cold reduces pain and edema after acute trauma and can help the patient tolerate the pain caused by acute inflammation, as in the case of gout or periarthritis, for example.

As a general rule, acute inflammatory lesions tend to improve with the application of local cold, while degenerative or "post-inflammatory" lesions tend to benefit from local heat. This general rule varies considerably, however, from one patient to the next, and it is better adopt a strategy of trial and error rather than a strict rule.

### Massages

Massages are often used to relieve muscle spasms, pain and stiffness. They are frequently associated with local heat, to facilitate muscle relaxation, or topical anti-inflammatories for superficial lesions.

### Home exercises and recreational activities

Maintaining and increasing the range of articular movements and muscle strength is a central goal in treating all forms of arthropathy, not only because this improves function, but also because it helps to prevent further destruction of the joint. Immobility, inflammation and pain cause early, accentuated loss of muscle strength. This will, in turn, contribute towards physical disability and progression of the arthropathy, as strong muscles are important to maintain joint stability and absorb mechanical impact. For these reasons, all rheumatic patients should be encouraged to perform regular physical exercise as appropriate to their condition.

Although physical therapy centers offer the ideal conditions for supervised, controlled treatment by movement, there are always useful exercises that the patient can and should do at home. Regular exercise makes an important contribution to mobility and vitality, while also increasing the patient's confidence in his or her physical capabilities and reinforcing his or her involvement in the treatment program. Assess exercise and its results regularly, in order to reinforce the patient's compliance and commitment.

The home exercise program must naturally be adapted to each patient's conditions, under the guidance of a doctor or therapist. Ideally, the patient should be given leaflets explaining the nature of the exercises and other means of protecting the joints. Some examples are shown in Figures 11.20. and 16.12. Videos of exercises for rheumatic patients, available in some countries, are also extremely helpful.

Whenever possible, patients should be encouraged to follow a general workout program to maintain and improve their physical condition. Certain sports and pastimes like walking, golf, aerobics classes, hydro-exercise and swimming are particularly suited to improving neuro-muscular function and are more enjoyable than repetitive therapeutic exercises. Contact sports like football, basketball and handball should generally be avoided.

### Physical therapy

Physical therapists use three main types of therapeutical exercise: range of movement, muscle strengthening and endurance exercises.

Range of movement exercises can be passive, active or assisted. Muscle strengthening can be achieved with isometrics (effort against resistance, without movement) or isokinetics (constant speed). Increased endurance is important in rheumatic patients, as it improves autonomy and the feeling of well-being and reduces pain, while helping rehabilitation. It usually involves a gradual increase in the intensity and duration of the exercises.

At a physical therapy center, these exercises are usually combined with other forms of physical treatment to facilitate relaxation and control the pain, such as application of heat or cold, hydrotherapy, massage, etc. Hot water is an important aid to exercise that the patient can also use at home before beginning exercise of any kind.

---

## EXERCISE AND RECREATIONAL ACTIVITIES
### MAIN POINTS

All patients with a chronic rheumatic disease should be encouraged to follow a consistent physical exercise program.

The main goals include maintaining joint mobility, reducing pain and fatigue, strengthening the muscles, improving general physical condition and improving autonomy.

The exercise program should be adapted to the patient's circumstances, including his or her cultural level, interests, and respiratory and cardiovascular capacity.

Low-impact recreational activities and swimming should be encouraged as back up for the exercise and to stimulate social interaction.

The application of heat or hot water facilitates exercise.

High-impact and contact sports should generally be avoided.

Ideally, exercises should be supervised by trained professionals, at least at the start, though patients should be encouraged to do them alone, within the scope of their abilities.

---

### Aids to daily life

There is currently a wide range of devices designed to facilitate the daily activities of patients with deformities and motor limitations. For example, a patient with deformed hands limiting grip can use wide-handled cutlery, adapted knives, special packet openers, etc. (Figure 29.1.). Walking may be made easier with a stick or walking frame, which can be personalized. In extreme situations you may have to recommend a motorized wheelchair in cases of significant limitations of the lower limbs.

Patients with limitations of the hip joints or knees may benefit from using raised seats in chairs or on the toilet. Handles in the bath may be crucial in preventing falls and fractures, etc. Occupational therapy laboratories are ideal places for learning to use these devices, but any

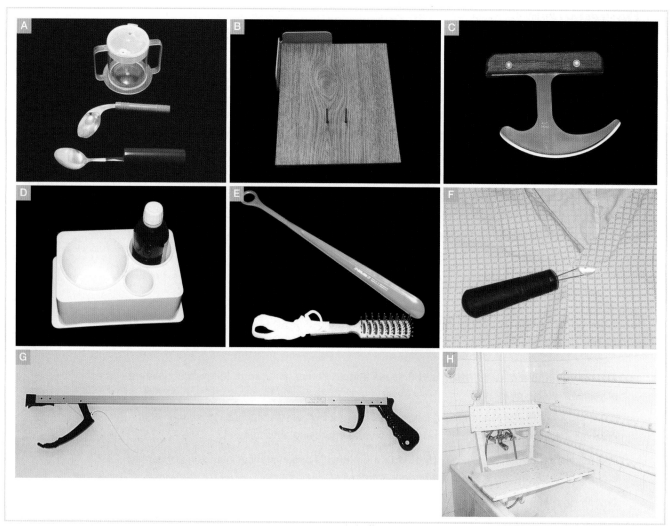

**Figure 29.1.** Daily life accessories. **A.** Glass and table gear with adapted handles. **B.** Fruit managing board. **C.** Cutter. **D.** Flask opener. **E.** Extended hairbrush and shoe horn. **F.** Button fastener. **G.** Long handled grabber. **H.** Bath seat and handles.

physician dealing with these situations should be sufficiently familiar with them to be able to advise his or her patient.

### Footwear and insoles

Foot pain caused by congenital or acquired deformities are a very important cause of suffering and disability. In patients with rheumatoid arthritis, for example, the feet can be the main cause of limitation to walking and social interaction. Ideally, it is possible to get the help of a specialist (a podiatrist) to design personalized footwear and insoles. If this is not possible, however, an informed physician can offer useful advice.

Generally speaking, patients with deformities of the feet should wear loose, supportive yet pliable shoes and to avoid areas of excess pressure that may exacerbate the pain and cause calluses and ulceration. The sole must be thick and flexible to absorb the impact of walking and the load on the structures of the foot. The sole should guarantee good adherence to the ground. The internal arch of the shoe should be elevated so as to broaden the support and distribution area of the pressure. Good-quality, carefully chosen trainers are often a simple, useful solution.

Marked deformities require personalized insoles or shoes. Some standardized models are, however, useful and can be prescribed with no great risk of error. Examples are the insoles for plantar fasciitis described in Chapter 14. When the pain is localized under the metatarsophalangeal joints, as in rheumatoid patients, for example, insoles with a metatarsal bar (placed just posteriorly to the painful joints) can help relieve local pressure and pain.

### Splints and orthoses

Splints and orthoses are used to stabilize a body segment. Stabilization may be essential to reduce the pain and prevent progressive deformity. Although there is a wide range of orthoses for different situations, some are in common use and can be prescribed by a GP. Examples are thumb splints (very useful in osteoarthritis of the trapezo-metacarpal joint or De Quervain's tenosynovitis – Figure 29.2.) or wrist splints for patients with painful arthropathy of the wrist (Figure 29.3.) or carpal tunnel syndrome.

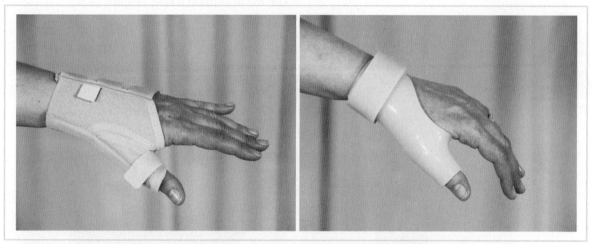

**Figure 29.2.** Thumb splints. Relieve pain from osteoarthritis of the 1st CMC joint and from De Quervain's tenosynovitis.

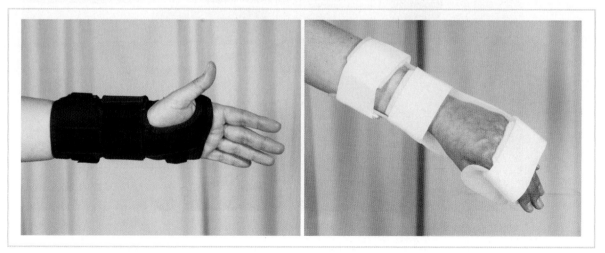

**Figure 29.3.** Wrist splints. Help relieve pain in wrist arthropathies.

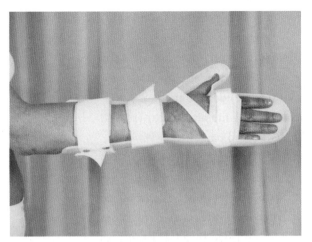

**Figure 29.4.** Firm hand and wrist splints are recommended for night use, aiming at preventing or correcting hand deformities such as ulnar deviation of the fingers in rheumatoid arthritis.

Night splints are prescribed to correct or prevent joint deformity and retraction, as in rheumatoid hands, for example (Figure 29.4.). They may be made of heat-molded material which allows easy adaptation according to change over time. Some splints may be dynamic and permit some movement of the joint. They must be made by specialized technicians.

Splints and orthoses must be empirically tested on each patient, as there is no hard and fast rule that identifies the patients who will benefit from them.

### *Walking aids*

Patients who have difficulty walking may benefit from using sticks or crutches with height and handles adapted to their condition, on the side opposite the dominant lesion (Figure 29.5.).

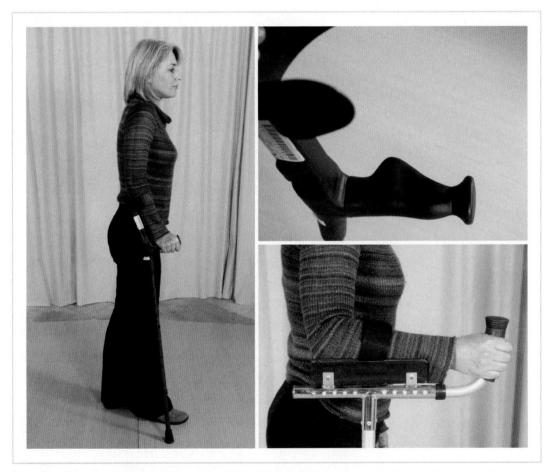

**Figure 29.5.** Different types of walking stick can make walking easier and safer. In the common model, the handle height should be adjusted to level with the great trochanter. Patients with concomitant hand deformities may benefit from adaptations of the handles.

# SURGERY

Orthopedic surgery is one of the greatest advances in the treatment of a variety of rheumatic diseases, and results in highly significant improvements in the functional capacity of many patients. Close collaboration between rheumatologists, GPs and orthopedists is essential if there is to be profitable, opportune use of the surgical methods available. In many patients, procedures like synovectomy, tenosynovectomy or arthroscopic articular debridement performed at the right time can avoid the need for more complex, less effective surgery at a later date.

It is not easy to establish clear rules on the ideal timing for a surgical procedure. Generally speaking, surgery is used as a resort when conservative treatment is unable to provide reasonable function and comfort. It is, however, important to remember that severe articular destruction can hinder the technical execution of the surgery and limit its therapeutic result. The surgical goal should always be focused on pain and function more than on aesthetic or structural correction.

Table 29.2. shows some of the most common surgical procedures and their indications.

| Procedure | Indications | Expected result |
|---|---|---|
| **Peripheral nerve decompression or transposition** | Peripheral nerve compression (e.g. carpal tunnel syndrome) | Reduction in pain and paresthesia |
| **Decompression of a nerve root or the spinal cord** | Symptomatic radiculopathy Compressive myelopathy | Pain reduction. Preservation of function |
| **Debridement of a joint** | Intra-articular free bodies. Septic arthritis | Mechanical improvement. Preservation of structure and function |
| **Reconstruction of ligaments, tendons and capsule** | Joint instability and subluxation Ruptured tendons (e.g. rheumatoid arthritis, ruptured knee ligaments) | Reduction in pain and instability. Preservation of structure and function |
| **Synovectomy and tenosynovectomy** | Synovial chondromatosis, hemophilia, persistent synovitis | Temporary elimination of joint inflammation Prevention of tendon rupture. Improvement in function |
| **Osteotomy** | Osteoarthritis of the hip and knee | Realignment Improvement in pain and function. Delaying joint destruction |
| **Joint prosthesis** | Advanced joint destruction of any cause (shoulders, elbows, hips and knees) | Pain relief Substantial improvement in function |
| **Arthrodesis (fusion of the joint)** | Advanced joint destruction of any cause, prosthesis not an option (wrist, subtalar joint, spine,…) | Reduction in pain. Improvement in function Risk of secondary alteration in neighboring joints |

**Table 29.2.** Common surgical procedures in rheumatic patients, their indications and expected results.

# DRUGS COMMONLY USED IN RHEUMATIC DISEASES

30.

J.A.P. da Silva, A.D. Woolf, *Rheumatology in Practice*, DOI 10.1007/978-1-84882-581-9_30,
© Springer-Verlag London Limited 2010

# 30. DRUGS COMMONLY USED IN RHEUMATIC DISEASES

This chapter describes some of the classes of drugs often used to treat rheumatic diseases, and addresses the basic rules for selecting, dosing and monitoring them. Other drugs with more specific indications, like immunosuppressants, osteoporosis treatment and gout medications have been dealt with in the appropriate chapters.

## ANALGESICS

Analgesics are very often used to relieve the pain caused by rheumatic diseases, as adjuvants to the disease-modifying treatment. Analgesics can be classified according to their strength (Table 30.1.). Traditionally, narcotic analgesics were avoided in this group of conditions, as their tendency to cause dependence made them unsuitable in treating relatively benign, chronic diseases. Meanwhile, improvements in the tolerance and safety of these drugs in recent years means that some of them are now part of the therapeutic arsenal for rheumatic diseases. Generally speaking, analgesics are used in flexible doses depending on the intensity of the pain and its response to treatment, within the limits of the maximum dose. However, some authors

| Analgesics | | | |
|---|---|---|---|
| **Drug** | **Doses** | **Side effects** | **Reservations contraindications** |
| Paracetamol | 1 g, 3–4 times a day | Excessive doses can cause hepatic or renal lesions | Liver or kidney disease. Alcohol abuse |
| Paracetamol and codeine | Paracetamol 600 mg + 30–60 mg codeine, 2–4 times a day | Constipation, dizziness, nausea, vomiting, tiredness and muscle weakness. Chronic treatment can cause psychological and physical dependence. | History of alcohol or drug abuse. Liver, kidney or thyroid disease. Asthma. Hypersensitivity to any of the constituents |
| Dextropropoxyphene | 65 mg, every 3–4 hours to a maximum of 390 mg/day | Dizziness, nausea and vomiting | History of depression. Concomitant use of anxiolytics or antidepressants |
| Tramadol | 50–100 mg, 2–4 times a day | Constipation, dizziness, nausea, insomnia and mental confusion, especially in the elderly | History of alcohol or drug abuse. Liver or kidney disease. Asthma |

**Table 30.1.** Analgesics most commonly used in rheumatic diseases.

advocate that once we decide to use an analgesic it should be given regularly. This is also our choice whenever painful muscle contraction seems to play an important role in maintaining the pain. In these circumstances, effective pain control is essential in breaking the vicious circle of pain and muscle spasm.

Provided that they are used properly, analgesics are sufficiently safe not to require any regular toxicity monitoring. They can, however, have side effects, particularly in the elderly, which it is important to be aware of.

### Additional treatment of pain

As we pointed out in Chapter 2, pain is a complex phenomenon involving not only the lesion responsible for the nociceptive stimulus, but also mechanisms of sensitization and central and peripheral amplification, not to mention the inherent psychological and social aspects.

An informed physician can also contribute towards the patient's progress by using drugs targeting other components of the pain phenomenon, depending on its probable significance in the case in question.

The presence of inflammation in the place of origin of pain means non-steroidal anti-inflammatory drugs or even local corticosteroids may be indicated to minimize the peripheral sensitivity induced by inflammatory mediators. In cases of neurogenic pain or manifestations of anxiety or secondary emotional disturbances likely to amplify the pain, patients may benefit from a local injection of anesthetic or from taking tricyclic antidepressants. These drugs not only have a modulating effect on the central pain amplification mechanisms, but also reduce the stress and anxiety associated with the pain.

Repeated application of ointments containing capsaicin has been shown to relieve pain in superficial joints, such as in osteoarthritis of the hands.

Some physical agents, like massage, heat and cold, can also help pain tolerance and control. Specialized centers can also provide additional support in cases that prove resistant to the above measures, including cognitive-behavioral techniques and a variety of specialized resources for controlling pain, such as local and epidural injections, nerve blocks, transcutaneous nerve stimulation, etc.

## NON-STEROIDAL ANTI-INFLAMMATORY DRUGS

These drugs are extremely widely used in the treatment of a variety of rheumatic diseases. The combination of their side effects, especially in the digestive tract, and their popularity has lead to something of a public health problem, demanding careful consideration on the part of the prescribing physician.

Anti-inflammatory drugs are effective in controlling inflammatory symptoms including pain, stiffness, swelling, redness and warmth. Note, however, that they have no modulating effect on the underlying pathological process. In other words, they cannot alter the course of the disease or prevent joint destruction or functional disability.

Although a reduction in pain may be noticeable in 30–40 minutes, the effects on the inflammation are not immediate, and only reach their maximum after 7–10 days of continued use in appropriate doses. It is therefore necessary to wait about 2 weeks before evaluating their efficacy.

There is a great variety of anti-inflammatory drugs on the market. Doctors are generally advised to familiarize themselves very well with a small number of drugs so that they know how to deal better with their specificities. Table 30.2. summarizes the characteristics of some of the most popular anti-inflammatory drugs.

| Common anti-inflammatory drugs | | |
|---|---|---|
| Drug | Half-life (hours) | Recommended dose |
| Aspirin | 0,25 | 500–1,000 mg, 1–4 times a day<br>Children: 75–90 mg/kg/day in divided doses |
| Ibuprofen | 2,1 | 400–600 mg, 3–4 times a day<br>Children: 35–45 mg/kg/day in divided doses |
| Naproxen | 14,0 | 250–500 mg, 2–3 times a day<br>Children: 15–20 mg/kg/day in divided doses |
| Sodium diclofenac | 1,1 | 50 mg, 2 times a day<br>or<br>75–100 mg, once a day (retard formulation) |
| Etodolac | 6,0 | 400 mg, 1–3 times a day. |
| Indomethacin | 4,6 | 25–50 mg, 2–4 times a day. |
| Nabumetone | 26,0 | 500–1000 mg, once or twice a day. |
| Meloxicam | 20 | 7.5–15 mg, once a day. |
| Etoricoxib | 17 | 60–90 mg, once a day. |
| Celecoxib | 13 | 100–200 mg, once or twice a day |

Table 30.2.
Some common anti-inflammatory drugs, duration of action and recommended doses. (The different colors identify different pharmacological groups).

### Individual variations

Although they act essentially by inhibiting the synthesis of prostaglandins, it has been demonstrated that the efficacy and tolerance of different anti-inflammatory drugs vary considerably from one patient to another. Not much is known about the mechanisms underlying this individual susceptibility, but they justify testing the efficacy and tolerance of several products on each patient until you find the most suitable one, i.e. that with the best efficacy/risk ratio.

## *Toxicity*

The toxicity of anti-inflammatory drugs is dominated by three main aspects:

### *1. Gastrointestinal (GI) toxicity*

These drugs are associated with an increased incidence of dyspepsia, gastritis, peptic ulcer, bleeding and gastroduodenal perforations. The lower GI tract may also be affected by ulcerous lesions and bleeding. About 3% of patients treated with anti-inflammatory drugs suffer clinically significant GI events per year, resulting in a high number of deaths. The risk is greater in elderly patients (>65), those treated concomitantly with corticosteroids or anticoagulants and those with a history of peptic ulcer or heavy smoking. The risk increases with the dose.

| **DIGESTIVE TOXICITY OF NSAIDS** |
| --- |
| *Risk factors* |
| History of ulcers or GI bleeding. |
| Age > 65. |
| Association with corticosteroids or anticoagulants. |
| Heavy smoking. |

Note that most of the events caused by anti-inflammatory drugs have no alerting symptoms, and prevention should be established in accordance with the risk.

The GI effects of anti-inflammatory drugs are mostly the result of systemic inhibition of type 1 cyclooxygenase. Altering the route of administration (e.g. rectal, intramuscular) does not, therefore, improve gastrointestinal safety. Topical use is associated with sufficiently low systemic absorption to offer greater safety. Administration of these drugs with meals reduces the incidence of dyspepsia, but not of more severe events.

We do not recognize any indications for the use of injectable anti-inflammatory drugs in the treatment of rheumatic diseases.

As a rule, the use of anti-inflammatory drugs should be seriously questioned in all patients at risk of gastropathy.

Should they prove indispensable, the following rules should be considered:

1. GI toxicity is not the same for all anti-inflammatory drugs, which should influence our choice (Table 30.3.).

2. Selective cyclooxygenase 2 inhibitors – COXIBs – have much less gastrointestinal toxicity than nonselective (Relative risk 0.41–0.55[1]).

3. The association of a proton pump inhibitor significant-

| Relative risk of gastrointestinal complications with Different anti-inflammatory drugs | | |
| --- | --- | --- |
| **Drug** | **Relative risk** | **Confidence interval 95%** |
| **Non-use** | 1,0 | |
| **Etodolac** | 2,2 | 0,4–11,3 |
| **Ibuprofen** | 2,5 | 1,9–3,4 |
| **Nabumetone** | 3,4 | 1,1–10,6 |
| **Meloxicam** | 3,6 | 0,8–17,2 |
| **Naproxen** | 4,0 | 2,8–5,8 |
| **Diclofenac** | 4,6 | 3,6–5,8 |
| **Indomethacin** | 5,2 | 3,2–6,3 |
| **Piroxicam** | 10,3 | 3,5–30,0 |

**Table 30.3.** Relative risk of upper gastrointestinal complications with different anti-inflammatory drugs versus non-use, considering perforations and clinically significant upper GI bleeding.[2]

[1]Hooper L, et al. The effectiveness of five strategies for the prevention of gastrointestinal toxicity induced by non-steroidal anti-inflammatory drugs: systematic review. BMJ 2004; 329(7472): 948.

[2]Garcia Rodriguez LA and Hernández-Diaz S. Relative risk of upper gastrointestinal complications among users of acetaminophen and nonsteroidal anti-inflammatory drugs. Epidemiology 2001; 12: 570–576.

ly reduces the digestive toxicity of classic anti-inflammatory drugs. (The efficacy of H2 antagonists or sucralfate has not been demonstrated.[1])

### 2. Renal toxicity

Anti-inflammatory drugs can cause nitrogen and especially fluid retention with the onset or exacerbation of peripheral edema, arterial hypertension and cardiac insufficiency.

> The risk is greater in elderly patients and those with kidney disease or previous edematous states of any origin or those being treated with diuretics or angiotensin converting enzyme inhibitors.

The use of short-acting drugs in order to leave some hours of the day free from the effects of medication tends to reduce this effect. This problem is not solved by selective cyclooxygenase 2 inhibitors. **In high-risk situations, it is advisable to monitor renal and cardiac function before and after prescribing the medication**.

### 3. Cardiovascular events

Studies with rofecoxib demonstrated a significant increase in the incidence of myocardial infarction and stroke with prolonged treatment. This medication was withdrawn from the market. These observations led to a careful review of the cardiovascular safety of all NSAIDs. At present, available data strongly suggests that the risk of myocardial infarction is increased in association with most NSAIDs, irrespective of the selectivity to Cox-2.

### 4. Drug interaction

Anti-inflammatory drugs exhibit a variety of interactions with other drugs, especially anticoagulants, oral antidiabetic drugs and anticonvulsants. Table 30.4. shows the most important interactions in current clinical practice

| Interaction of anti-inflammatory drugs with other drugs | | | |
|---|---|---|---|
| Affected drug | NSAID involved | Effect | Control |
| Oral anticoagulants | Virtually all | ↑ anticoagulant effect | Avoid anti-inflammatory drugs if possible. Strictly monitor coagulation times |
| Oral hypoglycemic drugs | Fenylbutazone, Oxyphenbutazone, Azapropazone | ↑ risk of hypoglycemia with sulfonylurea | Avoid these anti-inflammatory drugs if possible. Monitor glycemia |
| Phenytoin sodium valproate | Virtually all Aspirin (Valproate) | ↑ serum concentration ↑ risk of toxicity | Avoid anti-inflammatory drugs if possible. Monitor serum concentration of anticonvulsants |
| Antihypertensives diuretics | Virtually all anti-inflammatory drugs | ↓ therapeutic effect Exacerbation of cardiac insufficiency | Avoid anti-inflammatory drugs if possible. Monitor BP and heart function. Adjust treatment |
| Digoxin | All anti-inflammatory drugs | ↑ concentration and toxicity | Avoid anti-inflammatory drugs if possible Monitor serum concentration of digoxin |

**Table 30.4.** The most important interactions of non-steroidal anti-inflammatory drugs.

The condition of some patients with asthma may be exacerbated by taking anti-inflammatory drugs. Although this phenomenon is more common with salicylates, no drug is free of this risk. In these cases, start by trying a low dose in a protected environment. Hypersensitivity rash and elevation of liver enzymes are not uncommon with several of these drugs.

Particularly in elderly patients, it is not unusual for signs of anxiety and insomnia, tinnitus or mental confusion to occur. Hematological changes including thrombocytopenia, leucopenia and aplastic anemia should also be watched for.

### Topical anti-inflammatory drugs

Local application of anti-inflammatory drugs in the form of gels or ointments was distrusted for a long time. However, there is now evidence that they reduce pain associated with soft tissue lesions and osteoarthritis. Some of these products contain a mixture of anti-inflammatories and agents that induce slight local vasodilatation and warmth (rubefacients), whose clinical utility has also been demonstrated. It is not possible to rule out that part of the benefit from rubbing on these products is a placebo effect, but many patients appreciate the relief obtained. They have the additional advantage of involving the patients in their treatment and giving them greater control over their condition, as they apply the product to the painful areas whenever they feel the need. The GI side effects are negligible with this form of administration.

---

**Strategies for minimizing side effects of anti-inflammatory drugs**

1. Always consider whether an anti-inflammatory is indispensable.

2. Use the minimum necessary dose (consider associating with an analgesic).

3. Never combine anti-inflammatory drugs.

4. Assess the patient's risk factors.

   A – Age, previous peptic ulcer, corticosteroids, anticoagulants, heavy smoking.

   B – Advanced age, hypertension, edema, renal disease.

   C – High-risk co-medication.

   D – Asthma.

5. **Group A:**
   • Opt for a COXIB or associate a proton pump inhibitor.

6. **Group B:**
   • Choose short-acting drugs.
   • Monitor blood pressure, heart function and peripheral edema.

7. **Group C:**
   • See Table 30.4.

8. **Group D:**
   • Avoid the use of anti-inflammatory drugs or ensure close monitoring in the first days of treatment.

9. Regularly monitor the efficacy and safety of the medication.

### Monitoring treatment with anti-inflammatory drugs

Gastrointestinal toxicity is the main factor determining the need for monitoring. The patient should be informed of the aims and risks of the treatment and told to report the appearance of significant dyspeptic complaints and, especially, blood in stool or black stools or ankle swelling. A full blood count and urea and electrolytes should be performed regularly to screen for anemia due to occult GI bleeding or renal toxicity. Hypertensive patients should be advised to take their blood pressure more frequently after starting on anti-inflammatory drugs.

Patients at special risk of drug interaction or edema should be clinically monitored in the first weeks of administration. This includes performing the appropriate lab tests on a regular basis.

## GLUCOCORTICOIDS

Glucocorticoids are very often used in the treatment of a variety of rheumatic diseases, especially diffuse connective tissue diseases. Corticosteroids also play an important role in clinical practice for the treatment of rheumatoid and other chronic forms of arthritis.

These drugs are, in fact, highly effective in treating inflammatory and immunological processes, with a rapid, marked effect on the symptoms. The sometimes dramatic response makes their use extremely tempting. Your eagerness to provide relief to a rheumatic patient should, however, be carefully weighed against the following information:

- Response to glucocorticoids is nonspecific. They are beneficial to symptoms in such a wide variety of circumstances that response to treatment can be used as a diagnostic indicator only exceptionally. Hasty administration of corticosteroids may create more problems that it solves.

- The effects of glucocorticoids can minimize the manifestations of diseases that they actually exacerbate, such as infections. For example, the administration of a glucocorticoids to a patient with septic arthritis that we have mistaken for gout can relieve local and general symptoms, thus delaying the diagnosis of a serious condition and increasing its destructive potential.

- The administration of corticosteroids can result in the mitigation or alteration of clinical and laboratory manifestations that are crucial to a definite diagnosis and therefore to the correct treatment.

- The prolonged administration of corticosteroids or repeated administration of depot formulations is associated with a high prevalence of important side effects that can have a decisive impact on the patient's survival and quality of life. A treatment that appears to be immediately successful may open the door to much more harmful consequences at medium and long term. Generally speaking, the incidence of side effects is proportional to the daily and cumulative dose.

Preventing the side effects of glucocorticoid therapy usually means using these drugs only when absolutely necessary and always at the lowest possible dose.

Prolonged administration of glucocorticoids should be accompanied right from the start by measures to prevent osteoporosis (see Chapter 26.)

Table 30.5. shows the main side effects associated with long-term glucocorticoid therapy. Their incidence and severity generally increases with dose and duration of treatment. The prescribing physician is responsible for informing the patient of these potential risks and monitoring their possible development. Note that, with the exception of osteoporosis, these undesirable effects are not generally amenable to preventive treatment.

| Side effects associated with systemic corticotherapy | |
| --- | --- |
| **Metabolic** | Obesity and fat redistribution* |
| | Glucose intolerance/diabetes mellitus* |
| | Hydro-electrolytic imbalance |
| | Dyslipidemia |
| | Atherosclerosis |
| **Susceptibility to infection** | |
| **Musculoskeletal** | Osteoporosis* |
| | Myopathy |
| | Osteonecrosis |
| **Gastrointestinal** | Peptic ulcer (if associated with non-steroidal anti-inflammatory drugs) |
| | Pancreatitis |
| **Ocular** | Cataracts* |
| | Glaucoma |
| **Cutaneous** | Stretch marks* |
| | Atrophy* |
| | Facial ecchymosis |
| | Acne |
| **Central nervous system** | Anxiety, depression psychosis |
| **Delayed growth** | |
| **Depression of the hypothalamus-hypophysis-adrenal axis** | |
| * relatively common even at low dose (<10 mg/day Prednisone equivalent) | |

**Table 30.5.**
shows the .main side effects associated with long-term glucocorticoid therapy. Note that, with the exception of osteoporosis, these undesirable effects are not generally amenable to preventive treatment.

Depression of the hypothalamus-hypophysis-adrenal axis by corticosteroid treatment may leave the patient with acute adrenal insufficiency, if the medication is discontinued too suddenly. This "adrenal crisis" may be reflected by fever, generalized pain, profuse sweating and severe electrolyte imbalances which may even be fatal.

In view of these considerations, we suggest that GPs follow the rules below when prescribing corticosteroids to treat rheumatic diseases.

## SYSTEMIC GLUCOCORTICOIDS
### General rules for use in primary health care

Never start glucocorticoids without a definite diagnosis. If in doubt, consult a rheumatologist.

Never use depot formulations without asking for a specialist's opinion.

Always give careful consideration to the risk/benefit ratio in each particular patient.

Pay special attention to the following risk factors:
- presence or risk of osteoporosis
- concomitant anti-inflammatory drugs
- arterial hypertension, cardiac or renal insufficiency
- glucose intolerance or diabetes
- family history of glaucoma

Always use the minimum necessary dose for the shortest possible length of time.

Preferably use a single daily dose at breakfast.

Always accompany glucocorticoids with appropriate monitoring and toxicity prevention.

Whenever discontinuing chronic glucocorticoids medication, do so slowly and wean gradually to prevent adrenal insufficiency.

## Intralesional glucocorticoids
### Injections

Injections of corticosteroids into inflammatory articular and periarticular lesions are extremely useful in the treatment of a variety of forms of bursitis, tendonitis and arthritis, for which they are often the most effective treatment.

Given the huge prevalence of periarticular lesions in the community, injection into these structures should be part of the arsenal at the disposal of any GP, provided they have received adequate training. The intra-articular administration of corticosteroids should, in our opinion, be reserved for specialists, in that it requires a precise diagnosis and an integrated treatment plan that should involve a rheumatologist. GPs should, however, know the technique for arthrocentesis of some joints, in order to be able to take synovial fluid for testing.

It is important to bear in mind some general rules to guarantee maximum efficacy and safety.

Generally speaking, we recommend the use of prednisolone or methylprednisolone acetate for injection into soft tissue. Avoid intratendinous injection, as the resulting increase in pressure can lead to necrosis and rupture of the tendinous fibers. This risk is particularly important in high load-bearing tendons, like the Achilles. This is also why the volume of product for injection into tendons is limited to 0.5–1 cc.

Once you have gained enough experience to be sure that you are not injecting into a tendon, in some cases you can mix a local anesthetic and a corticosteroid. The anesthetic provides immediate relief, for which the patient will be grateful, and allows us to confirm the diagnosis and correct positioning of the injection.

Injection should be considered contraindicated if it is not possible to rule out the existence of infection in the path or neighborhood of the needle. If there are active skin lesions in the injection area, it is wiser to postpone the procedure. Anticoagulation is also a relative contra-indication.

Provided that you respect these rules, the risk of complications from local injection is minimal. The most common complication is local depigmentation of the skin if there is a reflux of the product along the path of the needle.

We suggest that you consider the following general rules for soft tissue injections:

1. Whenever possible, seek formal training in these techniques.

2. Do not perform the injection without guaranteeing as accurate a diagnosis as possible.

3. Form a mental image of the structures that you are going to inject and locate the anatomical points of reference in your patient.

4. Find a comfortable, stable position for you and the patient.

5. Prepare the material:

    5.a. Always use an aseptic technique. Sterile fields are not obligatory and even gloves and masks are dispensable. Wash and carefully disinfect your hands and the injection area.

    5.b. Carefully disinfect the lid of any reusable bottles (anesthetic, for example).

    5.c. Always use disposable syringes and needles.

    5.d. Replace the needle that you used to withdraw the product with a new one for the injection.

    5.e. Do not touch the injection needle or the end of the syringe.

6. Identify the insertion point of the needle to ensure optimal access to the structure and the whole painful area without having to insert the needle again (piercing the skin is painful).

7. Mark the insertion point (or points) on the skin (by pressing it with your fingernail, for example). Disinfect the area again if needed.

8. Use your free hand to support the one performing the injection. This simple gesture will increase your accuracy and reduce the patient's pain.

9. Insert the needle at right angles to the skin in a single movement.

10. Push the needle down to the structure in question. In some cases, passive mobilization of the tendon will help ensure that the needle is in the right place. Push the plunger gently. If it is inside a tendon or ligament you will feel strong resistance. Do not force it, as you do not want to inject into the tendon.

11. Pull the needle back a little at a time, repeating the above procedure at each step. Inject a small quantity at the first point in which you feel the resistance weaken – you should be in the neighborhood of the tendon, i.e. in the *peritendinum* or tendon sheath.

12. Pull the needle back until it is close to the skin and go forward to another injection point. Always try to visualize where the point of the needle is.

13. Repeat the above steps until you have covered the painful area.

14. Remove the needle and disinfect again. Cover with a dressing.

15. Gently mobilize the structure.

16. Advise the patient to immobilize the joint for 24 hours.

17. Warn him or her that the pain may be worse than it was in the next few days and recommend analgesics and local ice if necessary. Tell the patient to contact you if a postinjection flare persists beyond 3 days.

# INDEX

J.A.P. da Silva, A.D. Woolf, *Rheumatology in Practice*, DOI 10.1007/978-1-84882-581-9,
© Springer-Verlag London Limited 2010

# INDEX

# INDEX